Occupational Therapy
Examination Review Guide

THIRD EDITION

Caryn R. Johnson, MS, OTR/L, FAOTA
Academic Fieldwork Coordinator
Department of Occupational Therapy
Thomas Jefferson University
Philadelphia, Pennsylvania

Arlene Lorch, MS, OTR/L, CHES
Clinical Instructor
Department of Occupational Therapy
Thomas Jefferson University
Philadelphia, Pennsylvania

Tina DeAngelis, EdD, OTR/L, ABD
Clinical Assistant Professor
Department of Occupational Therapy
Thomas Jefferson University
Philadelphia, Pennsylvania

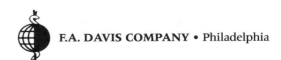
F.A. DAVIS COMPANY • Philadelphia

F.A. Davis Company
1915 Arch Street
Philadelphia, PA 19103
www.fadavis.com

Printed in the United States of America

Last digit indicates print number: 10 9 8 7

ISBN 13: 9780-8036-1481-9
ISBN 10: 0-8036-1481-0

Acquisitions Editor: Christa A. Fratantoro
Developmental Editor: Melissa Reed
Art and Design Manager: Carolyn O'Brien

Preface

The purpose of this workbook is to give occupational therapy students a general review of the profession and study tools to use while preparing to take the certification examination. It also will serve as an excellent review for occupational therapists reentering the field or changing areas of practice.

This workbook's format will encourage users to synthesize knowledge and become comfortable with the format of the National Board for Certification in Occupational Therapy (NBCOT) certification examination. The questions in the certification examination are designed to require the reader to call upon his/her knowledge of occupational therapy practice and to apply that knowledge to realistic practice situations. Questions in this book have been designed to simulate that. The reader will find that questions do not test basic knowledge alone, but require use of that knowledge to move through a reasoning process that leads to the best answer. While the majority of questions in the *Occupational Therapy Examination Review Guide* have been written in a style that simulates the examination, some have been written to maximize review of important content areas.

The textbooks cited as references for most answers are those most commonly required for purchase by students in occupational therapy programs across the United States. In some cases, the authors cite less well-known references because they provide the best rationales. Students can often access these books through their own occupational therapy libraries or libraries of other occupational therapy programs. In addition, many of the books cited are available from the Wilma West Library at AOTA headquarters.

Please keep in mind that this workbook will *not:*

- be a comprehensive guide to practicing as an occupational therapist,
- replicate the NBCOT Examination or any of the questions on the NBCOT examination.

This work book *will:*

- provide a general review of occupational therapy practice,
- help readers identify the strengths and weaknesses in their knowledge of occupational therapy,
- acquaint the reader with the format of questions used on the examination,
- provide the reader with opportunities to practice taking computerized examinations,
- help the reader organize and set priorities for study time, and
- provide the reader with a reference list from which further study may be pursued.

The Authors

Caryn Reichlin Johnson, MS, OTR/L, FAOTA, serves as Academic Fieldwork Coordinator and Assistant Professor in the Occupational Therapy Program at Thomas Jefferson University in Philadelphia, Pennsylvania, where she has taught since 1983. Caryn received her Bachelor's degree in Occupational Therapy from Tufts University in 1978 and an advanced Master's degree in Occupational Therapy from Thomas Jefferson University in 1991. In addition, she is president of Occupational Therapy Associates, a private practice specializing in aquatic rehabilitation. Past clinical experience includes working in the areas of adult physical rehabilitation and community mental health. Caryn's special interests include developing fieldwork opportunities in nontraditional community settings and in the development of professional behaviors in OT and OTA students. In her free time, Caryn works with a wide variety of craft media.

Arlene Lorch, MS, OTR/L, CHES, received a Bachelor of Science degree in Occupational Therapy from the University of Pennsylvania in 1976 and a Master of Science degree in Health Education from Arcadia University in 1995. She has practiced in acute care, rehabilitation, outpatient, long-term care settings, in home care, and has experience as an environmental accessibility consultant. Arlene has taught occupational therapy courses and labs in evaluation, intervention, occupation, older adult practice, group dynamics, and environmental adaptation as an instructor at Thomas Jefferson University since 1996, and currently supervises an innovative student fieldwork program at Riverview—the assisted living facility for the City of Philadelphia. Also a Certified Health Education Specialist, Arlene is interested in health promotion and safety programs. She is involved in a number of volunteer activities including providing wellness workshops in the community.

Tina DeAngelis, MS, OTR/L, ABD, is a practicing occupational therapist at Crozer Chester Medical Center in Upland, Pennsylvania, where she has been employed since 1991. She has experience in burn care, orthopedic and neurological conditions. She is currently a consultant to Thomas Jefferson University in Philadelphia, Pennsylvania, where she is assisting with the development of a post-professional OTD (occupational therapy doctorate) program. Tina received an Associate's degree in Occupational Therapy form Harcum College in 1987, a Bachelor's degree in Occupational Therapy from College Misericordia in 1992, and her advanced Master's degree in Occupational Therapy from Thomas Jefferson University in 1997. She is currently a doctoral candidate (ABD) in a Higher Education Leadership program at Widener University in Chester, Pennsylvania, where she is examining the impact of the entry-level OTD on the profession of occupational therapy. Tina is the mother of three children and also enjoys volunteering and fund-raising for local charities within her community.

Acknowledgments

The input and enthusiasm of many individuals have made this book possible. We especially want to thank Christa Fratantoro and Melissa Reed for their guidance and support. We also want to thank Janice Burke for her support and tolerance over the course of the work. Our deepest thanks to friends and family, for tolerating us, present and absent, while we lost ourselves to this project for the last year.

This book would have been impossible to complete without the tremendous support provided by our graduate assistants and alumni. For that contribution, we would like to thank Kristie Buechele, Erin Lynn, Ashleigh Rankin, Jaime Silberman, and finally, Andrea Pegg, who is capable of doing anything and everything.

Finally, we would like to recognize the efforts of those educators and practitioners from across the country who painstakingly reviewed, critiqued, and validated every question to ensure accuracy and appropriateness.

Tana Brown, PhD
University of Kansas Medical Center
Kansas City, Kansas

Cathy Dolhi, MS, OTR/L, FAOTA
Chatham College
Pittsburgh, Pennsylvania

Liane Hewitt, MPH, OTR/L
Loma Linda University
Loma Linda, California

Thomas Laster, MS, OTR/L
Midwestern University
Glendale, Arizona

MaryBeth Merryman, MS, OTR/L
Towson University
Towson, Maryland

Georgana Miller, MEd, OTR/L
Xavier University
Cincinnati, Ohio

Jaime Munoz, MS, OTR/L
Duquesne University
Pittsburgh, Pennsylvania

Marsha Neville-Smith, MS, OTR/L
Texas Women's University
Dallas, Texas

Neil Penny, MS, OTR/L
Alvernia College
Reading, Pennsylvania

Timothy Pulver
Pearl River Community College
Poplarville Campus
Poplarville, Mississippi

Carol Reinson, PhD, OTR/L
Universoty of Scranton
Scranton, Pennsylvania

Pat Sample, PhD
Colorado State University
Fort Collins, Colorado

Judy Vestal, PhD, OTR/L
Louisiana State University
Shreveport, Louisiana

Student Reviewers

Jennifer Lynn Illig, OTR/L

Melissa A. Lovins, OTR/L

Amy Janelle Perez, OTR/L

Kristine Steinhilper McBride, MOT, OTR

Contents

Preparing for the Examination

■ WHAT IS THE NBCOT EXAMINATION?

Successful completion of the certification examination is required for anyone who wants to practice as an occupational therapist. Passing the National Board for Certification in Occupational Therapy (NBCOT) examination is the culmination of academic and fieldwork study. The examination tests the student's depth of knowledge and ability to apply that knowledge to practice. The questions require the individual to apply knowledge of occupational therapy or synthesize bits of knowledge to select the correct answer. Questions on the certification examination are carefully constructed to test:

- your knowledge of occupational therapy practice and the skills performed by the occupational therapist.
- your grasp of background knowledge that supports practice.
- your ability to apply the your knowledge to practice situations.
- your ability to understand what the question is asking.
- your ability to select the correct answer based on correctly prioritizing the most significant issue presented in the question.

The purpose of the examination is to identify those candidates who demonstrate entry-level competence for practicing as an occupational therapist. Once candidates have successfully completed the examination, they are certified as occupational therapists. Examinations are given for both certified occupational therapy assistant (COTA) and registered occupational therapist (OTR) candidates.

The examination, which is computer-delivered, is offered at hundreds of centers around the country, as well as internationally, throughout the year. Students are eligible to take online practice examinations once they have registered for the NBCOT examination. More information on the NBCOT examination and practice examinations is available at www.nbcot.org.

■ WHO CAN TAKE THE NBCOT EXAMINATION?

The NBCOT oversees the certification examination and eligibility of candidates. Candidates must have graduated from an accredited occupational therapy education program and successfully completed the required fieldwork. Candidates are required to submit either an official transcript or the NBCOT Academic Credential Verification form from their occupational therapy programs.

In cases where graduation is not scheduled until after the examination date, students must be cleared for graduation (both academically and financially) by the institution's registrar. If complete official transcripts cannot be submitted, the student must have the "NBCOT Academic Credential Verification Form" completed by the registrar and submitted to the NBCOT. Deadlines are strictly enforced. An official transcript must be submitted *no later* than 90 days after the date of the examination. Failure to do so may result in loss of certification.

Individuals with a history of felony or some other types of criminal background history may not be eligible to take the NBCOT examination. For a fee, NBCOT will complete an "Early Determination Review" to determine eligibility.

■ ABOUT THE NBCOT CANDIDATE HANDBOOK

Students may access the most current version of the NBCOT Candidate Handbook online at www.nbcot.org. Detailed and critical information is included in the NBCOT Candidate Handbook, which the candidate should read from beginning to end before completing the application. Students also may request a hard copy of the Candidate Handbook by contacting NBCOT at (301) 990-7979.

The handbook includes a wealth of information necessary for completing the application to take the examination, such as eligibility criteria, information about test administration and scoring, special accommodations for individuals with disabilities, fees, testing locations, school codes, and special forms that may be necessary. *Read the handbook thoroughly.*

■ HOW TO APPLY FOR THE NBCOT EXAMINATION

Applications to take the examination may be submitted online or by mail. Applying online significantly reduces the possibility of submitting an incomplete application and is encouraged. The fee for taking the examination (at the time of this writing) is approximately $420 for an online application, and $470 for a paper application. NBCOT charges extra for practice examinations, to have reports of scores sent to state regulatory agencies, and for each notice of Confirmation of Eligibility the candidate requests. These items are frequently required in order to obtain a license or temporary license to practice.

Candidates should begin the application process early so that an "account" exists when required parts of the application begin to arrive, such as the academic transcript or academic credential verification form (ACVF). Candidates can check the status of their applications online. Those using a paper application may wish to send the application by certified mail to receive a "returned receipt" from the Post Office. Once the application is complete, NBCOT will mail or e-mail an authorization to test (ATT) letter to the candidate. Upon receipt of the ATT letter, the candidate may schedule a date to take the examination. The candidate must take the examination within 90 days, or a "reactivation" of the ATT will be required. Scheduling is done on a "first come, first served" basis, so to get the date and location of choice, candidates should be sure to apply early. It should be noted that some states require the applicant to take the examination within a certain period of time following graduation.

According to the NBCOT Web site (www.nbcot.org/WebArticles/articlefiles/111-asd_ppt_aota_conference.pdf), the most common problems experienced when applying to take the examination were:

- candidate did not request "Early Determination Review" when appropriate.
- candidate did not request academic transcripts or ACVF, or submitted them prior to their application account being opened.
- candidate changed his/her name, and different names appear on transcript, application, or other documents.
- candidate changed e-mail address.
- re-applicants created new accounts instead of using original account.
- incomplete payment.
- delays due to requests for special accommodations.

■ WHAT IS THE FORMAT OF THE NBCOT EXAMINATION?

The certification examination is composed of 200 multiple-choice questions that use the four-option format. No combination or "K" questions are used. Questions are designed as brief practice scenarios, and require candidates to decide what the therapist should *do* based on his/her application of occupational therapy *knowledge*. Candidates have 4 hours to complete the examination.

The questions for the examination are developed by the NBCOT Certification Examination Development Committee. The group consists of content experts, both occupational therapists and occupational therapy assistants, from a variety of treatment settings across the United States. The format of the new examination is based on the *2003 Practice Analysis,* which obtained information about current professional practice among recent OT and OTA graduates, and resulted in a new "examination blueprint."

Every time the examination is given, a new set of questions is drawn from a "pool" or "item bank." The item banks for the OTR and COTA examinations are separate. The questions on each examination correspond to the content outline for either OTR or COTA candidates. The content outline specifies how many items should be asked for each of the identified "domains." While some questions are easier and others harder, each item has the same weight in scoring, and every question on the examination has only one correct answer. There is not a penalty for guessing so you should *never* leave a question unanswered. Of the 200 questions, only 170 are actually scored; each test contains 30 questions that are being "pre-tested" to determine whether they meet the criteria to become real test questions in the future. The raw scores of correct answers are statistically converted to a "scaled score," which may range from 300 to 600 points. A scaled score of 450 or more is required to pass the examination. The score does not actually reflect how many questions the candidate got right or wrong. Approximately 80% of those who take the examination for the first time actually pass.

■ DOMAINS AND CONTENT AREAS

The 2003 Practice Analysis resulted in the identification of five domains of occupational therapy practice that describe what occupational therapy practitioners *do*. Each domain is accompanied by related tasks and knowledge areas the entry-level occupational therapy practitioner should be competent in. Certain concepts are emphasized throughout, such as the importance of being client-centered and occupation-based. These domains are summarized below.

■ Domain 1: Evaluation of Groups and Individuals

This area comprises approximately 25% of the examination, or about 50 questions. Few evaluations are actually referred to by name. These questions apply to tasks related to data collection such as:

- interviewing.
- observation.
- forming a hypothesis.
- screening and chart/record review.
- selecting assessments.
- use of standardized and nonstandardized evaluations.
- referring to other health professionals.
- integrating and interpreting results.
- developing conclusions from evaluation data.
- documenting results.

■ Domain 2: Intervention Planning

This area comprises approximately 21% of the examination, or about 42 questions. These questions apply to the ability to design treatment based on theory and will address tasks such as:

- prioritizing treatment needs.
- collaborating with the individual and relevant others.
- selecting frames of reference.
- establishing client-centered goals.
- selecting/designing goal-related interventions that establish or restore function, adapt or modify tasks or the environment, or prevent negative outcomes.
- selecting appropriate service delivery methods.
- determining frequency and duration of treatment.
- selecting appropriate environments and contexts.

- documenting treatment/intervention plans and goals.

■ Domain 3: Implementing Intervention

This area comprises approximately 41% of the examination, or about 82 questions—more than any other domain. These questions apply to tasks related to providing intervention to the individual and their caregivers and will address areas such as:

- collaboratively selecting intervention options.
- providing intervention within optimum environments, setting, and times.
- adaptation and grading of techniques/activities.
- adapting the environment to enhance participation.
- selecting therapeutic equipment, tools, objects, and assistive technology.
- adapting/grading therapeutic equipment, tools, objects, and assistive technology.
- teaching safe use of therapeutic equipment, tools, objects, and assistive technology.
- educating about health and wellness.
- educating about prevention.
- instructing in home programs.
- recommending equipment, strategies, and services.
- monitoring response to treatment.
- modifying the treatment plan as needed.
- documenting progress and response to treatment.
- assisting transition by recommending postintervention services.
- discharge planning and documentation.

■ Domain 4: Occupational Therapy for Populations

This area comprises approximately 6% of the examination, or about 12 questions. These questions apply to provision of occupational therapy to groups of people, not individuals, through preventive, supportive, or remediative services in select settings. Questions address tasks such as:

- identifying population-based needs for programs, agencies, schools, industry, at-risk populations, etc.
- recommending interventions for populations based on needs assessment data.
- developing specific population-based health, wellness, prevention, and educational programs.
- providing information, expertise, and consultation services for population-based programs.

■ Domain 5: Service Management and Professional Practice

This area comprises approximately 7% of the examination, or about 14 questions. Questions in this section apply to tasks relating to management, service delivery, and professional practice, such as:

- coordinating a variety of services.
- documenting services according to regulatory and funding guidelines.
- participating as a member of a team.
- understanding of and compliance with regulations, laws, policies, and procedures.
- engaging in professional development activities.
- maintaining competence.
- promoting occupational therapy.

■ THE DAY OF THE NBCOT EXAMINATION

The following checklist should help you manage on the day of the examination:

[✓] Double-check the date and time on your admission notice.

[✓] Be sure you know where you are going, how to get there, and where you will be able to park.

[✓] Arrive early.

[✓] Bring your admission notice.

[✓] Bring two forms of identification, including one photo ID with signature, that have the same name as the examination admission notice.

[✓] Bring a watch to help you stay on schedule during the 4-hour test. A clock option is available on each computer, but some find it distracting and prefer to turn it off.

The test area is divided into individual sections like cubicles in a library. You will be with other people in the room, and a proctor will monitor the examination. You may use earplugs provided by the facility to minimize distractions. Food and drinks, dictionaries, cell phones, and a host of other items are not permitted. Special permission is even required for bottled water. Lockers are provided for all items not permitted in the testing area. You have four hours to take the test, and no breaks are included. If you need to take a break, you may leave the testing room to use the bathroom, stretch, get a drink, etc., but the clock keeps running.

A tutorial will be offered at the beginning of the examination process. Be sure to take advantage of this. Students who take the tutorial do better on the examination.

■ WHAT HAPPENS AFTER THE NBCOT EXAMINATION?

Test results are mailed within 6 weeks after the certification examination. As previously stated, a score of 450 or higher is required to pass the certification examination. A grievance process is outlined in the NBCOT Handbook. If you experience difficulty with the testing conditions, wish to contest the content of any question, or have any other complaints about your experience taking the examination, you must report it immediately (within 72 hours) to NBCOT.

Candidates can request that results be sent to the licensing agency of the state(s) in which they will choose to practice. There is a fee for each report you request—no reports are sent free of charge. Almost all states require a copy of the report. It is recommended that the candidate complete an application for state licensure before taking the examination. Often, these applications require a notarized copy of transcripts from an accredited occupational therapy program, letters of reference, a picture identification, and so forth. Depending on the state licensure laws and facility requirements, OTRs may or may not be able to work with a temporary permit until examination results are received. Candidates should contact the licensing agency as soon as they know the state in which they will be practicing. Candidates should learn as early as possible what information will be necessary for licensure and when applications should be submitted.

Candidates who fail the examination and wish to retake it must retake the entire examination. There is no limit on how many times an individual may take the examination although there is a 90 day waiting period. In addition, failing the examination may affect employment status, and employers *must* be notified.

■ HOW TO USE THIS WORKBOOK

This workbook has four complete sample examinations of 200 questions each that simulate the actual NBCOT examination by asking application-oriented questions in a four-option multiple-choice format. Questions in the first three examinations are organized to allow candidates to assess their performance in each of the five domains. The questions in examination four are grouped by content area (pediatrics, mental health, physical disabilities, OT for populations, and service management/professional practice) allowing candidates to assess their competence with various age groups and diagnostic categories.

A complete set of answers follows each examination. In order to help the student as much as possible, the workbook provides a complete rationale for each answer, which explains why wrong answers are wrong and why the right answers are right. Hence, each question-answer unit is actually a mini-lesson on not one, but four concepts. In addition, each answer provides the reader with a reference from which further information may be obtained on the subject matter. A complete bibliography including primary textbooks that the reader is likely to own is located after the final chapter.

The section on "Developing Your Personal Study Plan" will help the reader identify his or her strengths and weaknesses and organize and set priorities for study time. At the end of the section is a tool for developing a study plan.

■ HOW TO USE THE ENCLOSED CD ROM

The CD ROM located on the inner back cover of this workbook is designed to allow the user to create **Personalized Examination Reviews.** Examination 5, which contains 200 randomized questions, is located on the CD. **The user also can create an unlimited number of randomized practice examination reviews to test their skills.** The questions in Examination 5 and the examination reviews the reader creates are presented in random order, simulating the format of the NBCOT examination. This arrangement is a bit more difficult and challenging in that it requires the reader to change domain and content areas frequently. These reviews enable the reader to evaluate how well he or she has retained and been able to implement the techniques recommended in this book. The mix of questions in each examination review covers the range of entry-level occupational therapy practice as determined by the examination blueprint, thus providing a general review of professional practice.

Using the CD ROM, the reader can select questions from a specific <u>content area</u> such as: pediatrics, mental health, physical disabilities, management/professional practice, and OT for populations. In addition, the user can focus upon a specific <u>domain</u> such as:

evaluation, treatment planning, intervention implementation, OT for populations, or management/professional practice. This allows the user to essentially "create a quiz" or, if so desired, simulate a full 200-question examination via the "pre-made quiz" option.

■ WHERE TO BEGIN

Viewed as one task, preparing to take the examination can seem overwhelming. Breaking the process into smaller parts makes it easier to manage. The first step is to identify your areas of strength and weakness. The **"Personal Study Plan Chart"** can help you through this process. Once you have completed this step, the second step is to complete your study plan. The final step is to pull all of the information together to take the practice examinations. It may be helpful to review the test-taking tips occasionally.

■ DEVELOPING YOUR PERSONAL STUDY PLAN

The question most frequently asked by occupational therapy students preparing for the examination is, "How do I start?" This *Examination Review Guide* was specifically developed to be a primary source for examination preparation. It will help you put all your educational preparation together and organize your study time. It also will make you comfortable with multiple-choice questions. All students preparing for the examination should have their coursework at their fingertips, including books, notes, handouts, etc. Once you have assembled the stacks of information you have accumulated over the years, the question arises, "Where do I start?"

One way to use this workbook is to develop a study plan based on your performance on the simulation examinations. Start by taking simulation Examination 1 and record how many correct answers you score in each Domain compared to the number of questions that will be on the certification examination in this area.

This will give you some idea of the Domains for which you need more concentrated review and study. The next step is to define your strengths and weaknesses. To do this, choose a Domain and then go through all the component parts of that area as well as the background knowledge areas suggested for review. Classify the areas in which you are weakest as

"D," and those in which you are strongest as "A." Assign "B" or "C," with "B" being stronger than "C," to the remaining practice areas. Within each letter grouping, identify the weakest subject with the number 4, and sequentially number through to the strongest subject—the higher the number, the higher your study priority. Once this has been completed, your individualized studying needs have been organized and priorities set for accomplishment.

After completing simulation Examinations 2 and 3, record the numbers of your correct answers for each Domain. This will further indicate areas for which you still need review.

Now that you have set your priorities for studying, set target dates for completing your review of each area or subject. For instance, you may choose to work on Domain No. 1 (evaluation) during the month of January. Another individual may choose to review evaluation the first week of January, treatment planning (Domain No. 2) the second week of January, and so forth. Design your study plan to meet your needs. Set target dates that are realistic and attainable.

Once your planning is complete, it is time for the studying to begin. Start with the area listed as "D4" (high priority for review) and work your way through to the last "D." Once this is finished, continue with the "C," "B," and "A" items. When you have reviewed all areas, you may choose to begin again at D4, or to reset priorities for your studying needs.

The Occupational Therapy Examination Review Guide CD, which is included on the back cover of this book, offers you a particular advantage in preparing for the NBCOT examination. It is available to you at any time during the process of reviewing, or when you have completed your review, and provides you with the opportunity to practice taking full-length simulated examinations. It also provides you with the option of selecting the specific kinds of questions you would like to practice. You may select questions that reflect the examination Domains of evaluation, treatment planning, implementing intervention, OT for populations, or service management/professional practice. Or you may select practice questions according to the content areas of physical dysfunction, mental health/cognition, or pediatrics. The flexibility of question selection offered by the CD allows you to target the high-priority areas you have identified in your study plan. Taking both the full-length examinations and the selected sections of the examinations can be very useful in measuring the effectiveness of your review as well as building your confidence.

The easiest part of this task will be defining the time frame in which to study specific topics. The toughest challenge will be implementing the examination review plan!

Table 1. PERSONAL STUDY PLAN CHART

Percentage of items on certification exam: 25%   Number of questions in each review exam: 50

Specific task areas	Self-rating of knowledge in each area of practice					
Questions test ability to apply OT knowledge to these therapy task areas	Pediatrics		Phys Dys		MH/Cognition	
	ABCD	1234	ABCD	1234	ABCD	1234
1. Interviewing skills						
2. Observing performance for data gathering						
3. Forming a hypothesis						
4. Screening methods and chart/record review						
5. Choosing appropriate assessments						
6. Administering standardized instruments						
7. Administering non-standardized tools and methods						
8. Referring to other health professionals						
9. Integrating and interpreting occupational performance findings based on frames of reference						
10. Developing conclusions from evaluation data for basis of intervention						
11. Documenting evaluation results professionally						

Background knowledge to review for the EVALUATION category

· Pathological conditions and resulting diagnoses, disabilities, injuries and conditions; ways they affect performance of occupations and development across the life span
· Influence of contextual factors (such as physical and social environments) that can affect how people perform occupations
· Normal and abnormal human development in sensorimotor, neuromusculoskeletal, and cognitive and psychosocial skill areas
· Progression of skill development in performance areas of ADL, work and productive activities, play and leisure, and social participation.
· Impact of disability and injury in terms of the individual's roles and occupational performance
· Impact of culture and diversity on the evaluation process
· Interviewing, screening, and observation techniques
· Selecting evaluations that are client-centered and appropriate for obtaining relevant evaluation findings
· Methods for safely performing and scoring screens, and standardized and non-standardized assessments
· Various types of assessments that represent commonly used frames of reference and are suitable for a variety of needs
· Team process, community resources, and circumstances when referrals to other professionals for evaluation are appropriate
· Clinical reasoning used in interpreting evaluation results for intervention, including knowledge of likely outcomes
· Impact medications, precautions, and contraindications may have on the evaluation process
· Writing of evaluation reports

Exam 1. Exam score _____/50   **Exam 2.** Exam score _____/50   **Exam 3.** Exam score _____/50

Table 2.	STUDY GUIDELINES: Intervention Planning Questions

Percentage of items on certification exam: 21%   Number of questions in each review exam: 42

Specific task areas	Self-rating of knowledge in in each area of practice					
Questions test ability to apply OT knowledge to these therapy task areas	Pediatrics		Phys Dys		MH/Psychosocial	
	ABCD	1234	ABCD	1234	ABCD	1234
1. Prioritizing treatment needs						
2. Collaborating with the individual and relevant others						
3. Selecting frames of reference						
4. Establishing client-centered goals						
5. Determining intervention approaches to restore skills						
6. Determining intervention methods to adapt activities and modify environments						
7. Selecting intervention methods and activities to meet goals						
8. Selecting environments that maximize abilities to achieve goals						
9. Determining frequency and duration of OT services						
10. Documentation of the plan and goals						

Background knowledge to review for the INTERVENTION PLANNING category

· Elements of an intervention plan
· Activity analysis
· Construction of long- and short-term goals based on effective OT interventions and methods for anticipated outcomes
· Issues related to developing client-centered, culturally appropriate intervention plans collaboratively, using appropriate communication skills
· Models of practice, theories, and frames of reference underlying intervention
· Principles of clinical reasoning for selection of intervention approaches to achieve goals
· Range of intervention methods for various pathological conditions and resulting diagnoses, disabilities, injuries, and conditions
· Selection of occupation-based interventions
· Activity adaptations and environmental modifications relative to planned interventions to facilitate occupational performance
· Impact of environments on performance
· Timing factors in intervention planning; estimating how long therapy should continue and how frequently therapy should occur to reach goals in relation to discharge process.
· Documenting intervention plans

Exam 1. Evaluation score ___/42	Exam 2. Evaluation score ___/42	Exam 3. Evaluation score ___/42

Table 3. STUDY GUIDELINES: Implementing Intervention Questions

Percentage of items on certification exam: 41%   Number of questions in each review exam: 82

Specific task areas	Self-rating of knowledge in each area of practice					
Questions test ability to apply OT knowledge to these therapy task areas	Pediatrics		Phys Dys		MH/Psychosocial	
	ABCD	1234	ABCD	1234	ABCD	1234
1. Collaboratively selecting intervention options						
2. Proving intervention within optimum environments, setting and times						
3. Adaptation and grading of techniques						
4. Adapting the environment to enhance participation						
5. Selecting therapeutic equipment, tools, objects and assistive technology						
6. Adapting and grading therapeutic equipment, tools, objects and assistive technology						
7. Teaching safe use of therapeutic equipment, tools, objects and assistive technology						
8. Educating about health and wellness						
9. Educating about prevention						
10. Instructing in home programs						
11. Recommending equipment, strategies, and services						
12. Monitoring response to treatment						
13. Modifying the treatment plan as needed						
14. Documenting progress and response to treatment						
15. Assisting transition by recommending post-intervention services						
16. Writing discharge notes						

Background knowledge to review for the IMPLEMENTING INTERVENTION category

· Principles of client centered intervention, collaborative strategies, and culturally sensitive care
· The effects of various physical, cognitive, and psychosocial disabilities on development and occupational performance
· Influence of environmental factors on development and occupational performance
· The use of activity analysis in implementing and grading interventions
· A variety of media, methods, modalities, and activities
· Frames of reference used to guide intervention and select interventions and related occupation-based activities and environment-based interventions
· Specific approaches and techniques to enhance motor and sensory skills, such as use of splints and orthotics; therapeutic exercise program and manual techniques; sensory re-education, desensitization and sensory processing techniques; motor learning and neurodevelopmental approaches
· Specific approaches and techniques to enhance process and cognitive skills such as cognitive rehabilitation techniques, training techniques and methods of assisting and cueing, compensatory methods used in dementia, such as task-breakdown, Allen's cognitive disabilities approach, perceptual rehabilitation techniques

(Continued on following page)

Table 3.   STUDY GUIDELINES: Implementing Intervention Questions (Continued)

· Specific approaches and techniques to enhance social/communication skills and psychosocial performance, such as strategies for dealing with behavioral issues; interventions which address living skills; coping skills and stress management; prevocational exploration; symptom management and relapse prevention
· Interventions for limitations in areas of occupational performance in ADL, work, education, play and leisure and social interaction
· Principles and application of compensatory strategies including the selection, use, and adaptation of assistive technologies, assistive and adaptive devices, environmental modification, assistance from others
· Activity adaptation principles and methods
· Therapeutic use of self; verbal and written communication methods
· Typical and atypical reactions that can be expected in response to intervention methods
· Clinical problem-solving related to client/patient response to intervention, reassessment of progress, and methods for adjusting intervention.
· Training, teaching, and educational methods for use with adults and children of varying developmental and cognitive abilities, and for caregivers and supervised personnel
· Group interventions and underlying group dynamics and strategies for use of group process to enhance performance and goal attainment; intervention techniques based on application of group process.
· Precautions and contraindications for intervention associated with various conditions; principles of safety during various intervention methods and in use of equipment.
· Knowledge of intervention possibilities in various settings, service delivery models, and reimbursement systems; resources in the community; and strategies and services that would support occupational performance relative to transition to other settings
· Techniques and methods for recording of treatment process; documentation of progress and outcomes; discharge planning and recommendations.

| Exam 1. Evaluation score ___/82 | Exam 2. Evaluation score ___/82 | Exam 3. Evaluation score ___/82 |

Table 4. STUDY GUIDELINES: OT for Populations Questions

Percentage of items on certification exam: 6%   Number of questions in each review exam: 12

Specific task areas	Self-rating of knowledge in each area of practice			
Questions test ability to apply OT knowledge to these therapy task areas	Children		Adults	
	ABCD	1234	ABCD	1234
1. Performing population-based needs assessments				
2. Recommending interventions based on needs assessment data				
3. Developing specific population-based health, wellness, prevention, and educational programs				
4. Providing information, expertise, and consultation services for population-based programs				

Background knowledge to review for the OT FOR POPULATIONS category

In addition to many of the knowledge areas previously mentioned, the following are particularly relevant to occupational therapy for populations:

· Typical occupations of populations at various development stages
· Pathological conditions and resulting diagnoses, disabilities, injuries, and conditions; ways they affect performance of occupations, development, health, and wellness across populations
· Methods of evaluating groups including use of assessment, observation, and interview for the purposes of data collection.
· Knowledge of intervention possibilities in various settings, service delivery models, and reimbursement systems; resources in the community
· Consultation techniques and roles of the consultant on teams
· Principles of program development, management, and evaluation for health, wellness, and prevention programs

Exam 1. Evaluation score __/12   **Exam 2.** Evaluation score __/12   **Exam 3.** Evaluation score __/12

Table 5.   STUDY GUIDELINES: Service Management and Professional Practice Questions

Percentage of items on certification exam: 7%   Number of questions in each review exam: 14

Specific task areas	Self-rating of knowledge in service management and occupational therapy promotion	
Questions test ability to apply OT knowledge to these therapy task areas	ABCD	1234
1. Coordinating a variety of services		
2. Documenting services according to regulatory and funding guidelines		
3. Participating as a member of a team		
4. Understanding of and ethical compliance with regulations, laws, policies, and procedures		
5. Engaging in professional development activities		
6. Maintaining competence		
7. Promoting and informing others about value of occupational therapy		

Background knowledge to review for the SERVICE MANAGEMENT category

· Collaboration methods and strategies for service management
· Knowledge of practice scope for OTR and COTA
· Guidelines for supervision of OT and non-OT personnel
· Role of the OT practitioners and other disciplines on teams
· Use and coordination of resources such as personnel, supplies, equipment, and time
· Cultural awareness concepts
· Relevant guidelines, standards, regulations, and laws that guide and regulate professional practice and how they are applied in practice situations
· Strategies to promote professional development
· AOTA Code of Ethics and how to apply to practice situations
· Safety issues in occupational therapy services and how to manage related liabilities
· Ways to promote the value and benefits of the profession to others and the public

Exam 1. Evaluation score ___/14   Exam 2. Evaluation score ___/14   Exam 3. Evaluation score ___/14

(Continued on following page)

Table 5. STUDY GUIDELINES: Additional Information About the Exam

The credentialing body for the profession of occupational therapy is the National Board for Certification in Occupational Therapy, Inc. (NBCOT). In developing the Certification Exam, NBCOT, Inc. has gathered information on entry-level occupational therapy practice by conducting a practice survey of occupational therapists entitled the, "Practice Analysis Study of Entry-Level Occupational Therapist Registered and Certified Occupational Therapy Assistant Practice," (NBCOT, Inc., 2004). The study results have been published in the journal, OTJR Occupation, Participation and Health, Volume 24, Supplement 1, Spring 2004. The information from this study provides a valid and detailed description of entry-level occupational therapy practice and is used by NBCOT, Inc. to provide a framework and basis for questions on the national Certification Exam. Basing the Certification Exam on the Practice Analysis ensures that exam questions accurately test the candidate's knowledge of frames of reference, evaluation, and intervention methods that are currently used within the practice of occupational therapy. The following data from the Practice Analysis indicates the most frequently reported responses by therapists in certain categories and should be carefully reviewed.

Most Frequently Seen Diagnoses
- Cerebral vascular accident
- Developmental disabilities
- Total hip/knee replacement
- Pervasive developmental disorders
- Cardiopulmonary
- Cerebral palsy
- General orthopedic injuries

Most Frequently Mentioned Frames of Reference
- Biomechanical
- Neurodevelopment approach
- Sensory integration
- Model of human occupation
- Rehabilitation frames of reference

Most Frequently Identified Assessment Methods
- Peabody scale
- Goniometer/range of motion
- Manual muscle testing
- Sensory testing
- Bruininks-Osterstky Test Motor Proficiency
- Visual-motor

Top 25 Most Frequently Reported Interventions (see Practice Analysis Study for full list)
1. Therapeutic activities
2. Fine motor coordination training
3. Strength and endurance training
4. Therapeutic exercise
5. Dressing
6. Gross motor coordination training
7. Functional mobility
8. Adaptive equipment recommendations/training
9. Grooming
10. Safety awareness/insight training
11. Visual motor training (hand-eye coordination)
12. Training for transfers
13. Toileting
14. Attention, orientation, and concentration training
15. Interventions based on motor learning
16. Bathing/showering
17. Caregiver skills
18. Eating
19. Interventions based on sensory integration theory
20. Interventions based on neurodevelopment treatment
21. Positioning and handling techniques
22. Functional communication skills (handwriting, typing, telephoning, augmented devices)
23. Visual perceptual skills training
24. Energy conservation training
25. Feeding

■ TEST-TAKING TIPS

■ Test-Taking Tip 1

Visit the NBCOT website periodically. You can access the candidate handbook and other vital information about the examination at the NBCOT Web site (www. nbcot.org). It is essential that you read the Candidate Handbook thoroughly and *more than once*—you'll pick up something new each time. This Web site has the most current information regarding test dates and locations and is updated frequently. It also has details about how the examination was developed and how it is scored.

■ Test-Taking Tip 2

Be prepared. The more prepared you are prior to the examination the more comfortable you will feel during the actual examination. Preparation includes studying the knowledge base of occupational therapy (in speaking with NBCOT representatives, we have learned that waiting too long to take the NBCOT examination actually decreases performance results), getting a good night's sleep and coming prepared to the examination. According to the NBCOT Web site (www.nbcot.org), items such as headphones, tissues, and an erasable board and marking pen are available at the test site. Test candidates are permitted to use earplugs and reading glasses during the examination, but are not permitted to bring snacks or cell phones into the examination room.

Although the examination is computerized, candidates do not necessarily need to have good computer skills. However, we have learned from NBCOT that students tend to do better if they take the tutorial offered at the beginning of the computer-delivered NBCOT Examination. When your studying is done, most of the preparation is complete. However, when asked to identify the single most important thing in preparing for the examination, a graduating class of students all agreed that the answer was getting a good night's sleep.

It also is a good idea to have directions to the test center location printed prior to your departure date and to remember to bring along two forms of personal identification, one being a government issued photo identification. Also, plan to arrive at the test site 30 minutes before the examination. Doing so will give you time to register, use the restroom, and become acclimated to your surroundings.

■ Test-Taking Tip 3

Prepare your body as well as your mind! Eating a well-balanced breakfast can actually help your performance on the examination. A breakfast high in carbohydrates and low in fat will increase your energy and not produce a sluggish feeling. Avoid caffeine, because its ultimate effect will be to leave you tired and drowsy in the middle of the examination. If possible, wear comfortable clothes in layers to allow you to adjust as necessary to the temperature of the room.

It also is important to be emotionally prepared for the examination. As a form of relaxation, the NBCOT Web site suggests slow, deep breathing as well as sitting in an upright position during the examination. Try to decrease any anxiety you might have by reminding yourself that you arrived at this day as a result of your hard work (passing fieldwork and coursework) and it is one of the last steps you must take on the road to working as an occupational therapy practitioner!

■ Test-Taking Tip 4

Pace yourself. The test is to be completed within 4 hours. Within this time frame, you have to answer 200 multiple-choice questions. Begin by familiarizing yourself with the computer test program and reading all of the instructions carefully. One technique for pacing the examination is to divide the test into four equivalent 50 question sections. You should aim to complete each of the four sections within 50 minutes to 1 hour. Understanding the format of the test and budgeting your time will help you work through the questions more efficiently and in the allotted time. Another pacing technique is to use a watch or the clock provided by the computer test program. At the end of every few pages of questions, briefly glance at the time to maintain a sense of your pace. If questions remain incomplete within the last 10 minutes of the examination, select one letter and fill in all of the remaining questions with that letter. *Remember, there is no penalty for guessing—only for leaving questions unanswered!* Another method is to wear a watch that can be set to signal on the hour. When the examination begins, set the watch for 12:00. Then you will know that at 4:00, the allotted time for taking the examination is up. Between 12:00 and 4:00, the watch will signal each hour so that you can check your pace without having to "watch the clock." The goal is to complete at least 25% of the examination, or 50 questions, within each hour. Avoid wasting time by looking frequently at your watch. If you find the computer test program clock too distracting, you have the option of turning it off. It also is important to remain calm if others complete the examination before you. According to NBCOT you do not need to leave the examination room until you have used all of the allotted examination time. If, for any reason, you experience problems during the examination, remain calm—a test center proctor will be available for your assistance.

■ Test-Taking Tip 5

Use key techniques to help select the correct answer.

1. *Follow your instincts when answering questions.* The first answer chosen is usually the correct one. Change an answer only if you later realize that it is absolutely correct.
2. *Ask, "What is this question about?"* Try to decipher what the question is testing by selecting the key terms in the questions and not being distracted by peripheral information. By sorting through the information provided to identify what the question is testing, you may be more likely to select the correct answer.
3. *Anticipate the answer.* Many times you may anticipate an answer while reading a question. If so, look for the anticipated answer among the options. However, it is important to read and consider all of the options to verify that the anticipated answer is the correct answer.
4. *Use logical reasoning.* A commonly used technique is the process of deduction—eliminating answers that are incorrect. Doing this allows you to concentrate on the options that remain.

As you complete the questions on the examination, remember these techniques and practice using them when you have difficulty answering a question.

■ Test-Taking Tip 6

There are no trick questions. Questions are designed to test entry-level, not advanced, knowledge and reason-

ing. Be careful not to read too much into the questions. However, most questions will have two answers that appear good. Many questions will ask for the "first" action the therapist should take, or the "best" or "most appropriate" choice. Make sure to note the qualifiers to help you determine the "best" answer. Also, remember that all NBCOT test answers on the examination are randomized. Do not look for patterns in the answers.

■ Test-Taking Tip 7

Use the enclosed CD ROM test program to your advantage. The enclosed computer test program allows you to "flag" a question similar to the format of the NBCOT examination so that you can go back to it later. It also allows you to identify unanswered questions and to change answers right up to the time you finally submit the test. The computerized practice examinations available from NBCOT are similar to the enclosed CD ROM practice examinations. As stated previously (please refer to: HOW TO USE THE ENCLOSED CD ROM), the user can select questions from specific **content areas,** such as pediatrics, mental health, cognition, physical disabilities, OT for populations, or service management/professional practice. Specific **Domains** also can be selected in areas such as evaluation, treatment planning, intervention implementation, OT for populations, or service management/ professional practice to essentially **create a personalized quiz** or to simulate a full 200-question examination.

■ BIBLIOGRAPHY

National Board for Certification in Occupational Therapy, Inc: A practice analysis study of entry-level occupational therapist registered and certified occupational therapy assistant practice. OTJR: Occupation, Participation and Health, volume 24, 2004.

Simulation Examination 1

Directions: Circle the correct answer to the following questions. When you have completed this examination, check your answers against the answer key that follows. As you will see, an explanation is given for each answer along with a reference for further study. The book author is listed as well as the chapter author. See the bibliography for complete references. Study the areas in which your comprehension was low then test yourself again by taking Simulation Examination 2.

■ EVALUATION

1.   When assessing an individual who is suspected of having carpal tunnel syndrome, the OT tests for Tinel's sign by gently tapping the median nerve at the level of the:

   A. elbow.
   B. mid-forearm.
   C. palmar crease.
   D. carpal tunnel.

2.   By using an interest checklist that includes a report of both interests and actual participation in activities, an OT practitioner will MOST likely collect information on an individual's:

   A. use of time.
   B. developmental level.
   C. mood and affect.
   D. communication skills.

3.   When evaluating a child who is at risk for shunt malfunction, it is MOST important for the therapist to observe for:

   A. increased tone.
   B. decreased tone.
   C. back pain.
   D. irritability and nausea.

4.   An OT practitioner working in a long-term care facility needs to evaluate the long-term memory of a resident. Which of the following methods is BEST for evaluating memory of personally experienced events (episodic memory)?

   A. Show the person a series of objects and ask him to recall the objects within 60 seconds.
   B. Ask the individual how he spent New Year's.
   C. Have the individual state the place, date, and time.
   D. Ask the client to remember to bring a specific item to the next therapy session.

5.   During assessment, an OT practitioner observes an individual who is able to place his dentures in his mouth, but has difficulty applying denture cream to the appropriate place on the dentures and attempts to place the cap on the tube backwards or on the wrong end of the tube. The OT is MOST LIKELY to interpret this as:

   A. constructional apraxia.
   B. ideomotor apraxia.
   C. dressing apraxia.
   D. unilateral neglect.

6.   As part of an initial evaluation, the OT practitioner is developing an occupational profile on a child with cerebral palsy. Which of the following BEST represents the OT's use of narrative clinical reasoning skills?

   A. Performing interviews with the child and family regarding daily routines, social, and child rearing practices
   B. Relying upon information gathered from the collaboration between the OT and the child/child's family
   C. Determining the child's performance level through an activity analysis task
   D. Focusing energy on the available social and financial resources of the family in order to identify the most appropriate intervention for the child

7.   An OT practitioner interviewing an individual diagnosed with Alzheimer's disease about his ADL performance realizes that the client is confabulating. Which of the following options is MOST appropriate?

    A. Complete the interview using closed-ended questions.

    B. Stop the interview and complete it the next day.

    C. Interview a reliable informant instead of the individual.

    D. Administer a written questionnaire using a checklist format.

8.   An OT practitioner documents that an individual exhibits elbow flexion strength of grade 1. According to the manual muscle test system of letters and numbers, the word that would be the equivalent of grade 1 would be:

    A. absent.

    B. trace.

    C. good.

    D. normal.

9.   During an initial visit with a 5-year-old child with a suspected learning disability, the OT practitioner observes the child run across the room, hop around on one foot, pick up a pencil, and draw a stick figure using a tripod grasp. When asked to complete a four-piece puzzle, the child gives up after several unsuccessful attempts. Which type of assessment would MOST effectively address this child's area of difficulty?

    A. Fine motor

    B. Gross motor

    C. Developmental

    D. Visual perceptual

10. A high school teacher diagnosed with a right-hemisphere CVA is given a paper with letters of the alphabet displayed in random order across the page and is instructed to cross out every "M." The individual misses half of the "M"s in a random pattern, which MOST likely indicates:

    A. a left visual field cut.

    B. a right visual field cut.

    C. functional illiteracy.

    D. decreased attention.

11. During an initial interview, parents describe their child as having severe difficulty communicating and interacting with others. The OT also observes that the child exhibits many repetitive and ritualistic behaviors. The behaviors described are MOST likely to be associated with:

    A. attention deficit hyperactivity disorder.

    B. childhood conduct disorder.

    C. obsessive-compulsive disorder.

    D. pervasive developmental disorder of childhood.

12. An OT practitioner is treating an individual who demonstrates progressive weakness and atrophy of the thenar muscles and numbness and tingling in the thumb, index, and middle fingers. The individual is not experiencing proximal upper extremity limitations so the practitioner will MOST likely suspect problems with which of the following?

    A. Ulnar nerve

    B. Median nerve

    C. Radial nerve

    D. Brachial plexus

13. The OT practitioner has just completed observing a child eating lunch. Which of the following statements BEST describes an objective observation?

    A. The child did not appear to like the food presented.

    B. The child demonstrated tongue thrust.

    C. The child was uncooperative and kept pushing the food out of her mouth.

    D. The child was obviously not hungry at the time.

14. An OT practitioner is preparing to complete an initial evaluation on an individual diagnosed with obsessive-compulsive disorder. Which strategy for modifying the environment is likely to be MOST effective while interviewing this individual?

    A. Limit the time available to answer each question.

    B. Instruct the individual to take her time and not rush.

    C. Utilize open-ended questions.

    D. Minimize environmental distractions.

15. An individual is able to complete the full range of shoulder flexion while in a side-lying position during an evaluation. However, against gravity, the individual is not quite able to achieve 75% of the range for shoulder flexion. This muscle should be graded as:

- A. good (4).
- B. fair (3).
- C. fair minus (3−).
- D. poor plus (2+).

16. An OT practitioner observes a child with a learning disability use an unusually tight grip when writing with a pencil. The child also frequently breaks the pencil point by applying too much pressure on the paper. This type of problem is MOST likely caused by inadequate sensory information from the:

- A. vestibular system.
- B. auditory system.
- C. somatosensory system.
- D. visual system.

17. During an initial evaluation, an OT practitioner documents that the individual's chart reveals a dual diagnosis from two mental health diagnostic categories. The individual MOST likely has a history of:

- A. Depression and substance abuse.
- B. Depression, mental retardation, and arthritis.
- C. Arthritis and peripheral vascular disease.
- D. Bipolar disorder, depression, and amputation.

18. Which of the following criteria must be met in order for an individual to be a candidate for a mobile arm support?

- A. Diagnosis of quadriplegia.
- B. Lateral trunk stability.
- C. Fair plus elbow flexion.
- D. At least 90 degrees of passive shoulder flexion and abduction.

19. An OT practitioner is evaluating an individual who has undergone a total hip replacement to determine compliance with hip precautions prior to discharge. When the individual is observed leaning forward and stopping at 90 degrees of hip flexion to use the long-handled shoe-horn, the therapist determines that the individual:

- A. demonstrates compliance with hip precautions.
- B. requires verbal cueing to observe hip precautions.
- C. requires a longer shoe horn.
- D. demonstrates cognitive deficits.

20. An OT practitioner is evaluating an adolescent with an attention deficit hyperactivity disorder. The therapist will be PARTICULARLY observant for behaviors such as:

- A. the individual becomes easily frustrated, cannot remain seated, and grabs tools from his peers.
- B. the individual frequently refers to himself as "the authority" and "the smartest" in the group.
- C. the individual uses profanities and strikes other students.
- D. the individual verbalizes anxiety about working on a project and expresses fear of failure.

21. An OT practitioner is treating an individual who has suddenly been diagnosed with a disabling condition. Which would be the adaptive response that would MOST likely pass in time without intervention?

- A. A dependency reaction
- B. A stress reaction
- C. A mourning response
- D. A desire to set unrealistic goals

22. An individual is unable to read a standardized evaluation because he does not have his glasses with him. Which of the following options is MOST appropriate?

- A. Instruct the individual to bring his glasses to the next session and complete the evaluation then.
- B. Ask the OT aide to read the evaluation to the individual and check off his answers.
- C. Include the individual in the group session that is about to begin and remind the individual to bring his glasses to the next session.
- D. Read the questions to the individual and check off his responses.

23. A toddler diagnosed with developmental delays does not finger-feed when presented with food in the clinic. The BEST way to obtain further information about his feeding skills is to:

- A. interview his parents to determine his favorite foods.
- B. observe him in his home during feeding time.
- C. review his chart for food allergies.
- D. repeat the observation in a quiet area to minimize distractions.

24. During evaluation, an individual who had a severe myocardial infarction 2 weeks ago displays good memory of information processed before the MI, poor recall of the first week after the MI, but good recall of information from the past week. The OT practitioner would MOST likely document this as:

- A. disorientation.
- B. long-term memory deficits.
- C. anterograde amnesia.
- D. retrograde amnesia.

25. An OT practitioner is performing a functional ROM assessment on an elderly individual with arthritis. How should the OT evaluate internal rotation?

- A. Ask the individual to touch the back of his neck.
- B. Use a goniometer to measure internal rotation in a supine position.
- C. Observe the individual touching the small of his back.
- D. Interview the individual regarding areas of pain and stiffness.

26. While developing an occupational therapy profile on a child with a pervasive developmental disorder, the OT practitioner meets with the child's primary caregiver. The OT should attempt to do which of the following FIRST:

- A. Ask the caregiver about the child's typical day and nighttime routines as well as strategies the child uses to communicate.
- B. Obtain permission to perform norm referenced testing on the child.
- C. Interview the child's teacher to determine developmental milestones the child has reached.
- D. Observe the child in daily activities within the child's home environment.

27. An OT practitioner is assessing an individual who has schizophrenia and appears to be experiencing positive symptoms of the disease. During the initial evaluation, the individual might exhibit:

- A. a toneless voice.
- B. very little facial expression.
- C. a false perception of reality.
- D. difficulty concentrating.

28. Upon completion of the initial interview and chart review, the NEXT step to be taken in the OT process is to:

- A. analyze the data.
- B. develop a treatment plan.
- C. perform selected assessments.
- D. select appropriate evaluation procedures.

29. An OT practitioner observes that a 10-month-old child is able to sit alone by propping himself forward on his arms, but consistently loses his balance when reaching for a toy. This behavior MOST likely indicates:

- A. a developmental delay.
- B. unintegrated primitive reflexes.
- C. normal development.
- D. advanced development.

30. An OT is evaluating attention through a cooking task with an adult client. Which of the following will the OT MOST likely focus on?

- A. Visual discrimination and the ability to locate single visual targets
- B. Orientation to time, place, and space
- C. Alertness, selective attention, and mental tracking
- D. Degree of awareness regarding impairment

31. An individual who recently experienced an MI has been referred to OT. To determine the individual's current endurance level, the OT practitioner plans to monitor performance of self-care activities. The FIRST step is to:

- A. take the individual's vital signs after performance of self-care activities.
- B. observe the individual for signs and symptoms of exhaustion during self-care activities.
- C. take the individual's vital signs at rest.
- D. take vital signs 5 minutes after the individual has completed self-care activities.

32. While assessing the motor skills of an 11-month-old child, the OT practitioner observes the child assume a quadruped position and then begin to rock back and forth. This behavior MOST likely indicates:

- A. perseverative tendencies.
- B. normal development.
- C. low muscle tone.
- D. limitation in movement repertoire.

33. Determining a developmentally disabled adult's level of cognitive function according to Allen's Cognitive Disability theory provides information about the person which is MOST helpful for:

- A. identifying the client's difficult behaviors that might interfere with intervention.
- B. planning a training program to improve prevocational skills.
- C. identifying the type of environmental supports that can maximize the client's level of function.
- D. developing an educational plan to improve social skills.

34. An OT practitioner is working with an individual who has dysphagia. The OT should anticipate that the individual will have difficulty:
   A. coordinating the two sides of the body.
   B. expressing him/herself orally.
   C. swallowing crushed ice.
   D. speaking clearly.

35. A child with significantly low muscle tone caused by Duchenne's muscular dystrophy is losing trunk control when sitting. The OT assesses the child's range of motion, strength, and endurance which indicates that the practitioner is MOST likely relying upon which frame of reference?
   A. Neurodevelopmental treatment
   B. Sensory integration
   C. Biomechanical
   D. Visual perceptual

36. In evaluating an adolescent with psychosocial problems, an OT practitioner would be MOST likely to begin the process by screening the adolescent's level of function in which areas?
   A. Play skills, overall development, and visual motor skills
   B. Socialization, task performance, daily living skills, and time management
   C. Interest in work and household management
   D. Motor skills and sensory processing

37. An OT practitioner is conducting a perceptual function screening with an individual who has had a CVA. Which of the following informal screening activities would the therapist ask the individual to perform in order to identify the presence of agnosia?
   A. Demonstrate common gestures such as waving
   B. Identify objects through touch only
   C. Identify or demonstrate the use of common household objects
   D. Read a paragraph and explain its meaning

38. An individual with a head injury is frequently observed watching the person next to her instead of performing her assigned task. The OT practitioner should document this as a problem with:
   A. memory.
   B. spatial operations.
   C. generalization of learning.
   D. attention.

39. When evaluating motor control in a beginning-level patient with TBI (Rancho Los Amigos Scale score of 1-3), the OT practitioner will MOST likely observe for:
   A. response to simple verbal commands.
   B. response to pain or temperature.
   C. tone, rigidity, and reflexes.
   D. eye contact.

40. During the evaluation of a 6-month-old baby, the OT practitioner gently pulls the infant from a supine position into a sitting position by the hands. The child demonstrates the ability to hold her head and trunk in alignment against gravity. This observable movement can MOST accurately be described by the practitioner as a(n):
   A. protective reaction.
   B. flexion righting reaction.
   C. body righting on body reaction.
   D. optical righting reaction.

41. A method that an OT practitioner can use to document total finger flexion without recording the measurement in degrees would be to measure the:
   A. passive flexion at each joint and total the numbers.
   B. distance from the fingertip to the distal palmar crease with the hand in a fist.
   C. active flexion at each joint and total the measurements.
   D. distance between the tip of the thumb and the tip of the fourth finger.

42. The OT is assessing sensory awareness in an individual who is s/p right CVA. Which of the following techniques is MOST appropriate?
   A. Establish a rapport with the individual, then test the affected side, followed by the unaffected side.
   B. Demonstrate the procedure on the unaffected extremity, then occlude the individual's vision and test the affected side.
   C. Occlude the individual's vision, demonstrate the procedure on the affected extremity, then unocclude vision and test both sides.
   D. Interview the individual and assess only the areas that he or she reports are impaired.

43. At a team meeting, a teacher reports that a child is having difficulty copying letters, doing mazes, and using scissors. This behavior MOST likely indicates a problem in which of the following areas?

- A. Visual-motor integration
- B. Visual acuity
- C. Visual tracking
- D. Visual perception

44. An OT practitioner has been working with an individual who sustained a deep laceration of the median and ulnar nerves, resulting in complete sensory loss. Upon re-evaluation, the therapist should FIRST expect to see return of:

- A. vibration and pain.
- B. temperature and pain.
- C. light touch and proprioception.
- D. tactile localization and proprioception.

45. In screening a child who has been referred to OT, the PRIMARY goal of the OT practitioner is to:

- A. obtain necessary information for an occupational therapy consultation with teachers or parents.
- B. test a wide variety of developmental behaviors.
- C. establish an information base for the occupational therapy treatment plan.
- D. determine the need for further evaluation.

46. When evaluating an individual with coronary artery disease for controllable risk factors, the OT practitioner should:

- A. determine the individual's age and gender.
- B. assess the individual's lifestyle and dietary habits.
- C. observe the individual for obesity and cholesterol levels.
- D. determine if the individual has a family history of heart disease.

47. A young child with a diagnosis of spina bifida has been referred for assessment. When collecting the initial data by interviewing the child's parent, the OT practitioner should focus PRIMARILY on:

- A. the parent's concerns and goals for the child.
- B. medical management.
- C. equipment needs.
- D. the physical layout of the home.

48. An OT practitioner is assessing the range of motion of an individual who actively demonstrates internal rotation of the shoulder to 70 degrees. The practitioner would MOST likely document this measurement as:

- A. within normal limits.
- B. within functional limits.
- C. hypermobility that requires further treatment.
- D. limited mobility that requires further treatment.

49. A woman who had a stroke tries unsuccessfully to put on a blouse using a one-handed technique. She states, "I can do it, I'm just not trying hard enough." The OT practitioner most accurately recognizes this as:

- A. denial.
- B. projection.
- C. rationalization.
- D. regression.

■ INTERVENTION PLANNING

50. An OT practitioner is working with a medically stable child who sustained bilateral upper extremity partial thickness burns 3 days ago while playing with a lighter. Which ADL intervention should the OT introduce first?

- A. Instruct the child to use adapted equipment for all ADLs.
- B. Encourage independent compression garment application.
- C. Perform bilateral upper extremity PROM exercises twice a day.
- D. Encourage independent ADLs with minimal reliance on adapted utensils and tools.

51. Following evaluation of an elderly individual, an OT practitioner determines that the individual no longer leaves home primarily because of fear of falling. The MOST important goal of treatment for this individual would be to:

- A. increase lower extremity strength.
- B. regain confidence in the ability to ambulate.
- C. modify the environment to reduce the risk of falling.
- D. reduce the use of medications that may be contributing to falls.

52. An OT practitioner is considering the use of classical sensory integration therapy for a child with a learning disability. Which of the following techniques would be MOST consistent with this approach?

    A. Include the child in a group of children using a program of sensory stimulation activities.

    B. Encourage the child to participate in activities that are passive and do not require adaptive responses.

    C. Design an individualized program directed at the underlying neurological deficit.

    D. Promote the development of specific motor skills, such as balance and coordination.

53. Which of the following activities would BEST represent an expected outcome for an individual who completes an energy-conservation program?

    A. Getting dressed without becoming fatigued

    B. Lifting heavy cookware without pain

    C. Doing handicrafts without damaging his or her joints

    D. Dusting and vacuuming more quickly

54. To effectively address the needs of a child with a pervasive developmental disorder, a teacher uses the Treatment and Education of Autistic and Related Communication Handicapped Children (TEACCH) curriculum. In keeping with the curriculum, the OT would MOST likely recommend to the teacher that the child engage in:

    A. large group, gross-motor obstacle courses.

    B. small group, fine-motor clay pinch pottery activities.

    C. unstructured group, collage poster projects.

    D. small group, unstructured games such as tag.

55. In establishing long-term goals for an individual with T4 paraplegia in a rehabilitation setting, the OT practitioner would MOST likely predict that the patient will attain what level of independence with bathing, dressing, and transfers?

    A. Complete independence with self-care and transfers

    B. Independence with self-care and minimal assistance with transfers

    C. Minimal assistance with self-care and moderate assistance with transfers

    D. Dependence with both self-care and transfers

56. An OT practitioner is running a sensorimotor group for individuals diagnosed with major depressive disorder who tend to withdraw from social activities. Which of the following would be the MOST appropriate opening activity?

    A. Group members take turns introducing themselves.

    B. Group members toss a ball to each other.

    C. Each group member describes his or her day.

    D. Group members pass around and feel different textured fabrics in a basket.

57. When developing play activities for a child with acute juvenile rheumatoid arthritis, which of the following precautions should the OTR follow?

    A. Avoid light touch.

    B. Avoid rapid vestibular stimulation.

    C. Avoid resistive materials.

    D. Avoid elevated temperatures.

58. An intelligent individual with a diagnosis of paranoid schizophrenia has been hospitalized in an acute care psychiatric setting and has just joined the OT program. Which initial activity would BEST engage this patient?

    A. Assembling a complex airplane model requiring the use of detailed directions

    B. Finishing and painting a preassembled wooden box

    C. Playing a competitive game of chess

    D. Engaging in a reminiscence discussion

59. Which individual would benefit the MOST from using a wrist-driven flexor hinge splint during a prehension activity?

    A. An individual with a C1 injury

    B. An individual with a C3 injury

    C. An individual with a C6 injury

    D. An individual with a T1 injury

60. To develop the MOST relevant goals and objectives for a child's OT program, the OTR should focus goals on:

    A. the child's priorities.

    B. the priorities of the parents or caregivers.

    C. the therapist's priorities for solution of problems identified in the OT evaluation.

    D. child, caregiver, and therapist priorities.

61. A long-term goal for an individual following a hip arthroplasty is independence in lower extremity dressing. The MOST relevant short-term goal for the OT practitioner to work on would be for the individual to:

A. increase standing tolerance to 10 minutes.
B. increase hip flexion to 90 degrees.
C. demonstrate appropriate hip precautions.
D. apply energy-conservation techniques during dressing activities.

62. An OT practitioner who selects the behavioral frame of reference for an individual with psychosocial issues is primarily seeking an approach which focuses on the:

A. level of skill required that is appropriate for the generally expected skills for that age.
B. symbolic potential and use of activities to explore personal meaning.
C. combined activity demands of sensations, perceptions, and motor skills.
D. observable analysis, measurable outcomes, and reinforcement for building specific skills.

63. An elderly individual who was hospitalized for a right cerebrovascular accident with left upper extremity flaccidity and decreased sensation is beginning to experience sensory return in the left upper extremity. Intervention strategies should now include:

A. remedial treatment, such as rubbing or stroking the involved extremity.
B. remedial treatment, such as the use of hot mitts to avoid burns.
C. compensatory treatment, such as testing bathwater with the uninvolved extremity.
D. compensatory treatment, such as using a one-handed cutting board to avoid cutting the insensate hand.

64. During an initial occupational therapy session with an individual in a psychosocial treatment setting, which of the following introductory statements would BEST reflect what is meant by a client-centered therapeutic relationship?

A. "The most important aspect of the therapy is the relationship that develops between the client and the therapist."
B. "We will be working together to achieve your goals."
C. "The process of therapy should be the beginning of a good friendship between us."
D. "Your situation is unfortunate and I hope that our relationship can improve the situation."

65. In planning a therapeutic dressing intervention for a first-grade child who is mentally retarded, the OT practitioner's FIRST consideration should be the need for:

A. adaptive equipment.
B. adaptive clothing.
C. proper positioning.
D. adapted teaching techniques.

66. An OT practitioner is working with an individual with AIDS who displays sensory loss and has become too weak to turn himself in bed. What should the therapist plan to do next?

A. Begin a strengthening program.
B. Begin a bed-mobility program.
C. Teach a caregiver how to lift and turn the client safely.
D. Provide an environmental control unit to the client.

67. A short-term goal of the treatment plan of a child with cerebral palsy is to inhibit flexor spasticity in his hands to improve the ability to manipulate objects during play. The activity that would be MOST appropriate in meeting this objective would be:

A. building a block tower.
B. active release of blocks into a container.
C. traction on the finger flexors.
D. weight bearing over a small bolster in prone.

68. An OT practitioner is treating an individual who has difficulty maintaining attention to a task, but is aware of the problem. The BEST example of a strategy that the therapist can teach the person to control effects of attention deficits would be:

A. simplifying the instructions given to accomplish the task so only one step is presented at a time.
B. learning the self-monitoring technique of asking oneself if any part of the task has been missed.
C. providing practice in shape and number cancellation worksheets.
D. removing unnecessary objects from around the task area to decrease distractions.

69. Which of the following children with neuromotor impairment would benefit MOST from using a prone scooter for exploratory play?

A. A child with cerebral palsy with predominant extensor tone
B. A child with low tone who is easily fatigued
C. A child with cognitive limitations and poor sensory awareness
D. A child with spina bifida with lower extremity paralysis

70. Which of the following is MOST important to include in the initial intervention for an individual with complete paralysis as a result of Guillain-Barré syndrome?

    A. ADL training

    B. Balance and stabilization activities

    C. Passive ROM, positioning, and splinting

    D. Resistive activities for the intrinsic hand muscles

71. An individual with right unilateral neglect is able to track from the left side to the midline of the body on paper-and-pencil tasks. The BEST treatment activity to promote crossing the midline to improve writing skills would be to:

    A. have the individual practice wheeling a wheelchair following a taped line on the floor.

    B. place commonly used self-care items on the left side.

    C. have the individual trace lines across the page with the right index finger from the left to the right side.

    D. place playing cards in a horizontal row from right to left in sequence.

72. An OT practitioner is planning treatment for a child after an assessment. The FIRST step in the general problem analysis of a child's occupational therapy evaluation is to:

    A. define and describe the child's problem.

    B. describe precautions associated with the problem.

    C. identify the critical elements of development and role performance for the age of the child.

    D. consider the effects of the problem on developmental tasks and performance.

73. An individual in the early stages of amyotrophic lateral sclerosis has been referred for OT in an outpatient setting. Which of the following interventions is MOST appropriate for this individual?

    A. Work simplification and energy conservation

    B. Progressive resistive exercises

    C. Splinting

    D. Active and passive range-of-motion exercises

74. A child with a physical disability and poor postural stability is developmentally ready for toileting. Which of the following elements of the treatment plan should be considered FIRST?

    A. Training in management of fasteners

    B. Provision of foot support

    C. Provision of a seatbelt

    D. Training in climbing onto the toilet

75. An OT practitioner is planning a vocational intervention program to assist an individual in a community mental health day program to develop skills needed for obtaining employment. Which of the following would be the MOST relevant intervention to include?

    A. Self-assessment of work habits and personality characteristics

    B. Activities focused on organizational and communication skills and practice of job-seeking strategies

    C. Educating the work supervisors about the individual's needs and offering environmental modifications to maximize performance

    D. Expressive activities such as making a collage with pictures of different types of jobs

76. An older adult with diabetes is working on a macramé project as a way of increasing standing tolerance. The MOST relevant safety factor to take into consideration is the:

    A. length of the cords to be used.

    B. thickness of the cords to be used.

    C. texture of the cords to be used.

    D. type of surface the individual will be standing on.

77. An individual with a history of anger self-control issues has met the goals of independently identifying anger-provoking stressors in his home and work life and identifying his typical behaviors in anger-provoking situations. The OT practitioner's NEXT action should be to:

    A. begin instruction in anger management strategies, such as relaxation.

    B. change the focus of treatment to developing self-assertiveness skills.

    C. provide activities, such as hammering, that provide outlets for anger.

    D. recommend discontinuation of occupational therapy services.

78. Which of the following activities should the OT practitioner suggest to promote prewriting skills for a child in kindergarten?

    A. Hammering objects into a Styrofoam board

    B. Having the child create his or her own books on specific topics

    C. Rolling clay into a ball

    D. Drawing lines and shapes using shaving cream, sand, or finger paints

79. An individual with an upper extremity fracture has asked how to maintain strength in her arm until the cast is removed. The activities that would BEST accomplish this goal are those which incorporate:

    A. isometric muscle contractions.

    B. isotonic muscle contractions.

    C. progressive resistance.

    D. passive movement.

80. An OT practitioner is planning group programming in an acute care psychiatry setting for severely mentally ill individuals who display disorganized thinking and difficulty functioning in many areas. The MOST appropriate type of group to use is a(n):

    A. activity group.

    B. psychoeducational group.

    C. neurodevelopmental group.

    D. directive group.

81. The OT is planning treatment to promote developmental acquisition for an infant in the neonatal intensive care unit. Which of the following actions will have the most PERMANENT impact?

    A. Modify the environment to protect the infant from additional stressful stimuli.

    B. Recommend early intervention referral to assess the infant upon discharge home.

    C. Complete the neurobehavioral assessment and identify interventions emphasizing developmental skill acquisition.

    D. Create a comfortable foundation for fostering parent skills through parent-therapist collaboration.

82. An individual has sustained a large, full-thickness burn to both upper extremities and is in the acute care phase of treatment. Which of the following BEST represents an acute care rehabilitation goal?

    A. Prevent loss of joint and skin mobility.

    B. Provide adaptive equipment.

    C. Provide compression and vascular support garments.

    D. Prevent scar hypertrophy through scar management techniques.

83. Which of the following community activities provides an appropriate level of challenge for a client beginning assertiveness training?

    A. Asking a department store salesperson for information about an item without buying it

    B. In a restaurant, requesting that food be sent back to be rewarmed

    C. Returning an item to a department store for cash with the receipt

    D. Questioning a waitress about whether a restaurant bill is accurate

84. The goal for a child with a neuromuscular disorder is to develop postural reactions. Which of the following activities would BEST address this goal?

    A. Pulley exercises to increase upper extremity strength.

    B. Direct the child to reach for a toy while sitting on a therapy ball.

    C. Encourage the child to engage in playdough activities while in the prone position.

    D. Request that the child practice figure-ground tasks in a supported seated position.

85. An OT practitioner is fabricating a splint for an individual who sustained a low-level ulnar nerve injury. The MOST appropriate splint for this individual is one that:

    A. prevents hyperextension of the PIP joints and allows PIP flexion.

    B. prevents hyperextension of the MCP joints and allows MCP flexion.

    C. allows hyperextension of the MCP joints and prevents MCP flexion.

    D. allows flexion and hyperextension of the MCP joints.

86. When planning treatment for individuals diagnosed with eating disorders, the OT practitioner's initial OT treatment goals would MOST likely address:

    A. increasing self-awareness through expressive activities.

    B. increasing awareness of nutritional issues.

    C. improving school performance skills.

    D. making recommendations or referrals for family therapy.

87. A 3-year-old child with a diagnosis of mental retardation is dependent in all areas of dressing. When using a developmental approach with this child, which skill should FIRST be addressed?
  A. Putting on garments with the front and back of clothing correctly placed
  B. Putting on a tee shirt
  C. Removing pants
  D. Buttoning and tying bows

88. An individual is experiencing edema in the right upper extremity and hand, and complains of joint stiffness. Which of the following should be implemented FIRST?
  A. Contrast baths, active and passive range of motion, and massage
  B. Ultrasound, electrical stimulation, and dynamic splinting
  C. Resistive exercises, weight bearing, and lifting
  D. Joint mobilization, serial casting, and dynamic splinting

89. An individual is participating in a work-hardening program after an accident resulting in physical limitations. The individual's goal is to return to his job as an auto mechanic. Which of the following BEST represents a work-simulation activity?
  A. Lifting weights
  B. Working on a mock car engine
  C. Visiting the work site garage
  D. Preparing a light lunch for mealtime

90. An OT practitioner is using a visual perceptual frame of reference to plan intervention for a child with visual perceptual problems. The FIRST activities planned should address which type of visual skills?
  A. Visual memory skills
  B. Visual attention skills
  C. General visual discrimination skills
  D. Specific visual discrimination skills

91. An OT practitioner is planning a meal preparation activity for an individual with cognitive deficits in the areas of attentional and organizational skills. The most appropriate activity to use FIRST in addressing sequencing skills is:
  A. setting the table.
  B. planning a meal.
  C. baking cookies using a recipe.
  D. preparing a shopping list.

92. An individual who previously worked as a cashier in a clothing store has been referred to a work-hardening program following knee surgery. Limitations are present in standing tolerance and balance. The activity that will BEST prepare this individual to return to work is:
  A. moving piles of clothing from one end of the clinic to the other.
  B. folding laundry and putting it in a basket while standing.
  C. washing dishes while standing.
  D. putting price tags on clothing while sitting.

■ IMPLEMENTING INTERVENTION

93. An individual with Parkinson's disease has particular difficulty with both starting and stopping movements. The BEST strategy for the OT to teach the individual and the individual's caregivers is to:
  A. encourage the individual to perform a deep breathing exercise when movement is "frozen."
  B. have the individual practice the starting phase of the movement repeatedly.
  C. have the individual mentally identify the series of steps needed to initiate the movement.
  D. provide a sensory cue, such as saying "stop!"

94. A child's short-term goal is to "demonstrate increased manipulation skills by opening a 3-inch screw-top jar independently." The MOST important tool for determining the child's progress is:
  A. a goniometer.
  B. a 3-inch screw-top jar.
  C. a dynamometer.
  D. a developmental fine-motor assessment.

95. The principles MOST important to include when training an individual in joint protection are:
  A. using the strongest joint and avoiding positions of deformity.
  B. preparing muscles and joints with massage before exercise.
  C. practicing vivid imagery and relaxation exercises during difficult functional activities.
  D. application of heat before treatment, and application of cold after range-of-motion treatment.

96. A child with an attention deficit disorder, hyperactivity type is receiving OT to increase his attention span. Keeping this in mind, the OT introduces a construction activity. When a puzzle with many pieces is placed in front of the child, the child sweeps many of them onto the floor and starts throwing the remaining ones around the room. How can the OT MOST effectively restructure the activity to facilitate a successful experience for this child?

    A. Use soft foam puzzle pieces.

    B. Provide puzzle pieces of one color only.

    C. Use larger interlocking puzzle pieces.

    D. Present only a few puzzle pieces at a time.

97. An individual is having difficulty getting around her home as a result of low vision. The MOST appropriate strategy the OT practitioner can recommend to improve accessibility would be to:

    A. instruct the individual to sit while performing ADL.

    B. provide strong color contrast at key areas to identify steps, pathways, etc.

    C. recommend the individual arrange to get assistance from another person when moving within the home.

    D. recommend training in white cane use for identifying obstacles in the home.

98. An OT practitioner is preparing for the discharge of a preadolescent child with limited strength and endurance. Which of the following home adaptations is MOST important to recommend?

    A. Mount lever handles on doors and faucets.

    B. Remove all throw rugs.

    C. Install nonskid pads on steps.

    D. Mount a table top easel for written homework.

99. An individual demonstrates flaccidity in the left upper extremity following a CVA. While performing PROM to the affected arm, the OT practitioner notes marked pitting edema of the left hand. The OT practitioner should:

    A. continue to perform PROM and then position and elevate the affected extremity.

    B. fabricate a resting splint for the affected extremity.

    C. take no action and wait for the edema to subside.

    D. have the individual attempt to squeeze a ball.

100. An OT practitioner is working with a teenager whose upper extremity physical disabilities and lack of head control limit the ability to independently read magazines. The BEST solution would be to:

    A. teach the student how to use a book holder and mouthstick.

    B. hire a human attendant to assist the student during school.

    C. purchase talking books.

    D. train the student to use an electrically powered page turner.

101. An individual is being discharged from inpatient rehabilitation following a CVA. The individual requires minimal assistance in advanced ADL, but is independent in transfers and most basic ADL, demonstrates continuing improvement in RUE function, and plans on eventually returning to work. Recommendations for continued OT services would MOST likely include:

    A. home health OT.

    B. outpatient OT.

    C. a work-hardening program.

    D. discontinuation of OT services.

102. During the clean-up portion of a cooking activity, an elderly woman with a diagnosis of depression and dementia begins to dry the plates and utensils she has already dried. The OT practitioner should:

    A. tell the client that the same dishes and utensils are being redried.

    B. put the dried dishes away and begin to hand her wet dishes.

    C. ask the client to stop the activity because it seems too difficult.

    D. ask the client to describe what she is doing.

103. An OT practitioner is demonstrating bathing techniques for a child with hypertonic muscle tone. Which of the following suggestions would be MOST appropriate for the OT to recommend to the child's parents?

    A. Avoid the use of adaptive equipment.

    B. Bathe the child quickly to avoid an increase in tone.

    C. Handle the child slowly and gently.

    D. Stand and lean over the tub to support and wash the child.

104. An OT is applying PNF techniques for weight shifting during an activity that requires an individual to use the right hand to remove groceries from a bag on the floor to the right. The MOST benefit would be gained from this activity by then placing the groceries:

A. on the counter directly in front.
B. on the counter to the left side.
C. in the upper cabinet to the right side.
D. in the upper cabinet to the left side.

105. An OT practitioner is working with an elderly patient with early stage dementia who was admitted to the hospital after accidentally setting fire to his kitchen. The MOST appropriate follow-up services to identify relative to this patient's meal-planning needs after discharge would be:

A. OT services to teach the patient to cook safely.
B. volunteer companion services to supervise cooking at home.
C. transportation services to bring the person to a community meal site.
D. home-delivered meal services.

106. An individual who is s/p total hip arthroplasty is working on independence in lower extremity dressing. Which of the following instructions is MOST important to convey to this individual regarding safety?

A. Sit during dressing activities.
B. Avoid internal rotation and adduction of the involved hip.
C. Use a long-handled shoe horn and dressing stick.
D. Wear shoes with elastic laces.

107. The OT practitioner is working with a child with low muscle tone who has difficulty engaging in activities against gravity. The OT also wants to encourage the child to play. To address these issues, the OT would MOST likely position the child:

A. long sitting along a wall.
B. side-lying on a mat.
C. supine on a large wedge.
D. prone over a bolster.

108. A patient with poor visual acuity is about to be discharged after completing a rehabilitation program following a total hip replacement. The MOST appropriate environmental adaptation to ensure that the individual can go up and down stairs safely is:

A. installing a stair glide.
B. installing handrails on both sides of the steps.
C. marking the end of each step with high contrast tape.
D. instructing the patient to take only one step at a time when going up or down.

109. An OT practitioner is seeing a home health-care client who is in the middle stages of Alzheimer's disease and whose memory loss is now interfering with the performance of daily self-care activities. The MOST relevant OT intervention at this point would be:

A. memory retraining activities for the client.
B. ADL retraining program for the client.
C. instructing caregivers in task breakdown.
D. leisure activity planning.

110. Which of the following would the OT practitioner MOST likely recommend an individual use at home after discharge following a total hip arthroplasty?

A. A wire basket attached to a walker
B. A padded foam toilet seat 1 inch in height
C. A short-handled bath sponge
D. A long-handled bath sponge

111. The OT practitioner has fitted a 6-year-old child for an adapted seat for use in the home for mealtime and other tabletop activities. Which of the following instructions is MOST appropriate to convey to the parents?

A. Change the seat as needed.
B. Bring the seat in for each weekly therapy session in order to adjust it according to the child's growth.
C. Bring the seat in for reevaluation within 6 months.
D. Keep the seat until the end of the IEP.

112. While performing endurance training activities, an individual on a cardiac rehabilitation unit begins to slow down, using progressively smaller movements to perform the activity. Which of the following is the MOST appropriate action for the OT practitioner to take?

A. Stop the activity.
B. Upgrade the activity for the next session.
C. Modify the activity to make it less challenging.
D. Replace the activity with isometric exercises.

113. An individual who sustained a mild head injury continues to have difficulty with remembering appointments and activities. Which external compensatory memory devices would be appropriate for the OT practitioner to recommend to assist this person with memory following discharge to home?

    A. visual imagery techniques

    B. Calendars

    C. Mnemonics

    D. Repetition

114. An individual with Parkinson's disease reports recently having "an accident" when unable to make it to the bathroom in time. When the home health OT recommends a bedside commode, the idea is immediately rejected. Which of the following actions should the OT practitioner take FIRST?

    A. Identify options and the consequences of each option.

    B. Document the individual's reasons for rejecting the bedside commode.

    C. Practice with a "demo" bedside commode.

    D. Allow time for the individual to think about the bedside commode.

115. Setting up an unstructured obstacle course that provides several options for allowing a child to choose the direction he will take would be MOST appropriate if the OT wished to encourage:

    A. exploratory play.

    B. symbolic play.

    C. creative play.

    D. recreational play.

116. Which one of the following is the BEST bathing technique for an individual with chronic obstructive pulmonary disease and low endurance?

    A. Tub bathing with hot water

    B. Standing for a quick shower

    C. Using a bath chair and leaving the door open

    D. Tub bathing using lukewarm water

117. A 16-year-old boy with juvenile rheumatoid arthritis is ready to begin shaving, but has difficulty as a result of limited range of motion in his shoulders and elbows. Which of the following is the BEST adaptation for him to use?

    A. Electric razor attached to universal cuff

    B. Safety razor with built-up handle

    C. Safety razor with extended handle

    D. Safety razor attached to universal cuff

118. An OT practitioner observes that an individual who had been doing well on a pureed diet has demonstrated a gurgle, or wet voice, after swallowing a second time. The MOST appropriate recommendation for the therapist to make is for this person to have a:

    A. videofluoroscopy.

    B. diet change to include thin liquids.

    C. tracheostomy tube.

    D. regular diet.

119. A young individual with neurological deficits has been unable to carry over skills learned previously in therapy, and has exhibited the inability to learn new information. The MOST appropriate strategy to suggest to the patient's mother to improve ADL functioning would be to recommend:

    A. repetitive practice of simple ADL under the OT practitioner's guidance.

    B. environmental adaptations and assistance for ADL.

    C. ADL training in the familiar home environment.

    D. forward or backward chaining techniques.

120. A child with a diagnosis of athetoid CP would like to be able to dress herself independently. Which of the following clothing features could the OT practitioner recommend that would be MOST useful in facilitating self-dressing?

    A. Mini tee shirts made of elasticized fabric

    B. Dresses with side zippers and zipper pulls

    C. Oversized tee shirts and elastic top pants

    D. Shirts with front closures, such as snaps or large buttons

121. An unmarried patient with a spinal cord injury is on a rehab unit and constantly flirts with the OT. The MOST appropriate action for the OT practitioner to take would be:

    A. firmly reject the patient's advances.

    B. acknowledge the patient's actions and mildly flirt back in order to promote the patient's self-esteem.

    C. request that the supervising OTR discuss the effects of SCI and sexual functioning with the patient.

    D. set personal boundaries appropriate to the therapist-patient relationship.

122. An OT practitioner is planning to begin work on self-care activities with an individual who recently had a traumatic brain injury, and who has cognitive and visual perceptual impairments. The MOST effective way for the practitioner to present directions during the activity would be to:

    A. tell the patient about the activity he will be working on and ask him to begin.

    B. rely on facial expressions and body gestures, rather than words, to get the patient started.

    C. state simple, concrete directions allowing time for delayed responses.

    D. provide a written list of steps with pictures for the patient to follow.

123. An OT practitioner places a 6-month-old infant in the supine position and arranges attractive toys overhead to provide an opportunity to work against gravity. This position will MOST likely encourage:

    A. shoulder flexion and protraction.

    B. shoulder extension and retraction.

    C. head control.

    D. trunk control.

124. An OT practitioner is working with an individual who recently had a myocardial infarction and fatigues easily. His long-term goal is to be able to dress independently while applying energy conservation techniques. Which statement is the BEST example of a short-term goal?

    A. "The patient will demonstrate energy conservation techniques during performance of all ADLs."

    B. "The patient will perform lower extremity dressing with assistance for shoes and socks."

    C. "The patient will perform lower extremity dressing with verbal cueing for energy conservation techniques 50% of the time."

    D. "Instruct patient in the use of energy conservation techniques that apply to dressing."

125. An individual exhibits no awareness of functional limitations resulting from his recent head injury, attempts to perform transfers unsafely without assistance, and says that he doesn't see the need for therapy. To promote awareness and insight, the OT practitioner is MOST likely to:

    A. have the individual explain why he believes he is not impaired.

    B. provide the individual with a checklist of skills he must have to perform various activities and review these.

    C. have the individual predict his performance before an activity, then have him self-evaluate the performance.

    D. disregard the individual's perceptions and proceed with therapy.

126. In order to promote tenodesis when performing PROM, the OT practitioner should position the wrist in:

    A. the neutral position to promote finger flexion and extension.

    B. flexion to promote finger flexion and extension.

    C. extension to promote finger flexion, and flexion to facilitate finger extension.

    D. flexion to encourage finger flexion, and extension to promote finger extension.

127. The BEST recommendation for activities to reduce the physical symptoms of muscle tension associated with anxiety disorder would be:

    A. sewing and handcrafts.

    B. aerobic exercise.

    C. line dancing.

    D. woodworking projects.

128. An OT is working with the mother of a child who has an oral structural problem related to a recessed tongue. When bottle feeding, the OT suggests that the mother use:

    A. a wide nipple.

    B. a single hole nipple.

    C. a broad-based nipple.

    D. a long, thin nipple.

129. Which of the following devices is required for an individual with C7-C8 quadriplegia when performing oral hygiene activities?

    A. Mobile arm support with utensil holder

    B. Universal cuff

    C. Toothbrush with built-up handle

    D. Wrist support with utensil holder

130. The PRIMARY functions of an OT practitioner leading a therapeutic group in the beginning stages of group development are to:

   A. observe, set the climate, and model desired behaviors.
   B. require group members to observe each other, set the climate, and model desired behaviors.
   C. aid group members in separation and reinforce gains made in the group.
   D. work individually with group members until each is ready to join group activity.

131. The MOST appropriate adaptation for gardening for a individual with a back injury would be:

   A. ergonomically correct hand tools.
   B. a wheelbarrow with elongated handles.
   C. a 12-inch-high seat with tool holders.
   D. a raised-bed garden.

132. In a social skills group, members have learned about social skills and their components, and the OT practitioner has spent time in modeling and demonstrating ways to perform social skills. Which of the following would be the NEXT step in the process of learning social skills?

   A. Practicing how to self-evaluate one's social behavior
   B. Independent practice in real life situations
   C. Role-playing of social situations
   D. Providing feedback on the client's hygiene and physical appearance

133. An OT is discharging a 4-year-old child with athetoid cerebral palsy from a rehabilitation setting to home. The MOST appropriate instructions for the OT to provide to the family for maintaining correct jaw control while feeding the child from the side are:

   A. "jaw opening and closing are controlled with your index and middle fingers; place your thumb on the child's cheek."
   B. "jaw opening and closing are controlled with your index and middle fingers; place your thumb on the child's larynx for stability."
   C. "jaw opening and closing are controlled with your whole hand on the child's jaw."
   D. "jaw opening and closing are controlled with your index and middle fingers; place your thumb on the child's ear for stability."

134. An OT practitioner is fabricating a dynamic splint for an individual who sustained a low-level radial nerve injury while slicing lunchmeat. The splint should be designed to:

   A. provide wrist extension, MCP flexion, and thumb flexion.
   B. prevent wrist extension, MCP extension, and thumb extension.
   C. prevent wrist extension, MCP flexion, and thumb flexion.
   D. provide wrist extension, MCP extension, and thumb extension.

135. An OT practitioner is discussing skills that can help a client with substance abuse problems to develop an alcohol-free lifestyle. The area that the practitioner is MOST likely to address first with the client is:

   A. work or job performance.
   B. self-care skills.
   C. use of leisure time.
   D. medication management.

136. Poor impulse control has been identified as the primary deficit in a 12-year-old boy with conduct disorder. Which of the following is the MOST effectively written functional OT goal?

   A. Within 6 months, the client will participate in classroom activities for 1 hour without disruptive outbursts, twice a day.
   B. Within 6 months, the client will attend to an activity for 30 minutes, demonstrating improved impulse control.
   C. The client will show a 50% reduction in the frequency of disruptive outbursts within 6 months.
   D. When presented with a new activity, the client will follow directions without protest, four out of five times, within 6 months.

137. When fabricating a splint for an individual with swan-neck deformities, the splint should be designed to prevent further:

   A. hyperextension of the PIP and DIP joints.
   B. hyperextension of the PIP joint and flexion of the DIP joint.
   C. flexion of the PIP joint and hyperextension of the DIP joint.
   D. hyperextension of the MP joint and flexion of the PIP joint.

138. An individual with mental illness has accepted a secretarial position, but is concerned that her high levels of distractibility may interfere with concentration and job performance. Which of the following interventions is MOST appropriate for this individual?

    A. Arrange for the individual to have a job coach.

    B. Ask the employer to provide more frequent breaks.

    C. Explain the problem of distractibility to the employer.

    D. Ask the employer to provide an isolated cubical as the work space.

139. An OT practitioner is working with a withdrawn child whose OT objectives include increasing the ability to express feelings and conflicts. Which of the following activities will MOST effectively promote this skill?

    A. Drawing a picture entitled "This is me"

    B. Playing soccer with a small group of children

    C. Playing a board game, such as "Monopoly" with two classmates

    D. Singing folk songs in a group

140. An OT practitioner is performing an assistive technology intervention with an individual who demonstrates severely impaired motor performance. The FIRST function of the therapist in this process is to:

    A. identify the most appropriate commercially available forms of assistive technology.

    B. identify the individual's abilities, needs, and goals.

    C. select the appropriate method of accessing the technology.

    D. modify the assistive technology device to meet the needs of the client.

141. An individual in an adult day program who is interested in obtaining employment is observed grabbing tools from others, acting out of turn, and rejecting feedback. Which of the following occupation-based interventions is MOST appropriate for addressing this individual's limitations and preparing him for a work environment?

    A. Operating the photocopy machine in a clerical group

    B. Handing out trays and utensils in a food service group

    C. Placing books back on the shelves in a library group

    D. Balancing the books at the end of the day in a thrift store group

142. An individual with multiple sclerosis reports she is exhausted after cleaning her house, but that she cannot afford a house cleaner. Which of the following strategies is MOST appropriate to recommend to this individual?

    A. Convince the individual to hire a house cleaner.

    B. Prescribe activities that will increase strength.

    C. Use the largest joints available for the task.

    D. Alternate tasks that require standing with those that can be performed sitting.

143. An individual with depression refuses to participate in an initial evaluation. He sits away from the other clients, does not make eye contact with anyone, and states he just doesn't "feel like doing anything right now." Which of the following actions is the MOST appropriate to take?

    A. Leave the individual alone until he begins to make eye contact, indicating his readiness to participate.

    B. Approach the individual briefly several times throughout the session without making any demands on him.

    C. Inform the individual that his doctor will need to be notified of his refusal to participate.

    D. Explain to the individual that once he lets you evaluate him, you'll be able to help him more effectively.

144. An OT practitioner is instructing the parents of a newborn infant regarding the facilitation of the suck-swallow reflex. Prior to feeding the infant a bottle, the OT encourages the parents to perform which of the following?

    A. Stroke the infant's cheek before feeding her a bottle.

    B. Gently touch the infant's lips to encourage her to open her mouth and begin sucking motions.

    C. Softly stimulate the infant's gums before bottle feeding.

    D. Gently rub the infant's gums and cheek simultaneously before feeding the baby her bottle.

145. An OT practitioner is fabricating a resting pan splint for an individual with extremely fragile skin. Which of the following areas will the OT have to inspect most carefully for signs of skin breakdown?

A. Metacarpal heads, pisiform, and, trapezium

B. Volar PIP joints, medial fifth digit, and thumb MP joint

C. Ulnar styloid, distal head of radius, and thumb CMC joint

D. Thumb PIP joint, pisiform, and hamate

146. When working with an individual who is severely depressed and demonstrates psychomotor retardation, it is MOST important to:

A. encourage more rapid responses.

B. provide extensive visual and auditory sensory stimulation.

C. give simple directions and patiently wait for responses.

D. provide activities involving large groups.

147. An OT is working on discharge plans for a child with paraplegic spina bifida who has just started using a powered wheelchair. The community resource that would be recommended as MOST critical for this child is:

A. the local social service agency.

B. a local wheelchair equipment vendor.

C. the family physician.

D. an early intervention program.

148. To improve written communication, an OT practitioner would be MOST likely to recommend a large keyboard to enhance computer access when an individual:

A. has limited UE range of motion, but adequate fine coordination.

B. fatigues rapidly when reaching for the keys.

C. uses only one hand to access the keyboard.

D. has good UE range of motion, but difficulty accessing small targets.

149. An individual with an anxiety disorder has been placed on new antianxiety medication. While monitoring the individual over the next few days, the OT practitioner should be particularly observant for which of the following side effects?

A. Akathisia

B. Decreased arousal and drowsiness

C. Extrapyramidal syndrome

D. Tardive dyskinesia

150. An OT practitioner is planning intervention for an individual with limited shoulder abduction and external rotation. The craft activity that would provide the desired upper extremity movement at the lowest level of challenge is:

A. macramé with short cords.

B. macramé with long cords.

C. macramé with fine cords.

D. macramé with thick cords.

151. A school-age child has Duchenne's muscular dystrophy. Although he is able to use a manual chair for distances between classes, he is tired on arrival. What would be the BEST recommendation the OT could make for wheelchair use at school?

A. Retain the manual chair to build up strength.

B. Change to an ultralight sports model because it requires less strength.

C. Change to a power wheelchair to reduce effort.

D. Encourage walking with a walker to alternate mobility methods.

152. An OT practitioner is educating the family of an individual admitted to the ICU after sustaining full-thickness dorsal hand burns. Which of the following MOST accurately explains the purpose of burn hand splints?

A. Burn hand splints decrease pain and allow for active range of motion.

B. Burn hand splints prevent hypertrophic scarring.

C. Burn hand splints prevent the need for skin grafting.

D. Burn hand splints prevent stress on the tendons and ligaments, while decreasing edema.

153. A 48-year-old roofing contractor experienced extrapyramidal syndrome side-effects after being placed on neuroleptic medications in the hospital. If this individual is to continue taking the medication after discharge from the hospital, it would be MOST important to educate him about the need to:

A. limit sun exposure as much as possible.

B. avoid use of power tools and sharp instruments.

C. get up slowly from a standing, sitting, or lying position.

D. be aware of the dehydrating effects of caffeinated drinks and alcohol.

154. To avoid overstimulation when handling a stable, 12-week premature infant in the Neonatal Intensive Care Unit setting, the OT practitioner must FIRST:

    A. provide gentle human touch to enable the infant to slowly respond to intervention.

    B. establish a calm state by utilizing an infant musical mobile.

    C. rock and then swaddle the infant in a blanket to provide containment and warmth to assist with self-regulation.

    D. establish a bond through visual orientation to the therapist's face.

155. Which of the following is the BEST example of the plan section of a discharge summary when using the SOAP note format?

    A. "The patient reports intentions to continue to practice proper body mechanics at work."

    B. "The patient demonstrates independence in performing the home exercise program."

    C. "The patient expressed a desire to return to work, but does not yet demonstrate the capacity for the required sitting tolerance."

    D. "Recommend the use of lumbar support and regular performance of home program."

156. Which of the following is the BEST support group to recommend to a husband who describes having difficulty in coping with the ups and downs of his wife's bipolar disorder?

    A. Al-Anon

    B. Family therapy

    C. National Alliance for the Mentally Ill

    D. Recovery, Inc.

157. An individual with a low back injury lives alone and must be able to do laundry independently. To prevent reinjury, the OT practitioner should instruct the individual to:

    A. place the clean laundry basket on the floor next to a chair and sit for folding.

    B. stop the activity when pain becomes severe.

    C. divide the laundry into several small loads for carrying.

    D. carry the laundry in one or two large loads.

158. A child with athetoid cerebral palsy is learning to use augmentative communication and is frustrated because it takes so long to produce a sentence. Which of the following is the BEST solution for this problem?

    A. A larger monitor

    B. A voice output tool

    C. Word prediction software

    D. Masking inappropriate keys

159. An OT practitioner is performing a home evaluation for an individual with paraplegia who uses a standard manual wheelchair, and notes that the entrance to the bathroom is 32 inches wide and the toilet is 15 inches high. Which of the following recommendations will BEST facilitate use of the bathroom for this individual?

    A. Widen the doorway.

    B. Raise the toilet.

    C. Widen the doorway and raise the toilet.

    D. Widen the doorway and lower the toilet.

160. When adapting a toilet for use by a child with poor postural control, the OT practitioner should pay PRIMARY attention to which of the following issues?

    A. Can the toilet paper be reached without a major weight shift?

    B. Is the flush handle easy to manipulate?

    C. Can the child's feet reach the floor?

    D. Is a nonskid mat placed on the floor to prevent slipping?

161. Which one of the following individuals would MOST likely need to use a transfer board?

    A. An individual who is unable to follow commands.

    B. An individual who cannot bear weight on the lower extremities.

    C. An individual who has good lower extremity strength, but is fearful of fatigue.

    D. An individual who is able to perform a stand pivot transfer.

162. The OT is working with a patient who needs to be independent in medication management prior to discharge. The MOST effective technique for the OT to teach the patient to remember whether he has taken his medications is to:

    A. establish a routine of taking medications the same time every day.

    B. keep the medications in a special, labeled location.

    C. use a diary to record each dosage after it is taken.

    D. arrange for a caregiver to remind the patient when medications should be taken.

163. A child diagnosed with ataxic CP exhibits tremors in the upper extremities. When she feeds herself, the tremors cause most of the food to fall off her spoon before it can reach her mouth. Which of the following adaptations should the OT practitioner recommend?

    A. Replace the spoon with a blunt-ended fork.
    B. Build up the handle of the spoon.
    C. Give the child a swivel spoon.
    D. Bend the spoon handle 45 degrees.

164. An OT practitioner is working with a patient with a C4 spinal cord injury to determine the best method of input access for a powered wheelchair. The MOST effective recommendation would be to use a:

    A. joystick.
    B. sip and puff switch.
    C. single-switch digital control.
    D. mouth stick.

165. A child has mastered brushing her teeth with the OT practitioner giving verbal and physical cues. In order to progress with the process of reducing the intrusiveness of cues, the OT should NEXT provide:

    A. verbal cues only.
    B. verbal and gestural cues only.
    C. physical cues only.
    D. verbal and physical cues only.

166. In order for an individual sitting in a wheelchair to achieve maximal postural positioning, the OT practitioner should position the individual's pelvis in a:

    A. moderate posterior tilt.
    B. neutral position.
    C. slight anterior tilt.
    D. slight posterior tilt.

167. An OT practitioner is training an adult worker with a developmental disability to put a pencil in a box before putting a score pad in the box for a game packaging task in a sheltered workshop assembly line. Which of the following reinforcement schedules would MOST likely achieve the goal of learning this task sequence?

    A. Intermittent reinforcement with correct responses
    B. Reinforcement every 10 minutes
    C. Reinforcement for every fourth correct response
    D. Continuous reinforcement of correct responses

168. A first-grade child has difficulty with finger isolation and handwriting. The MOST appropriate activity for the OT practitioner to recommend to the child's teacher is:

    A. crayon drawing on sandpaper.
    B. copying shapes from the blackboard.
    C. rolling out "Play Doh" with a rolling pin.
    D. picking up raisins with pair of tweezers.

169. An individual with a short below-elbow amputation lacks sensation in the residual limb. The MOST appropriate intervention would be for the OT practitioner to teach the patient:

    A. techniques of tapping, rubbing, and application of textures to the residual limb.
    B. to routinely inspect the skin closely for signs of skin breakdown.
    C. to perform deep massage on the residual limb.
    D. the necessary procedures of proper skin hygiene.

170. A preteen with a history of TBI is relearning to prepare simple foods, but has been having difficulties with sequencing. The OT has provided the patient with a chart of steps to follow and he has just learned to prepare his favorite sandwich without "losing his place" in the process. He continues to require occasional verbal cues to look at the chart and to ensure safety. At this point, the patient's level of independence would be documented as:

    A. independent.
    B. independent with setup.
    C. supervision.
    D. minimal assist.

171. A patient with a fractured radial head has the arm immobilized from above the elbow to below the wrist. The patient has requested exercises that will help maintain strength in the elbow and forearm muscles while awaiting permission to move the arm. In response, the OT practitioner should provide instructions to perform:

    A. isometric exercises.
    B. isotonic exercises.
    C. progressive resistive exercises.
    D. passive exercises.

172. A therapist is discussing discharge plans with the parents of a 7-year-old child with sensory defensiveness problems. The MOST appropriate activity the OT could recommend to provide proprioceptive input for this child would be to:

    A. walk barefoot on textured surfaces.
    B. rock over a large therapy ball.
    C. play in a large box full of Styrofoam pellets.
    D. perform slow push-ups against the wall.

173. Upon discharge, an individual will be performing sliding board transfers with assistance from family members. When ordering a wheelchair, which features will be MOST important to include?

    A. One-arm drive and low backrest
    B. Reclining backrest and elevating footrests
    C. Swing-away footrests and removable armrests
    D. Elevating footrests and removable armrests

■ OCCUPATIONAL THERAPY FOR POPULATIONS

174. An OT practitioner is designing a stress management series for individuals who have multiple sclerosis. The first step of the stress management process to be integrated into the program format should be:

    A. teaching time management techniques.
    B. providing a method for guided self-assessment.
    C. providing aerobic exercise.
    D. teaching how to perform progressive resistive exercise.

175. Which of the following BEST represents a school-based consultive relationship between the OT practitioner and school teacher?

    A. The teacher identifies a child's classroom needs so the OT can follow up with appropriate intervention within the child's home environment.
    B. Cooperative partnership between two disciplines.
    C. Minimal interaction between the two disciplines, occasionally touching base at IEP meetings.
    D. One discipline identifies goals while the other discipline carries out intervention techniques.

176. Which of the following activities would be MOST appropriate to recommend for vocational skills training of high school students with severe learning disabilities?

    A. Stocking the shelves at a local grocery
    B. Packaging items in a local sheltered workshop
    C. Cleaning the school cafeteria after lunch
    D. Reading help wanted ads and role playing interviews

177. An OT practitioner needs to determine the most relevant focus of wellness programming for individuals with hemiplegia in a community center. Which method of data gathering would be MOST effective and efficient for determining perceived needs of a broad number of the targeted population?

    A. Review of records and demographic statistical data concerning the population
    B. Written questionnaires sent to the groups' members
    C. Individual interviews with each member
    D. Group meeting in formats such as community forum or focus groups

178. An OT practitioner is preparing a presentation for a business with a high incidence of workers diagnosed with cumulative trauma disorders. The therapist should explain that the MOST significant risk factors are associated with:

    A. repetition, high force, and awkward joint postures.
    B. progressive resistive exercise, joint mobilization, and weight bearing.
    C. inflammation, swelling, and pain.
    D. fatigue, muscle cramps, and paresthesias.

179. An OT practitioner consulting in a supervised living environment is teaching the residential staff strategies to help minimize the effect of hallucinations for residents with schizophrenia. Which of the following would be the MOST effective suggestion for the OT practitioner to offer?

    A. Teach staff not to disturb persons while they are experiencing the hallucinations.
    B. Suggest moving persons experiencing hallucinations to areas where they can be completely isolated from other people.
    C. Attempt to provide meaningful activities that will engage attention.
    D. Move the persons experiencing hallucinations to more stimulating environments.

180. An OT practitioner is developing a prevention program for a local company with many workers who have developed tendonitis, nerve compression syndromes, and myofascial pain. A primary focus of the prevention program should be to:

    A. educate company workers about osteoarthritis disorders.
    B. develop a pamphlet on peripheral vascular disease.
    C. produce a flyer identifying risk factors for cumulative trauma disorders.
    D. offer screening for neuroma-related conditions

181. The administrator of an assisted living facility has asked an OT practitioner to help implement programming that will decrease the number of residents needing to move from the assisted living facility to nursing homes. The MOST important area for the practitioner to address is:

    A. adaptive equipment needs.
    B. fall prevention.
    C. meaningful use of leisure time.
    D. balancing work, leisure, and rest.

182. Prevention of cumulative trauma disorders (CTD) in the workplace is the primary focus of an OT practitioner working as an industry consultant. The OT suggests that the MOST appropriate way to reduce risk of CTD in an industry where there is heavy keyboard use is to:

    A. teach employees to identify the symptoms of cumulative trauma disorder early.
    B. educate employees about ergonomic adaptations including correct typing techniques, posture, hand positioning, and equipment modification.
    C. provide inexpensive resting splints to employees to rest hands and wrists at night if symptoms appear.
    D. instruct employees in exercise routines to increase strength in weak upper extremities.

183. An OT practitioner is planning a program to address the needs of persons with Alzheimer's disease, and their families, as part of a hospital outreach program. The focus of the program that would be MOST beneficial to maintaining safety and supporting function at home for people in the advanced stages of Alzheimer's is:

    A. strength and endurance activities.
    B. cognitive rehabilitation techniques.
    C. environmental modification.
    D. assertiveness skills.

184. An OT practitioner provides consultation to a school district to help maximize the learning environment for students with attention deficit disorder. Which environmental adaptation recommendation would BEST promote optimal learning for students with attention deficit disorder, without affecting other students?

    A. Use dim lighting and reduce glare by turning down lights.
    B. Remove all posters and visual aids to reduce visual distractions.
    C. Provide a screen to reduce peripheral visual stimuli.
    D. Restructure classroom activities into a series of short-term tasks.

185. An OT practitioner is developing a factory onsite work-hardening program protocol for workers returning to light duties following musculoskeletal work-related injuries. Which of the following would be MOST relevant to include in the design of the program?

    A. Pain management techniques
    B. Achieving a balance between work and leisure
    C. Energy conservation techniques
    D. Vocational counseling

186. An agency placing individuals with mental health conditions in a municipal jobs program has hired an OT practitioner to make recommendations for ADA accommodations. Which of the following areas would be MOST essential to assess in order to make these recommendations?

    A. Work environment, structure of work tasks, rules, and supervision
    B. Architectural barriers within the work site
    C. Work aptitudes and interests of the persons to be placed in the work program
    D. Capacity of the individuals to perform specified work tasks

■ SERVICE MANAGEMENT AND PROFESSIONAL PRACTICE

187. When ordering a wheelchair for an individual who has Medicare, part B, the OT practitioner must be sure the wheelchair:

    A. will increase functional independence.
    B. is medically necessary.
    C. will maintain patient function.
    D. will reduce deformity.

188. A homebound individual has been receiving OT for self-care and home management training and PT for ambulation and stair training following a stroke. The individual reported to the OT practitioner on the last visit that she walked to the bus stop alone. This statement is significant in that it indicates that the individual:

A. is making progress toward her goals and home therapy should be continued.

B. has achieved her PT goals.

C. has achieved her OT goals.

D. is no longer homebound.

189. During a group community outing, one day-program member complains of chest pain. The OT practitioner determines the individual's resting heart rate is 120 bpm, and blood pressure is 220/180 mm Hg. The MOST appropriate action for the practitioner to take is to:

A. continue the community re-entry outing.

B. immediately return the rest of the clients to the day program.

C. help the patient lie down and wait until his vital signs return to normal.

D. call 911.

190. The administrator of a nursing home asks the OTR who works there to help develop a job description so they can hire a second OTR. An OT job description would MOST likely contain:

A. previously established mutual goals, quality of patient care, achievement of predicted outcomes, and evidence of relationship building.

B. a summary of primary job functions, references, and job requirements.

C. the organizational relationships, personality characteristics desired in a job candidate, and accomplishments of the candidate.

D. the title of the job, employer's expectations, how much productivity is expected, and how the employee's performance will be measured.

191. The OT practitioner is seeking a site that will assist a developmentally delayed client to develop basic work skills. The community vocational service that adults with developmental disabilities are MOST commonly referred to are:

A. adult activity centers.

B. supported employment.

C. fast-food restaurants with supervision from job coaches.

D. sheltered workshops.

192. An OT practitioner is supervising an OT aide. The MOST appropriate kinds of activities and level of supervision for the aide include:

A. selected tasks in which aides have been trained, with close supervision.

B. various intervention activities with routine supervision.

C. completing ADL training with a patient without supervision.

D. selecting adaptive equipment from a catalog with general supervision.

193. The term that BEST describes the mandate of confidentiality of patient information and also holds the practitioner to remain faithful to the patient's BEST interest is:

A. informed consent.

B. fidelity.

C. beneficence.

D. nonmaleficence.

194. An OTR/COTA team need to report discharge information and document the information in the patients' chart. At what level does the COTA participate in making discharge recommendations?

A. An entry-level COTA may perform the task independently.

B. An intermediate-level COTA may perform the task independently.

C. A COTA contributes to the process, but does not complete the task independently.

D. A COTA cannot perform the task.

195. An OT practitioner completing a home assessment has recommended a hospital bed, lightweight wheelchair, bedside commode, reachers, long-handled sponge, shower chair, and hand-held shower. The family states they can only afford the items that can be billed as durable medical equipment. The OT practitioner should:

A. explain to the family that they will need to pay for all items.

B. order only the reachers and long-handled sponge.

C. order only the shower chair and hand-held shower.

D. order only the lightweight wheelchair and hospital bed.

196. An OT working in an outpatient setting has completed ROM measurements on an individual who is s/p hand surgery. After bandaging the open wounds, what should the OT do with the stainless steel goniometer?

   A. Place it in a plastic bag and label it with the individual's name.

   B. Sterilize it before using it again.

   C. Store it with the other goniometers, and sterilize them all at the end of the day.

   D. Wash it with hot, soapy water before using it again.

197. An OT public relations campaign is being instituted in your state. It was suggested by the OT state representative that a committee be formed in order to externally educate potential consumers of OT. Which of the following BEST represents an appropriate form of external marketing?

   A. Community newsletter

   B. Departmental open house

   C. In-service to all rehabilitation nurses

   D. Participation in conference

198. An OT practitioner is filling out an incident report regarding a patient who was seen on the rehabilitation unit. Which of the following scenarios is the MOST likely to be the subject of an incident report?

   A. The patient complained of nausea during a standing activity.

   B. A patient with a spinal cord injury indicated that his hand splints were uncomfortable.

   C. A patient who had a total hip replacement did not follow precautions while completing dressing activities but did not complain of discomfort.

   D. A patient with the diagnosis of a CVA and left neglect caught his left arm in the wheel of the wheelchair, resulting in a cut and bruise.

199. A COTA frequently administers the Allen Cognitive Level Test and then discusses it with the supervising OTR. Which of the following MOST accurately describes the OTR's role during these discussions?

   A. Determine the COTA's service competency.

   B. Collect data on the patient's performance.

   C. Interpret the results based on data collected by the COTA.

   D. Develop the treatment plan.

200. The OT program manager of a local hospital must determine the cost effectiveness of services provided. Which of the following methods would MOST effectively obtain this information?

   A. Outcomes measurement

   B. Utilization review

   C. Program evaluation

   D. Cost-benefit analysis

Answers for Simulation Examination 1

1. (D) carpal tunnel. Testing for a Tinel's sign involves tapping over the median nerve at the level of the carpal tunnel. In addition to a positive Tinel's sign (tingling along the nerve distally when tapped), symptoms would include pain and parasthesias along the median nerve distribution. Individuals also frequently complain of hand swelling and increased symptoms at night. See Reference: Mackin, Callahan, Skirven, et al. (eds). Evans, RB: Therapist's management of carpal tunnel syndrome.

2. (A) use of time. By comparing interests and actual participation, the OT practitioner may identify discrepancies between interests and actual play and leisure behavior. This information can help address the individual's use of time, and facilitate temporal organization. The issues in answers B, C, and D are not directly addressed using this method. See Reference: Case-Smith (ed). Cronin, AF: Psychosocial and emotional domains.

3. (D) irritability and nausea. The major signs of shunt malfunction in children are irritability, nausea, and vomiting. In addition to this, the therapist may observe changes in behavior or school performance, fever, pallor, visual perceptual difficulties, and headaches. Answers A, B, and C are incorrect. See Reference: Solomon (ed). Parker, GE: Other common pediatric disorders.

4. (B) Ask the individual how he spent New Year's. The ability to recall autobiographical events from one's past is one aspect of delayed memory called "episodic memory." It is commonly assessed through verbal interviews and informal testing, such as a question about an individual's recall of personal events. Other aspects of delayed memory include semantic memory which includes, "Recall of knowledge such as major world events, famous people, and general facts" (p. 410). The category of delayed memory also includes recall of information from any time after 20 minutes and can be determined by giving the individual information and asking about the same information at least 20 minutes later. If a person is asked to recall information immediately (within 60 seconds) as in answer A, immediate memory is being tested. Orientation is determined by asking about the current time and date (answer C). Asking a person to bring an object to the next session (answer D) would be a way to assess prospective memory or the "Ability to respond to cues, such as an alarm, that remind the client to perform a particular activity at the future time" (p. 410). See Reference: Crepeau, Cohn, and Schell (eds). Golisz, KM and Toglia, JP: Perception and cognition.

5. (A) constructional apraxia. An individual with constructional apraxia (answer A) may have full sensory awareness of the affected side of the body, but still may be unable to perform the assembly of one or more objects onto each other to carry out a verbal command or don clothing (answers B and C) in the proper sequence or position. Unilateral neglect (answer D) occurs as the individual neglects the affected side of the body and performs activities toward or with the unaffected side. An example would be an individual's only combing one side of his hair or shaving one side of his face. See Reference: Trombly and Radomski. Quintana, LA: Assessing abilities and capacities: vision, visual perception, and praxis.

6. (A) Performing interviews with the child and family regarding daily routines, social, and child rearing practices. According to Schell in Mulligan (2003), "clinical reasoning is a multifaceted, cognitive process used by occupational therapists to plan, direct, perform, and reflect on their client serv-ices" (p. 3). According to Mulligan (2003), "occupational therapy evaluations and interventions will be most effective when you use narrative reasoning first because understanding the client's life story (family and child priorities, concerns, lifestyle, medical history, etc.) will help you focus on what is most important" (p. 3). Thus, answer A would be correct. Answer B, relying upon the collaborative processes between the OT and the child/family is most representative of the interactive facet of clinical reasoning. While answer C, activity analysis, is used by the OT to define specific "client diagnosis-related problems" when engaging in the procedural component of clinical reasoning (p. 4). Answer D, determining the family's social and financial available resources, is a task most related to the pragmatic or practical side of clinical reasoning. See Reference: Mulligan. Mulligan, S: Pediatric Occupational Therapy Evaluation.

7. (C) Interview a reliable informant instead of the individual. Individuals who are unable to think clearly, or who are experiencing memory loss, are often disturbed or frightened by this change, and may confabulate stories or answers to cover themselves. When an individual is unable or unwilling to provide accurate information, it may be necessary to use a reliable informant (answer C). This is often someone who lives with the individual and is able and willing to provide the necessary information. Using closed-ended questions (answer A) with this individual would not necessarily yield more accurate information, but can be useful when specific information is being sought, or to more effectively structure or control an interview situation. This individual is unlikely to do any better with a written questionnaire than an oral interview. However, written questionnaires (answer D) may be used effectively with individuals with the requisite cognitive skills. There is no reason to think the individual would be any more reliable the next day (answer B). See Reference: Early. Data collection and evaluation.

8. (B) trace. Trace muscle strength equals a 1 on the numerical scale of muscle testing. The other answers would be incorrect since answer A, absent strength, would equal 0, answer C, good strength, would equal a 4, and answer D, normal strength, would equal a 5. See Reference: Pedretti and Early (eds). Pedretti, LW: Muscle strength.

9. (D) Visual perceptual. Running, hopping, using a tripod grasp, drawing a stick figure, and putting together a 10-piece puzzle are all developmentally appropriate skills for a 5-year-old child. Although the child cannot put together the 10-piece puzzle, the gross and fine motor skills that doing a puzzle require have been observed. No fine motor evaluation (answer A) is indicated because the child demonstrates a tripod grasp. No gross motor evaluation (answer B) is necessary because running and hopping skills are evident. Because the child's abilities appear developmentally appropriate, developmental evaluation (answer C) is not indicated. Because gross, fine, and developmental skills appear to be appropriate, visual perception should be evaluated. See Reference: Case-Smith (ed). Case-Smith, J: Development of childhood occupations.

10. (D) decreased attention. An attention deficit (answer D) is indicated if the individual recognizes a letter and marks it accurately on both the right and left sides of the page but misses letters in a random pattern. A visual field cut (answers A and B) is evidenced by missed letters appearing close together in one area, on either the left or right side of the page. Illiteracy (answer C) is unlikely because the individual is a high school teacher. See Reference: Trombly and Radomski. Assessing abilities and capacities: cognition.

11. (D) pervasive developmental disorder of childhood. This disorder "is characterized by severe and complex impairments in social interaction, communication, and behavior" (p. 164). Children with ADHD (answer A) display behaviors of inattention, hyperactivity, and impulsivity. Children with childhood conduct disorder (answer B) display repetitive and persistent antisocial behavior. Obsessive-compulsive disorder (answer C) is characterized by obsessive thoughts and displayed in compulsive behaviors such as hand washing. See Reference: Case-Smith (ed). Rogers, SL, Gordon, CY, Schanzenbacher, KE, and Case-Smith, J: Common diagnosis in pediatric occupational therapy practice.

12. (B) Median nerve. The median nerve passes through the carpal tunnel at the wrist. Impingement in this region causes sensory changes in the thumb, index finger, long, and half of the ring finger. Prolonged impingement in the carpal tunnel results in atrophy of the thenar eminence and weakness of the opponens pollicis. Injury to the radial nerve (answer C) in the wrist area causes sensory damage only. Damage to the ulnar nerve (answer A) at the wrist causes decreased grip strength and complete or partial loss of sensation over half of the fourth digit (ring finger) and all of the fifth digit (little finger), plus the proximal hypothenar region. A brachial plexus injury (answer D) may result in damage to any or all of the UE peripheral nerves. This may cause motor and/or sensory impairments. See Reference: Pedretti and Early (eds). Belkin, J: Orthotics.

13. (B) The child demonstrated tongue thrust. "Tongue thrust" is an objective, well-defined term. The other answers are less objective. Answer A infers the child's emotional reaction. Answer C implies voluntary control and judges behavior. Answer D interprets data based on insufficient evidence. See Reference: Creek (ed). Creek, J: Assessment.

14. (A) Limit the time available to answer each question. Individuals with OCD frequently experience time consuming compulsions having to do with thoughts and/or actions and may not be "appropriate candidates for interviews or should be interviewed only in highly structured situations" (p. 287). Limiting the time available to answer questions (answer A) will help these individuals structure their time and be able to more effectively complete the evaluation process. Open-ended questions (answer C) are useful for eliciting more information, but are more difficult to time limit than closed ended questions. Instructing the individual to take as much time as necessary (answer B) may be beneficial for a highly anxious individual. Individuals with attention deficits would most likely benefit from limiting environmental distractions (answer D). See Reference: Crepeau, Cohn, and Schell (eds). Henry, AD: Introduction to evaluation and interviewing Section II: The interview process in occupational therapy.

15. (C) fair minus (3−). The definition of fair minus (3−) is the grade given when an individual moves a part through incomplete range of motion (=50%) against gravity, or through complete range of motion with gravity eliminated against slight resistance. A grade of good (4), answer A, indicates ability to move through full range of motion against gravity and to take moderate resistance. A fair grade (3), answer B, would be the ability to move through the full range of motion against gravity, but not take any additional resistance. A grade of poor plus (2+), answer D, would move through full range of motion with gravity eliminated and take minimal resistance before suddenly relaxing. See Reference: Pedretti and Early (eds). Pedretti, LW: Muscle strength.

16. (C) somatosensory system. Many children who use an excessively tight grip on the writing tool and press too hard with the pencil on the paper have poor proprioceptive awareness (somatosensory). Answer A, vestibular system, is not the correct answer because, although it is difficult to completely separate one sensory system from another, the vestibular system primarily affects balance and general motor coordination. Answer B, the auditory system, is not the correct answer because the auditory system interprets sound for use in language. Answer D, the visual system, is not correct because although the visual system can monitor motor control such as pencil grip and pressure, the use of a pencil requires unconscious awareness of body position and pressure at times when the task is not monitored visually. See Reference: Case-Smith (ed). Amundson, SJ and Weil, M: Prewriting and handwriting skills.

17. (A) Depression and substance abuse. Examples of dual diagnostic categories are mental health and mental retardation and mental health and substance abuse (answer A). "Multiply-handicapped" is the coexistence of physical and mental health types of problems such as answers B and D, whereas answer C would reflect physical diagnostic categories. See Reference: Cottrell (ed). Jacobs, B: Dual diagnosis: A parent's perspective.

18. (B) Lateral trunk stability. Criteria for use of an MAS include adequate power from neck, trunk, shoulder girdle, or elbow muscles; adequate motor control; 0–90 degrees PROM in shoulder flexion and abduction, as well as adequate PROM in internal and external rotation, elbow flexion, and pronation; trunk stability; motivation; and a supportive environment. An individual with fair plus (3+) elbow flexion (answer C) would be able to stabilize the elbow on the table to bring the hand to the mouth and would have enough strength to move the arm without the mobile arm support. While individuals with quadriplegia often meet these criteria (answer A), so do individuals with muscular dystrophy, Guillain-Barré, ALS, and polio. See Reference: Trombly and Radomski. Deshaies, LD: Upper extremity orthoses.

19. (A) demonstrates compliance with hip precautions. Precautions following total hip replacement include no hip flexion past 90 degrees, no internal rotation, and no adduction past midline. Flexing the hip to 90 degrees (answer A) is acceptable. Individuals with poor short term memory, impulsivity, or poor judgment may require verbal cueing (answers B and D) to remember hip precautions. A longer shoehorn (answer C) may be necessary for an individual who is not able to put on shoes safely with the shorter shoehorn. See Reference: Trombly and Radomski. Bear-Lehman, J: Orthopaedic conditions.

20 (A) the individual becomes easily frustrated, cannot remain seated, and grabs tools from his peers. The behaviors described in answer A exemplify the excessive fidgeting and restlessness, inattention, and impulsiveness characteristic of ADHD. Although some of the symptoms of overactivity and impulsiveness can be classified as part of a mood disorder of the manic type, such as the behaviors described in answer B, these behaviors are typically linked with symptoms of grandiosity and inflated self-esteem. The use of profanity and striking another student (answer C) exhibit interference with the basic rights of other children or societal rules and is most related to conduct disorders, while answer D is typical of a child with an anxiety disorder where the student shows signs of uneasiness, apprehension, or dread associated with the anticipation of danger. See Reference: Crepeau, Cohn, and Schell (eds). Florey, L: Psychosocial dysfunction in childhood and adolescence.

21. (C) A mourning response. Mourning (answer C) is an adaptive mechanism used for dealing with a disabling condition because a loss of function has occurred. Dependency, stress reactions, and unrealistic goals (answers A, B. and D) are responses that would not normally pass with time. They also can interfere with the recovery process when they are present in the extreme, as with mourning. See Reference: Pedretti and Early (eds). Yerxa, EJ: The social and psychological experience of having a disability: implications for occupational therapists.

22. (D) Read the questions to the individual and check off his responses. It may be necessary to adapt the administration of some standardized tests to accommodate individuals with visual deficits. When this occurs, it is important to read the instructions and information to the individual exactly as it is written on the evaluation. It also is important to describe any modification to the assessment when documenting the evaluation results. In this case, it would be better to read the evaluation (answer D) to the individual than to waste a day of inpatient hospitalization (answer A). It would not be appropriate to begin treatment (answer C) before the evaluation is complete, goals set, and a treatment plan developed. Administering an evaluation (answer B) is beyond the scope of what an aide may do. See Reference: Crepeau, Cohn, and Schell (eds). Golisz, KM and Toglia, JP: Perception and cognition.

23. (B) observe him in his home during feeding time. "Considering the context of the child's environment is a critical process in occupational therapy assessments" (p. 167). The reason he does not feed himself may be environmental; for instance, his parents may have taught him not to touch food with his fingers or he may not have learned to feed himself because his grandmother always feeds him. In addition, the child may not be able to transfer skills learned at home to the clinic; that is, he may believe that "the place to eat is home, not the clinic." Although answers A and C provide useful information for treatment planning, they do not address feeding skills. Answer D does not put the skill to be assessed into an environmental context. See Reference: Case-Smith (ed). Stewart, KB: Occupational therapy assessment in pediatrics.

24. (C) anterograde amnesia. Anterograde amnesia is the inability to recall events after a trauma. Retrograde amnesia (answer D) is the inability to recall events prior to trauma. Long-term memory (answer B) is the storage of information for recall at a later time. Disorientation (answer A) is a problem in the awareness of person, place, and time. See Reference: Trombly and Radomski. Radomski, MV: Assessing abilities and capacities: cognition.

25. (C) Observe the individual touching the small of his back. Touching the small of the back requires shoulder abduction and internal rotation. Reaching the back of the neck (answer A) requires external rotation. Functional evaluations are best performed by observing movements during functional activities. A goniometer would be used when formal joint measurement is required (answer B). An interview (answer D) will provide useful information concerning pain, stiffness, and limitations in occupational performance, but is not a reliable method for assessing ROM. See Reference: Trombly and Radomski. Kohlmeyer, K: Evaluation of sensory and neuromuscular performance components.

26. (A) Ask the caregiver about the child's typical day and nighttime routines as well as strategies the child uses to communicate. Asking the caregiver about the child's daily activities would be the first thing the OT practitioner should do when compiling an occupational therapy profile. A caregiver can provide valuable information not obtained in the classroom/therapy environment. Answers (B and D), performing testing on the child and observing the child in the home, would be something the OT practitioner would most likely do after speaking to the child's parent/primary caregiver. Answer (C), meeting with the child's teacher, is not considered to be part of the interview with the primary caregiver. See Reference: Miller-Kuhaneck. Clark, G, Miller-Kuhaneck, H and Watling, R: Evaluation of the child with an autism spectrum disorder.

27. (C) a false perception of reality. The symptoms of schizophrenia are generally classified as either negative or positive. Answer C, a false perception of reality, or hallucinations, is representative of a positive symptom. "Positive symptoms are those that are conspicuously disturbing to others...the individual experiences bizarre delusions and insulting or commanding auditory hallucinations" (p. 855). Negative symptoms (answers A, B, and D) tend to persist after the positive symptoms, which are treated with medications. See Reference: Crepeau, Cohn, and Schell (eds). Ward, J: Adults with mental illness.

28. (D) select appropriate evaluation procedures. An OT evaluation begins with the initial interview and chart review, which guide the OT practitioners in deciding on a frame of reference and the identification of specific evaluation procedures or assessments. Assessments are then performed (answer C) to gather information to identify problem areas and plan treatment. After the assessments are complete, the OTR uses clinical reasoning skills to analyze data (answer A) and to identify the person's strengths and weaknesses. The treatment plan (answer B) is developed after the individual's problems have been identified and evaluation data have been analyzed. Finally, specific interventions are selected. See Reference: Pedretti and Early (eds). Pedretti, LW and Early, MB: Occupational therapy evaluation and assessment of physical dysfunction.

29. (A) a developmental delay. Typically, developing children (answer C) should be able to sit unsupported for several minutes by the age of 8 to 9 months; therefore, this child demonstrates delayed development (answer A). The ability to sit while propped forward on his arms indicates primitive reflexes have been integrated (answer B). Sitting unsupported earlier than 8 months could indicate advanced development (answer D). See Reference: Case-Smith (ed). Case-Smith, J: Development of childhood occupations.

30. (C) Alertness, selective attention and mental tracking. According to Golisz and Toglia (2003), "attention incorporates far more than the quantitative measure of length of time a client can concentrate. It is a multidimensional capacity that involves several components: alertness, selective attention, sustained attention, shifting attention, and mental tracking" (p. 402) (answer C). Answer A refers to areas within visual processing, answer B is most representative of orientation skills, and answer D is related to insight and awareness of disability. See Reference: Crepeau, Cohn, and Schell (eds). Golisz, K and Toglia, J: Evaluation of performance skills and client factors.

31. (C) take the individual's vital signs at rest. First, vital signs should be taken at rest (answer C). The individual should then perform a self-care activity while being monitored by the OT practitioner for any signs or symptoms of exhaustion (answer B). The third step is to take vital signs again immediately after completion of the activity (answer A). The final step is to retake vital signs after the individual has rested for 5 minutes (answer D). This process provides the OT practitioner with baseline information about the individual's endurance level. See Reference: Crepeau, Cohn, and Schell (eds). Doherty, RF: Cardiopulmonary dysfunction in adults.

32. (B) normal development. Proximal movement on a fixed distal limb component, that is, on hands and knees, is an example of the development of mobility superimposed on stability. This stage is essential in the development of coordinated anti-gravity movement. The development of this type of movement in the quadruped position occurs between the ages of 7 and 12 months. This pattern is typical of normal development and does not indicate answers A, C, or D. See Reference: Case-Smith (ed). Nichols, DS: Development of postural control.

33. (C) identifying the type of environmental supports that can maximize the client's level of function. A cognitive level assessment will not give information on difficult behaviors specifically (answer A), though it may provide insight into how the person reacts to cognitive challenges. Answers B and D are incorrect because the cognitive level assessment evaluates how a person processes information cognitively within the framework of functional activity, rather than evaluate specific prevocational skills or level of social interaction skills. Answer C is correct; "the most effective use of cognitive levels is in determining what type of environmental and/or social support is indicated to facilitate a client's best ability to function. See Reference: Crepeau, Cohn, and Schell (eds). Grant, S: Cognitive disability frame of reference.

34. (C) swallowing crushed ice. Dysphagia refers to difficulty with or inability to swallow. Answer A is representative of bilateral integration or the ability to coordinate both sides of the body. Aphasia, answer B, is the inability to express one's self orally, and answer D, the inability to speak clearly, or dysarthria, is best described as slurred speech secondary to cerebral lesions. See Reference: Crepeau, Cohn, and Schell (eds). Evaluation of performance skills and client factors.

35. (C) Biomechanical. According to Colangelo, "The biomechanical frame of reference is applied when a person cannot maintain posture through appropriate automatic muscle activity because of neuromuscular or musculoskeletal dysfunction" (p. 257). This child's physical status has changed with decreasing postural control. Adaptive support devices need to be considered, and a biomechanical frame of reference provides this approach. Answer A is not correct because the neurodevelopmental treatment frame of reference is concerned with improving

posture and movement, and supportive equipment is prescribed for that purpose. Answer B is not correct because the sensory integration frame of reference is concerned with sensory input in relation to posture and movement in children with sensory integration disorders, whereas Duchenne's disease is a neuro-muscular disorder. Answer D is not correct because the visual perceptual frame of reference is concerned with guiding and compensating for visual perceptual problems, not postural delays. See Reference: Kramer and Hinojosa (eds). Colangelo, CA: Biomechanical frame of reference.

36. (B) Socialization, task performance, daily living skills, and time management. Evaluation of children/adolescents who have psychosocial problems is centered on behavioral, affective, or interpersonal areas with visual motor and motor assessment following when screening suggests the need. However, specific emphases in evaluation vary according to the age of the client. Answer B, socialization, task performance, daily living skills, and time management are key areas of adolescent occupational performance which can be affected when psychosocial problems are present. Answer A reflects primary evaluation areas for toddlers and preschoolers. Answer C is more consistent with adult populations. While teenagers with psychosocial disorders also may have problems with motor skills and sensory processing, answer D usually reflects evaluation priorities for teenagers with neurological, rather than psychosocial, dysfunction. See Reference: Crepeau, Cohn, and Schell (eds). Florey, LL: Psychosocial dysfunction in childhood and adolescence.

37. (C) Identify or demonstrate the use of common household objects. Answer C is correct because visual agnosia is the inability to recognize common objects and demonstrate their use in an activity. Asking the individual to demonstrate common gestures such as waving (answer A) is a technique to screen for apraxia or the inability to perform purposeful movement on command. Answer B, asking the individual to identify objects through touch only would be used to evaluate stereognosis, which is the ability to identify an object by manipulating it with the fingers without seeing it. Asking the individual to read a paragraph and explain its meaning (answer D) would be a screening method for alexia or the inability to understand written language. See Reference: Pedretti and Early (eds). Wheatley, CJ: Evaluation and Treatment of Perceptual and Perceptual Motor Deficits.

38. (D) attention. Attention which is impaired can involve losing one's focus because of other stimuli. Memory (answer A) is the ability to recall knowledge and past events. Problems with spatial operations (answer B) are generally observed when individuals attempt to fit objects into specific spaces. Generalization of learning (answer C) may be observed by asking the client to use existing knowledge in a new situation. See Reference: Pedretti and Early (eds). Wheatley, CJ: Evaluation and treatment of cognitive dysfunction.

39. (C) tone, rigidity, and reflexes. Motor control includes the components of decorticate and decerebrate rigidity, hyper- and hypotonicity, and reflexes. Response to verbal commands (answer A) pertains to evaluation of cognition. Response to pain or temperature (answer B) pertains to evaluation of sensation. The ability to make eye contact (answer D) pertains to evaluation of vision. See Reference: Pedretti and Early (eds). Gutman, SA: Traumatic brain injury.

40. (B) flexion righting reaction. The flexion righting reaction (answer B) is correct because "the development of antigravity neck strength is first associated with the ability to maintain the head aligned with the body when pulled to a sitting position" (p. 273). Answer A is incorrect because protective reactions are elicited through displacement (such as falling forward), and these reactions protect infants from falls. Answer C is incorrect because the body righting on body reaction is represented by the rotation between trunk segments (also a rotational righting reaction). Answer D is incorrect because the optical righting reaction incorporates vision and allows the child to right the head against gravity (this also is referred to as a vertical righting reaction). See Reference: Case-Smith (ed). Nichols, DS: Development of postural control.

41. (B) distance from the fingertip to the distal palmar crease with the hand in a fist. The distance from the fingertip to the distal palmar crease with the hand fisted may be measured in either inches or centimeters. This measures how close the fingertip comes to the palm. A person who has full flexion would have a measurement of zero. Answers A and C are incorrect as actively or passively measuring the flexion at each joint and totaling them are measurements taken with a goniometer and recorded in degrees. Answer D, measuring the distance between the tip of the thumb and the fourth phalanx, is incorrect because it is a measurement of opposition. See Reference: Mackin, Callahan, Skirven, et al. (eds). Cambridge-Keeling, CA: Range of motion measurement of the hand.

42. (B) Demonstrate the procedure on the unaffected extremity, then occlude the individual's vision and test the affected side. The pre-

sentation of stimuli in sensory evaluation is extremely important. Because of the compensation that may occur with vision, it is necessary to occlude the individual's vision. Also, the unaffected extremity should be assessed before the affected extremity, the opposite of answer A, to reduce anxiety in the individual. Stimuli should be presented in a random proximal-to-distal pattern. A rapport (answer C) should be established before beginning any evaluation procedure, also to reduce anxiety. An individual may not be aware of any deficit areas (answer D) so the whole extremity should be assessed to ensure accuracy. Picture cards are helpful in assessing individuals with expressive aphasia. See Reference: Trombly and Radomski. Bentzel, K: Assessing abilities and capacities: Sensation.

43. (A) Visual-motor integration. Visual-motor integration skills (answer A) "require coordination of eyes with hands...such that the eyes guide complex, precise movements" (p. 277). Visual acuity (answer B) refers to the ability to see clearly. A child with poor visual acuity would be observed bringing objects and papers close to his eyes in order to see them better. Visual tracking (answer C) is the ability to follow targets with smooth eye movements. "Children who have poor visual tracking skills often lose focus while trying to follow or find an object" (p. 276). Visual perception (answer D) refers to "the capacity to interpret sensory input, recognize similarities and differences, and assign meaning to what is seen" (p. 276). Limitations in this area may result in difficulty matching and sorting (object perception); finding figures hidden in pictures, such as "Where's Waldo?" (figure-ground perception); and moving through small spaces (position in space perception). See Reference: Solomon (ed). Jones, LMW: Occupational performance areas: Daily living and work and productive activities.

44. (B) temperature and pain. The sensations of pain and temperature are carried along small, unmyelinated nerve fibers, which recover more rapidly than senses carried by larger, myelinated fibers. The sensations of pain and temperature also are part of the protective or primary sensory systems, which are the receivers of simple information. More complex information is carried through the discriminative or epicritic system. The senses carried on this system are vibration, light touch, proprioception, and tactile localization. See Reference: Trombly and Radomski. Bentzel, K: Assessing abilities and capacities: Sensation.

45. (D) determine the need for further evaluation. The purpose of screening is to determine whether further assessments are needed, and if so, which tests would be appropriate for that child. A screening test is not designed for planning programs (answer C) or consultation (answer A), and they do not test any skills (answer B) in a comprehensive way. See Reference: Solomon (ed). Peralta, AM and Kramer, P: General treatment considerations.

46. (B) assess the individual's lifestyle and dietary habits. Controllable risk factors include: smoking, cholesterol level, hypertension, sedentary lifestyle, obesity, diabetes, and psychological stress. OT practitioners have expertise in working with individuals to address goals associated with lifestyle performance and dietary habits (answer B) that can help to prevent heart disease. While obesity can be observed, cholesterol levels cannot (answer C). Age, gender, and family history (answers A and D) are all uncontrollable risk factors associated with heart disease. See Reference: Trombly and Radomski. Huntley, N: Cardiac and pulmonary diseases.

47. (A) the parent's concerns and goals for the child. The caregiver's concerns are essential in planning effective intervention within the context of the family. Medical management (answer B), equipment needs (answer C), and the physical layout of the home (answer D) are important issues as well, but can be addressed at a later time. See Reference: Case-Smith (ed). Stewart, KB: Occupational therapy evaluation in pediatrics.

48. (A) within normal limits. Normal range of motion for internal rotation is 70 degrees (answer A). Rotation can be assessed with the humerus adducted against the trunk or with the shoulder abducted to 90 degrees. If the humeral movements for internal or external rotation are observed during the performance of activities and found to be adequate for performance of functional activities, range of motion may be noted as WFL (answer B). The OT practitioner may choose not to perform a formal joint measurement if the joint is WFL, even though the end of the range may be lacking a few degrees, because the loss of movement may not be significant to the individual. Hypermobility (answer C) at a joint is motion past the average range of motion, which at the shoulder would be past 70 degrees of internal rotation. If hypermobility is caused by an unstable joint as might occur after a surgical repair or a disease process, then splinting or another form of stabilization or immobilization can be used to correct the problem. If the practitioner observes hypermobility during range of motion, they should compare the range of motion to that on the individual's opposite side in order to assess normal range. A limitation of internal rotation (answer D) at the shoulder would be less than 70 degrees of motion. If a limitation is

apparent, the rehabilitation team may choose not to treat it unless it interferes with the function of the upper extremity. See Reference: Trombly and Radomski. Trombly, CA and Podolski, CR: Assessing abilities and capacities: range of motion, strength, and endurance.

49. (A) denial. "Defense mechanisms or defenses are used unconsciously by the person's ego in order to keep anxiety-producing thoughts, information or wishes out of consciousness" (p. 372). This individual may be having difficulty accepting her stroke and is using denial to avoid dealing with it (answer A). Projection (answer B) is a process by which a "...person attributes to another person the unacceptable thoughts and feelings he/she is having" (p. 372). Rationalization (answer C) is when an individual makes excuses for unacceptable behavior. Regression (answer D) is when an individual reverts to infantile or childlike behavior as a way of dealing with a difficult situation. See Reference: Bruce and Borg. Appendix H: Styles of defense.

50. (D) Encourage independent ADLs with minimal reliance on adapted utensils and tools. Encouraging independent self-feeding and dressing skills with minimal use of adapted utensils and tools is the most appropriate ADL intervention. It is important to avoid an overreliance on adapted equipment so the child can experience full active range of motion when engaged in ADL. Answer A, instruct the child to use all adapted equipment, may interfere with the achievement of reaching full AROM when engaging in ADL. Answer B, encourage independent compression garment application, is typically contraindicated with open wounds and is not implemented until wound closure. Answer C, perform bilateral upper extremity PROM exercises twice a day, is not considered an ADL intervention. See Reference: Crepeau, Cohn, and Schell (eds). Rivers, EA: Skin system dysfunctions: Burns.

51. (B) regain confidence in the ability to ambulate. Fear of falling may result in reduction of activity, which may result in even further loss of mobility skills and decreased participation. "The goal of treating fear of falling is to help these people regain confidence in their ability to achieve safe, independent mobility" (p. 280). Strategies to achieve that goal may include reducing factors that contribute to risk of falls such as poor lower extremity strength (answer A) and balance, eliminating environmental hazards (answer C), and reducing the use of medications that may be contributing to falls (answer D). See Reference: Bonder and Wagner (eds). Tideiksaar, R: Falls.

52. (C) Design an individualized program directed at the underlying neurological deficit. Sensory integration is a complex treatment modality that is a highly individualized form of treatment carried out by a therapist with advanced training and understanding in the area of neuroscience. Answer A is incorrect because the child's program is not being "individualized," but is included in a group program. Answer B is not correct because sensory integration treatment is active and requires an adaptive response from the child. Answer D is not correct because sensory integration is directed at improving underlying neurological functioning rather than skill development. See Reference: Bundy, Lane and Murray (eds). Bundy, A: The process of planning and implementing intervention.

53. (A) Getting dressed without becoming fatigued. Prevention of fatigue is the primary purpose of energy conservation. Energy conservation techniques may often result in slower, not faster (answer D), performance. Using proper body mechanics may enable an individual with back pain to lift heavy cookware without pain (answer B). Using joint protection techniques may prevent further joint damage to arthritic hands when the patient is doing handicrafts (answer C). See Reference: Pedretti and Early (eds). Buckner, WS: Arthritis.

54. (B) small group, fine-motor clay pinch pottery activities. According to Pape and Ryba (2004), "many teachers who have children with autism spectrum disorders in their classrooms incorporate instruction techniques from the TEACCH curriculum. At the preschool level this involves having children learn individually or in small groups, with an emphasis placed on structuring the environment to increase development of communication and social skills, fine-motor and gross-motor development, and self-help skills" (p. 239). Thus, answer B, small group pinch pottery activities, would be the best choice for intervention. Answers A, C, and D would not be appropriate choices because of the use of large group and/or unstructured activities that would most likely frustrate a preschool child with a PDD. See Reference: Pape and Ryba. Chapter 7: The pervasive developmental disorders.

55. (A) Complete independence with self-care and transfers. An individual with T4 paraplegia will have sufficient trunk balance, upper extremity strength, and coordination to complete self-care and transfers independently. Individuals with high cervical injuries are likely to be dependent in self-care and transfers (answer D). Individuals with low cervical and high thoracic injuries require assistance with transfers and some self-care (answers B and C). See Reference: Pedretti and Early (eds). Adler, C: Spinal cord injury.

56. (D) Group members pass around and feel different textured fabrics in a basket. Using sensory stimuli, such as touch, helps arouse an individual's attention and increase their level of participation. Individuals with severe depression tend to have difficulty initiating a physical activity such as throwing a ball (answer B); therefore, having a warm-up activity is useful. These individuals also are likely to have difficulty initiating conversations (answers A and C), and these activities are not consistent with a sensorimotor format. However, they may be effective activities for individuals functioning at a higher level. See Reference: Early. Cognitive and sensorimotor activities.

57. (C) Avoid resistive materials. For a child with acute juvenile rheumatoid arthritis, the OT should always use techniques for joint protection and energy conservation. Activities requiring the manipulation of highly resistive materials (answer C) such as clay, leather, and copper sheets should be avoided; the pressure applied to the joints could exacerbate the condition. Avoiding light touch (answer A) is a precaution more relevant for the treatment of a child with tactile defensiveness. Rapid vestibular stimulation (answer B) is contraindicated for a child who is prone to seizures. The need to avoid above-normal body temperature (answer D) is more relevant to a client with multiple sclerosis, because high temperatures exacerbate the symptoms. See Reference: Case-Smith (ed). Rogers, SL, Gordon, CY, Schanzenbacher, KE, Case-Smith, J: Common diagnosis in pediatric occupational therapy.

58. (A) Assembling a complex airplane model requiring the use of detailed directions. Assembling a complex airplane model would be the best choice, because it has many of the activity characteristics that appeal to a person with paranoid schizophrenia (e.g., it is complicated enough to engage the person intellectually and sustain his interest), and it uses controllable materials and requires organization to complete. Answer B, finishing and painting a reassembled wooden box, would be insufficiently challenging. Answer C, playing a game of chess, is intellectually challenging, but presents an element of competition that can be threatening to a person with this diagnosis. Answer D, engaging in a reminiscence discussion, requires a degree of self-disclosure through the sharing of previous experiences and feelings that might prove disturbing for this patient. See Reference: Early. Responding to symptoms and behaviors.

59. (C) An individual with a C6 injury. An individual with C6 quadriplegia has some use of the abductor pollicis longus, extensor pollicis longus, extensor digitorum communis, and extensor carpi ulnaris. The extensor tone of the muscles in conjunction with the splint will operate the power for prehension force. Individuals with C1 or C3 injuries (answers A and B) have higher level lesions and lack the wrist extension strength needed to operate the wrist-driven flexor hinge splint. An individual with a T1 injury (answer D) is able to grasp and manipulate utensils without difficulty or need for assistance. See Reference: Trombly and Radomski. Atkins, MS: Spinal cord injury.

60. (D) child, caregiver, and therapist priorities. The problems established in the OT evaluation are not the only basis for writing OT goals and objectives. The child's priorities, as well as the caregiver's needs and concerns, must be addressed so that immediate needs are met and there is a commitment on everyone's part to the success of the program. See Reference: Case-Smith (ed). Richardson, PK and Schultz-Krohn, W: Planning and implementing services.

61. (C) demonstrate appropriate hip precautions. The ability to stand for 10 minutes (answer A) or to increase hip flexion to 90 degrees (answer B) is not necessary for independence in dressing. However, the use of appropriate hip precautions (answer C) is mandatory in order for the individual to perform activities safely. Energy-conservation techniques (answer D) are appropriate for individuals who demonstrate very low endurance levels, and may be appropriate for some individuals following hip arthroplasty, but hip precautions would need to be observed during energy conservation activities in order to prevent dislocation of the prosthesis. See Reference: Trombly and Radomski. Bear-Lehman, J: Orthopaedic conditions.

62. (D) observable analysis, measurable outcomes, and reinforcement for building specific skills. Observation and analysis of problem behaviors as well as identifying specific measurable outcomes which will indicate change in behaviors are characteristic of the behavioral frame of reference, as is the use of reinforcement methods (applied reward systems) to develop desired behaviors and skills. Answer A is linked to developmental frames of reference, answer B is linked to psychoanalytic frames of reference, and answer C is linked to sensory integrative frames of reference. See Reference: Bruce and Borg. Behavioral frame of reference—objective perspective.

63. (A) remedial treatment, such as rubbing or stroking the involved extremity. When sensation begins to return, it is appropriate to initiate remedial activities for sensory retraining. Stimulating the involved extremity by rubbing or stroking (to provide tactile input), or through weight-bearing activities (to provide proprioceptive input), are examples of remedial activities. Compensatory activities, which are essential for individuals with decreased or absent sensation, would have been part of the original treatment plan. Answers B, C, and D are all examples of compensatory strategies. See Reference: Pedretti and Early (eds). Iyer, MB and Pedretti, LW: Evaluation of sensation and treatment of sensory dysfunction.

64. (B) "We will be working together to achieve your goals." The client-centered relationship that an OT practitioner develops with a client is "...one in which the therapist tries to determine what is important to the client and tries to involve the client in the decision-making process" (p. 56), as exemplified by the statement in answer B, which reflects a collaborative therapeutic partnership. Answer A suggests that the central focus of OT treatment is the development of the therapeutic relationship. This relationship is instrumental in the therapy process, but not the central focus of the therapy. Although it shares a few characteristics of friendship, the therapeutic relationship is significantly different because it requires the OT practitioner to understand the client's needs and values, as well as to understand and manage the OT practitioner's own reactions. Therefore, answer C is incorrect. Empathy, rather than sympathy, is recommended in therapeutic relationships, so the statement in answer D also is incorrect. See Reference: Bruce and Borg. Bases for best occupational therapy practice.

65. (D) adapted teaching techniques. Answer D is correct because a child with this type of disability characteristically has learning problems that require teaching methods, such as "chaining" or behavior modification. Answers A, B, and C are of secondary importance because physical coordination may be impaired, or there may be other physical limitations, such as abnormal muscle tone or significant problems with balance. These additional problems may require adaptive equipment, clothing, or techniques. However, all aspects of dressing depend on the child's ability to learn procedures of dressing; therefore, it is necessary to consider task analysis and teaching approach first. See Reference: Case-Smith (ed). Shepherd, J: Self-care and adaptations for independent living.

66. (C) Teach a caregiver how to lift and turn the client safely. Individuals unable to move themselves, especially those with sensory loss, are susceptible to the development of decubiti. Skin damage results from pressure on the skin over a prolonged period of time. The skin over bony prominences is particularly prone to the development of decubitus ulcers. Frequent position changes are essential for these individuals to prevent skin breakdown and the risk of serious infection. If the patient were already involved in a strengthening program (answer A), it may be appropriate to change it to a maintenance program at this point. A bed-mobility program (answer B) and an environmental control unit (answer D) would be appropriate if the individual has potential in these areas, but instructing a caregiver in how to reposition the patient is the most important modification. See Reference: Trombly and Radomski. Coperman, LF, Forwell, SJ, and Hugos, L: Neurodegenerative diseases.

67. (D) weight bearing over a small bolster in prone. Weight bearing on the arms can help with overall inhibition of tone before participating in hand skill activities. Inhibition of flexor spasticity occurs through slow joint compression from weight bearing, as well as facilitation of ulnar to radial function in the hand. Answers A and B are incorrect because they require voluntary control of the release of objects without inhibition. Answer C is incorrect because traction on the finger flexors would increase spasticity in the flexor muscles, and make opening of the hand more difficult. See Reference: Case-Smith (ed). Exner, CE: Development of hand skills.

68. (B) learning the self-monitoring technique of asking oneself if any part of the task has been missed. Teaching the client to self-monitor is an example of a strategy to control the tendency to miss details involved in the task process. Answer A, simplifying instructions, is an example of the method of adapting the amount of information presented during the task. Answer C, practicing shape and number cancellation worksheets, is an example of a remedial skill training activity. Answer D, removing unnecessary objects from the task area to decrease distractions, is an example of adapting the environment to compensate for attention deficits. See Reference: Crepeau, Cohn, and Schell (eds). Toglia, JP: Cognitive-perceptual retraining and rehabilitation.

69. (D) A child with spina bifida with lower extremity paralysis. Typically, a child who has spina bifida (answer D) has enough upper extremity coordination and strength to propel himself on a scooter on which the lower extremities are supported. A child with spina bifida will usually have the cognitive and sensory awareness to negotiate a scooter in its environment. Prone scooters may be contraindicated for the children described in answers A, B, and C. The neck hyperextension required for

exploratory play on a prone scooter could cause further increase in the abnormal tone of the child with CP (answer A). A child with low tone who is easily fatigued (answer B) may be unable to maintain this very exhausting position for very long and is likely to become even more tired. Because the child lacks the sensory feedback and cognitive skills, the child with cognitive limitations and poor sensory awareness (answer C) would be at risk of injury. See Reference: Case-Smith (ed). Wright-Ott, C, and Egilson, S: Mobility.

70. (C) Passive ROM, positioning, and splinting. The initial phase of treatment for the individual with Guillain-Barré syndrome includes PROM, splinting, and positioning to protect weak muscles and prevent contractures. This should be followed by gentle, non-resistive activities and light ADLs (answer A) as tolerated. Resistive exercises and balance and stabilization activities (answers B and D) should be implemented later after strength begins to improve. See Reference: Pedretti and Early (eds). Lehman, RM and McCormack, GL: Neurogenic and myopathic dysfunction.

71. (C) have the individual trace lines across the page with the right index finger from the left to the right side. A person who follows a line when wheeling a wheelchair (answer A) is focusing on midline positioning, not crossing the midline. Placing objects commonly used on the unaffected side (answer B) is a compensatory technique that does not involve crossing the midline. The individual with midline problems would need cueing to avoid starting at the midline when attempting to lay cards out from the right to left side (answer C). Also, the person would have difficulty accurately completing a sequencing task on the neglected side, making it difficult to complete the midline crossing successfully. However, when tracing a line across the page, the individual receives the same proprioceptive input from the movement, and uses the same amount of space in the visual field, as when writing on paper. This task makes the transfer of skills easier when performing writing. See Reference: Trombly and Radomski. Quintana, LA: Optimizing vision, visual perception and praxis abilities.

72. (C) identify the critical elements of development and role performance for the age of the child. Answer C is correct because it is the necessary step to understanding delays in development and the needs of the child. Next, the therapist defines and describes the child's problem, which includes course and outcome. Finally, in general problem analysis, the effects of the problem on tasks and performance (including the components of performance) are considered. This process can begin with referral of a child and continue through evaluation to the planning of intervention. See Reference: Case-Smith (ed). Richardson, PK, and Schultz-Krohn, W: Planning and implementing services.

73. (A) Work simplification and energy conservation. In the first stage of ALS, mild limitations in function and endurance begin to develop. The individual becomes easily fatigued so work simplification and energy conservation techniques are the most beneficial. Progressive resistive exercises (answer B) may cause cramping and fatigue, and therefore are not recommended for individuals with ALS. Splinting (answer C) will be required in later stages to prevent contractures, support weak muscles, and assist with function. Active range of motion and PROM activities (answer D) also will be required later as the disease progresses to prevent contractures and maintain strength. See Reference: Pedretti and Early (eds). Schultz-Krohn, W, Foti, D, and Glogoski, C: Degenerative diseases of the central nervous system.

74. (B) Provision of foot support. Adequate foot support (answer B) should be the first concern of the practitioner in order for the child to feel secure and stable on the toilet as well as be positioned for bowel control. Answer A is not correct because management of fasteners can be developed later after positioning for stability has been achieved. Answer C is not correct because provision of a seatbelt may not be necessary if foot support (or back support) is provided. Answer D is not correct because climbing onto the toilet independently may be developed later (as occurs with normal developmental progression). See Reference: Case-Smith (ed). Shepherd, J: Self care and adaptations for independent living.

75. (B) Activities focused on organizational and communication skills and practice of job-seeking strategies. There are several aspects and phases to vocational programming but answer B, activities focused on organizational and communication skills and practice of job seeking strategies, are relevant activities for building job hunting skills at the level of the community mental health setting. Answer A, self-assessment of work habits and personality characteristics, is a prevocational evaluation method used to help determine the individual's potential for work readiness rather than develop skills. Answer C, educating the work supervisors about the individual's needs and offering environmental modifications to maximize performance, might occur after employment is obtained. Expressive activities, such as making a collage with pictures of different types of jobs, answer D, provides opportunities for exploration of ideas about job possibili-

ties, but would not directly develop job seeking skills. See Reference: Cara and MacRae (eds). Vocational programming.

76. (C) texture of the cords to be used. Coarse materials like jute may shred and cause splinters or injure the skin on hands and fingers. This is particularly important for individuals with diabetes who frequently have poor sensation and circulation in their extremities. Skin damage must be avoided because healing is compromised. The length of the cord (answer A) would be significant for an individual with limited range of motion. The thickness of the cord (answer B) would be significant for an individual with limited hand function. The type of surface the individual stands on (answer D) would be important to an individual with back pain. See Reference: Breines. Folkcraft.

77. (A) begin instruction in anger management strategies, such as relaxation. Beginning instruction in anger management techniques such as relaxation, conflict resolution, and empathizing would be the next step in a plan to address anger management because the individual has accomplished the first step of identifying key stressors leading to his anger and of defining his typical response to such stressors. Answer B, modifying treatment to focus on self-assertiveness, would not be an appropriate emphasis. Answer C, providing activities as outlets for anger, may have the effect of "actually increasing anger" (p. 468). Though the individual has made some progress toward goals, he has not achieved competence in anger management skills; therefore, answer D, recommending discontinuation of services, is also incorrect. See Reference: Early. Responding to symptoms and behaviors.

78. (D) Drawing lines and shapes using shaving cream, sand, or finger paints. The best activity to encourage prewriting would be drawing lines in different sensory media (answer D). Answer B, having the child create his or her own books, is useful for increasing orientation to printed language. Answers A and C, rolling clay into a ball and hammering are recommended for improving the ability to regulate pressure during hand activity. See Reference: Case-Smith (ed). Amundson, SJ: Prewriting and handwriting skills. Exner, CE: Development of hand skills.

79. (A) isometric muscle contractions. Isometric muscle contraction involves contracting the muscle without joint movement or a change in muscle length. Isotonic contractions (answer B) shorten the muscle length with accompanying joint movement. Progressive resistance (answer C) is a type of isotonic exercise that uses an increase in weight during consecutive exercise repetitions. A person who has a cast obstructing movement would be unable to perform either type of isotonic exercise. Passive movements (answer D) are performed by an outside force to the arm and involve joint motion, but no muscle contraction. Passive movement could not be performed with a casted joint. See Reference: Pedretti and Early (eds). Breines, E: Therapeutic occupations and modalities.

80. (D) directive group. Directive groups have a highly structured approach and are often used in acute care psychiatric settings for patients with psychoses who display disorganized thinking and disturbed functioning. Activity groups (answer A) require a higher level of task behavior and ability to engage in occupation to enable skill development. Psychoeducation groups (answer B) which are based on cognitive behavioral theory and focus on teaching information and techniques require a level of learning capacity that may be impaired during acute mental illness. Neurodevelopmental groups (answer D) use gross motor activity and sensory stimulation techniques to enhance sensory integration in persons with long histories of chronic schizophrenia. See Reference: Cara and MacRae (eds). Groups.

81. (D) Create a comfortable foundation for fostering parent skills through parent-therapist collaboration. All four answers describe possible ways for the OT to impact an infant's developmental outcome. However, the most permanent action would capitalize upon developing family centered mutual collaboration. With this approach, communication is the key to creating a relationship that will foster parental skill development and expertise. This then provides the parents with effective tools to best nurture and care for their infant at any time and in any environment, and has a permanent impact on the developmental outcome for the infant. See Reference: Case-Smith (ed). Hunter, JG: Neonatal intensive care unit.

82. (A) Prevent loss of joint and skin mobility. During the acute stage, when burn wounds are partial or full thickness in nature, maintenance of joint range of motion and skin mobility is the primary goal of intervention. Providing adaptive equipment (answer B) is typically performed during the subacute, surgical or postoperative stage, and compression and vascular garments (answer C), and the prevention of scarring (answer D) are goals most commonly implemented during the rehabilitation phase. See Reference: Pedretti and Early (eds). Reeves, SU: Burns and burn rehabilitation.

83. (A) Asking a department store salesperson for information about an item without buying it. Intervention to develop assertive behavior is a process of gradually empowering clients to make their own decisions, request assistance, avoid being taken advantage of, and provide constructive criticism when it is warranted in a variety of situations. Activities to assist in this process need to be graded for success by starting with situations that are less threatening to the client. Answer A, asking for information about an item without buying it, requires a request for information, but one which is well within the expectations of a department salesperson, making it a suitable exercise for beginning assertiveness training. Answers B, C, and D each require the client to make a special request, and question or criticize a service, which requires more skill and confidence. See Reference: Stein and Cutler. Leisure-time occupations, self-care, and social skills training.

84. (B) Direct the child to reach for a toy while sitting on a therapy ball. By placing a child in the sitting position on a therapeutic ball, "the therapist can facilitate postural reactions using activities that displace the center of gravity and require corrective or protective responses" (p. 284). The addition of the reaching activity will cause the child to change his or her center of gravity during the reaching phase, which will require a further postural response to compensate for the change of position. Answers A, C, and D are not necessarily related to postural reaction development, rather, strengthening, decreasing tactile defensiveness, and visual-perception. See Reference: Case-Smith (ed). Nichols, D: Development of postural control.

85. (B) prevents hyperextension of the MCP joints and allows MCP flexion. An ulnar nerve splint's primary purpose is to support the hand secondary to ulnar intrinsic muscle paralysis. This splint also allows for MCP flexion. Answers A, C, and D are all inappropriate techniques for fabricating an ulnar nerve splint. See Reference: Pedretti and Early (eds). Karsch, MC and Nickerson, E: Hand and upper extremity injuries.

86. (A) increasing self-awareness through expressive activities. Increasing self-awareness would be an initial goal area because people with eating disorders are often out-of-touch with their bodies as well as their psychological and social needs. Expressive activities address psychosocial needs to increase self-awareness by providing opportunities for emotional self-expression and self-assertion (answer A). Answer B is incorrect because preoccupation with "good" versus "bad" nutrition may be part of the eating disorder. Answer C is incorrect because school performance tends to be unaffected when individuals have eating disorders unless they are physically ill. Family therapy referrals are typically performed by other disciplines on the team at the time of discharge so answer D also is incorrect. See Reference: Crepeau, Cohn, and Schell (eds). Ward, JD: Psychiatric diagnoses and related intervention issues.

87. (C) Removing pants. Answer C is correct because, according to most developmental scales, children first learn to remove garments, especially socks. Answer A is not correct, because the ability to put garments on with the front and back correctly placed is a skill that is developed later. Buttoning and tying bows (answer D) is incorrect for the same reason. Answer B is incorrect because children are typically able to remove garments before they are able to put them on. See Reference: Case-Smith (ed). Shepherd, J: Self-care and adaptations for independent living.

88. (A) Contrast baths, active and passive range of motion, and massage. Contrast baths, active and passive range of motion, and massage are all initial techniques considered for the management of edema and joint stiffness. Answers B and D, ultrasound, electrical stimulation, dynamic splinting, and joint mobilization, are all considered treatment techniques for more established joint stiffness. Answer C, resistive exercises, weight bearing, and lifting, could all potentially contribute to increasing joint stiffness and pain. See Reference: Pedretti and Early (eds). Kasch, MC and Nickerson, E: Hand and upper extremity injuries.

89. (B) Working on a mock car engine. Working on a mock car engine provides a work simulation that would be required by the client's job. This activity also would assist with increasing his endurance, strength, and productivity. Answer A, lifting weights, is not a work hardening goal when performed in isolation of a simulated work task. Answer C, visiting the work site, would not be a work hardening activity, but rather part of the onsite analysis that is typically completed by the practitioner and vocational retraining counselor. Answer D, meal preparation, is not considered to be a demand required by this particular vocation. See Reference: Pedretti and Early (eds). Kasch, MC and Nickerson, E: Hand and upper extremity injuries.

90 (B) Visual attention skills. According to Todd, answer B is correct because development of visual attention skills should be worked on first as they prepare and provide foundation skills for other aspects of visual perception. Answer A is incorrect because visual memory skills can only be developed after visual attention skills are established. Answers C and D are incorrect because general and specific visual perceptual skills develop after visual memory. See Reference: Kramer and Hinojosa (eds). Todd, VR: Visual information analysis: Frame of reference for visual perception.

91. (C) baking cookies using a recipe. Baking cookies (answer C) is a well delineated meal-preparation activity that provides structure with a specific sequence of tasks. Setting a table or preparing a shopping list (answers A and D) do not necessarily require sequencing of tasks. Planning a meal (answer B) involves a great deal of organizational ability, and would not be an appropriate choice for an initial activity to address goals relating to sequencing tasks. See Reference: Creek (ed). Creek, J: Treatment planning and implementation.

92. (B) folding laundry and putting it in a basket while standing. Work-hardening programs prepare individuals to return to work by combining work simulation, strengthening, and behavioral components. A cashier stands during the job, removes clothing from a hanger, folds it, puts it in a bag, runs price tags through a scanner, operates a cash register, and makes change. Putting price tags on clothing while seated (answer D) does not include standing, a critical component of the job. Washing dishes while standing (answer C) incorporates the standing aspect of the client's job, but not the other aspects. Moving piles of clothing from one end of the clinic to the other (answer A) involves walking, not standing. The activity that incorporates the most components of the client's job is folding laundry and putting it in a basket while standing (answer B). See Reference: Pedretti and Early (eds). Burt, CM: Work evaluation and work hardening.

93. (D) provide a sensory cue, such as saying "stop!" The use of auditory, visual, or tactile sensory cues (answer D) can help the person with Parkinson's disease change the motor program in which they are engaged. Deep breathing exercises (answer A), practicing movements (answer B), and mentally reviewing steps in the sequence of movement (answer C) will not provide the sensory information needed at the moment to evoke movement or change a "frozen" movement pattern. See Reference: Pedretti and Early (eds). Schultz-Krohn, W: Parkinson's disease.

94. (B) a 3-inch screw-top jar. Since the goal was written as a functional behavioral objective, the OT should collect information about the functional progress the child has made in performance areas. Assessing progress by measuring range of motion with a goniometer (answer A), the strength of grip using a dynamometer (answer C), or degree of coordination using a fine motor scale assessment (answer D) may provide useful information of individual performance components addressed; however, none of these will provide sufficient information to measure progress of a functionally written goal. See Reference: Case-Smith (ed). Richardson, PK and Schultz-Krohn, W: Planning and implementing services.

95. (A) using the strongest joint and avoiding positions of deformity. The significance of using these principles for individuals with preexisting joint conditions and adverse musculoskeletal changes may help to restore function as well as prevent further impairments. Answers B, C, and D involve common muscle relaxation and stress management techniques not always associated with joint protection techniques. See Reference: Pedretti and Early (eds). Buckner, WS: Arthritis.

96. (D) Present only a few puzzle pieces at a time. Similar to other children with attention deficit disorder, this child most likely has poor impulse control and experiences great difficulty completing a task. By presenting a few puzzle pieces at a time (answer D), the OT can help the child focus on a few relevant stimuli and make it possible to complete a short-term task successfully. This experience will then help the child increase attention span. Soft foam puzzle pieces (answer A) are less likely to cause injury if thrown, but their use is not likely to help increase the child's attention span. Providing puzzle pieces of only one color (answer B) may reduce visual stimulation somewhat, and using larger interlocking puzzle pieces (answer C) may make manipulation of the pieces easier, but the overwhelming stimulus caused by presenting all the puzzle pieces at once would make these strategies irrelevant. See Reference: Case-Smith (ed). Cronin, AS: Psychosocial and emotional domains.

97. (B) provide strong color contrast at key areas to identify steps, pathways, etc. Using contrast is a key environmental adaptation strategy for people with visual impairments. The more contrast, the easier it is to locate objects, steps, entrances, and pathways, thereby improving accessibility by maximizing remaining vision. Instructing the individual to sit during ADL (answer A), or recommending human assistance (answer C), would not directly address accessibility. Answer D, recommending training in white cane use, is a method of improving mobility for a person who is blind. See Reference: Christiansen and Matuska (eds). Golembiewski, D: Living with vision loss.

98. (A) Mount lever handles on doors and faucets. For children with reduced strength and endurance, using less complex movements and less force results in energy conservation. Lever handles require less energy than knob handles on doors, faucets, and appliances. Answers B and C are environmental adaptations recommended to minimize the danger of slipping and falling for children with incoordination or postural instability. Answer D is contraindicated, because work at a vertical surface against gravity requires more energy than movement in a horizontal plane. See Reference: Case-Smith (ed). Shepherd, J: Self-care and adaptations for independent living.

99. (A) continue to perform PROM and then position and elevate the affected extremity. Positioning, the use of a compression glove, edema massage, and PROM exercises are all effective methods for reducing edema and preventing further edema. The goal is to promote the movement of fluid back into normal circulation, rather than allowing it to collect in one area or body part. Gentle PROM is necessary to help maintain joint structure and provide nutrients to the joint. The actual movement of the extremity may serve as a "pump" to assist in moving excess fluid back into the body. These techniques are contraindicated for individuals who have deep vein thrombosis. Edema is caused in part by the loss of movement in an extremity because there is no contraction of muscles, which helps to pump the fluid to the heart. Splinting (answer B) is effective in preventing deformity, but elevation and compression gloves are more effective in reducing edema. Taking no action (answer C) could result in permanent damage to the tissue of the involved extremity. Having the individual attempt to squeeze a ball (answer D) would be inappropriate because the left arm is flaccid. See Reference: Trombly and Radomski. Woodson, AM: Stroke.

100. (D) train the student to use an electrically powered page turner. According to Cook and Hussey, "access to books, magazines, and other reading material is important for the acquisition of information for school, work, or leisure" (p. 380). Answer D, an electric powered page turner would be the most effective solution for this student since answer A, a book holder and mouthstick would require a significant degree of head control. Answers B and C (use of a human attendant and/or talking books) would not address the student's desire to independently read magazines. See Reference: Cook and Hussey. Technologies that aid manipulation and control of the environment.

101. (B) outpatient OT. Outpatient therapy is appropriate for individuals who are "medically stable and able to tolerate a few hours of therapy and a trip to an outpatient clinic" (p. 35). A patient with such high levels of function is not an appropriate candidate for a home health referral (answer A). Work-hardening programs (answer C) are for individuals who are severely deconditioned as a result of disease or injury, or for those who have significant discrepancies between their symptoms and objective findings. If the individual has potential for further functional improvement, continuation rather than discontinuation (answer D) of services is indicated. See Reference: Pedretti and Early (eds). Matthews, MM and Tipton-Burton, M: Treatment contexts.

102. (B) put the dried dishes away and begin to hand her wet dishes. Compensating for mistakes helps to increase the sense of self-worth and integrity of individuals with dementia. This approach is preferable to drawing attention to errors, especially in situations in which safety is not an issue. Answers A, C, and D all draw attention to the individual's errors. See Reference: Early. Responding to symptoms and behaviors.

103. (C) Handle the child slowly and gently. Answer C is correct because the child with hypertonicity will be most relaxed and easier to handle if tone is inhibited by slow and gentle handling of the body. Answer A is incorrect because adaptive equipment is frequently needed to provide a child with a sense of security during bathing. Answer B is incorrect because bathing the child too quickly could increase hypertonicity. Answer D is incorrect because it provides the parent with a poor model of good body mechanics; the child's parent should kneel by the tub or sit on a stool while bathing the child. See Reference: Case-Smith (ed). Shepherd, J: Self-care and adaptations for independent living.

104. (D) in the upper cabinet to the left side. Placing the groceries in the upper cabinet to the left side will promote the greatest degree of weight shift to the affected side. Putting groceries on the counter directly in front of the person (answer A), or in the upper cabinet to the right side (answer C), would not cause enough weight to be shifted to the affected side, and would even shift weight away from that side. When placing groceries on the counter to the left side (answer B), minimal weight shift occurs. See Reference: Pedretti and Early (eds). Pope-Davis, SA: Proprioceptive neuromuscular facilitation approach.

105. (D) home-delivered meal services. Answer A, continued OT services to teach the patient to use the kitchen safely, is incorrect because individuals diagnosed with dementia tend to decline over time, and interventions aimed at improvement are unrealistic. Volunteer companions (answer B) provide companionship to elders at home, but not skilled supervision of activities. Transporting to a community site for meals (answer C) on a daily basis could be inconvenient, overly challenging, and taxing for an elder with beginning dementia. Answer D, in-home meal delivery services such as Meals-on-Wheels, would be the best and safest option for providing consistent access to food in the home. See Reference: Aitken, MJ and Goldstein-Lohman H: Health care systems: Changing perspectives.

106. (B) Avoid internal rotation and adduction of the involved hip. Following hip arthroplasty, positions such as flexion of the hip past a prescribed range (usually 60 to 90 degrees), internal rotation, and adduction can result in dislocation of the hip. Therefore, answer B, avoid internal rotation and adduction of the involved hip, is the priority set of instructions to convey. OT practitioners instruct individuals in hip precautions and provide them with adaptive equipment so they can safely perform self-care, work, and leisure activities. Answers C and D may help an individual comply more easily with hip precautions. Sitting during LE dressing (answer A) also is recommended. See Reference: Pedretti and Early (eds). Coleman, S: Hip fractures and lower extremity joint replacement.

107. (B) side-lying on a mat. According to Wandel (2000), "Side-lying is a good positioning choice for children whose muscle tone becomes too high or low in prone or supine positions. Side-lying positions also give children a stable, midline head position and keep their hands in their line of vision; hands remain free to reach for and manipulate objects without having to resist the pull of gravity" (p. 354). Answer A, long-sitting, answer C, supine positioning, and answer D, prone positioning, all require the child to work against gravity, and would most likely be too difficult for the child to maintain while engaging in play activities secondary to low tone. See Reference: Solomon (ed). Wandel, JA: Positioning and handling.

108. (C) marking the end of each step with high contrast tape. Difficulty in seeing contrast and color are two forms of decreased visual acuity that cannot be addressed by corrective lenses. Two effective environmental adaptations to these deficits are increasing background contrast and illumination. Using tape or paint to make the edge of each step contrast sharply with the rest of the step is an inexpensive way to adapt the environment. Installing a stair glide or handrails (answers A and B) are more costly adaptations that do not address the problems of decreased visual acuity. Instructing the patient to take only one step at a time (answer D) may cause the individual to be unnecessarily slow, and does not address the problems of decreased visual acuity. See

Reference: Pedretti and Early (eds). Warren, M: Evaluation and treatment of visual deficits.

109. (C) instructing caregivers in task breakdown. Instructing the client's caregivers in task breakdown, or breaking down tasks into simple steps and then providing step-by-step instructions, will allow the client to perform activities as capabilities decline. At this stage of the disease, memory retraining (answer A) and ADL retraining (answer B) will probably not be effective. Leisure activities (answer D) structured to meet the needs of the client with Alzheimer's disease could be helpful, but will not address the primary problem of performance of self-care activities. See Reference: Pedretti and Early (eds). Schultz-Krohn, W, Foti, D, and Glogoski, C: Degenerative diseases of the central nervous system.

110. (D) A long-handled bath sponge. A person with a total hip arthroplasty must avoid hip flexion of 80 degrees or greater, hip adduction, and internal rotation. A long-handled bath sponge (answer D) would allow the person to adhere to the precautions stated above by providing an extended reach during bathing of the lower extremities. A wire basket attached to the walker (answer A) would not allow the person to come close to a counter without having to step sideways, which causes hip adduction. A padded foam toilet seat 1 inch height (answer B), or a short-handled bath sponge (answer C), would be inadequate in that they would cause the person to flex the hip past 80 degrees while performing self-care tasks. See Reference: Trombly and Radomski. Bear-Lehman, J: Orthopaedic conditions.

111. (C) Bring the seat in for reevaluation within 6 months. Fit and function of seating and mobility should be reassessed every 6 months to account for the child's growth, as well as any changes in posture. Parents should not make unsupervised adaptations (answer A), because improper positioning could harm the child. Weekly adjustment (answer B) are usually not necessary, and transporting the seat every week would be unnecessarily inconvenient. The end of the IEP (answer D) may be more than 6 months away and, therefore, too long to wait. See Reference: Case-Smith (ed). Wright-Ott, C and Egilson, S: Mobility.

112. (C) Modify the activity to make it less challenging. The OT should recognize subtle signs of fatigue, such as frustration, slowing down, hurrying to finish, lessening range of motion, and use of substitution movements, which indicate the training level was too difficult and should be downgraded. Other signs include the individual's heart rate exceeding the target heart rate; increase of more than 20 bpm above resting pulse; failure to return to resting heart rate after a 5 minute rest; and systolic pressure that does not increase at all, or that increases more than 20 mm Hg from baseline. Stopping the activity (answer A) is necessary if the individual experiences symptoms such as dyspnea, chest pain, lightheadedness, or diaphoresis. The activity should be upgraded (answer B) only when the individual is able to perform the activity without signs of fatigue or cardiac symptoms. Isometric exercises (answer D), which interfere with blood flow through the muscles and create a heightened demand on the cardiovascular system, should not be used in individuals with cardiac conditions. See Reference: Dutton. Introduction to biomechanical frame of reference.

113. (B) Calendars. An external memory device uses environmental adaptations or structure to assist an individual in remembering specific information. Examples include setting an alarm clock to wake up in the morning, labeling drawers according to contents, and using a log or calendar to keep track of events and activities. An internal memory device would be the use of internalized memory techniques to structure information. Visual imagery techniques (answer A), mnemonics (answer C), and repetition or rehearsal (answer D) are all examples of internal memory devices. See Reference: Pedretti and Early (eds). Wheatley, CJ: Evaluation and treatment of perceptual and perceptual motor deficits.

114. (A) Identify options and the consequences of each option. Individuals are frequently resistive to changes that will affect the familiar home environment, such as moving furniture or adding medically necessary equipment. To accept change, the feelings and cultural attitudes and beliefs of the client must be recognized. Then the following steps can be implemented to encourage acceptance of change: (1) identify options and the consequences of each option; (2) allow time for reflection and consideration of options (answer D); (3) practice with a "demo" device (answer C); (4) reassess the decision; (5) if acceptable, order the equipment; and (6) if rejected, document the steps taken and the reasons for rejection (answer B). See Reference: Bonder and Wagner (eds). Hunt, LA: Home health care.

115. (A) exploratory play. Exploratory play (answer A) provides children with experiences that develop body scheme, sensory integrative and motor skills, and concepts of sensory characteristics and actions on objects. Therefore, the unstructured obstacle course is an example of exploratory play. Symbolic play (answer B) is associated with the development of language and concepts (e.g., use of "dress-up" materials). Creative play (answer C) and interests are characterized by refinement of skills in activities that allow construction, social relationships, and dramatic play (e.g., finger painting). Recreational play (answer D) is leisure experiences that allow the exploration of interests and roles such as arts and crafts or sports. See Reference: Case-Smith (ed). Morrison, CD and Metzger, P: Play.

116. (C) Using a bath chair and leaving the door open. The best bathing method for a person with COPD considers the energy demands of the task, as well as the effect of water temperature, in light of the individual's functional status. People with COPD have difficulty breathing when the environment is hot or humid, or when there is a high degree of steam. Answer A is incorrect because the energy demand of transferring into a tub and the use of hot water may cause difficulty breathing. Answer B, standing for a quick shower, also is incorrect because even if brief, standing would be more energy demanding than sitting, and an overhead shower can increase humidity. A lukewarm tub bath (answer D) would provide lower humidity by using the coolest water temperature, but the need to transfer in and out of the tub may make the task very energy demanding. See Reference: Trombly and Radomski. Huntley, N: Cardiac and pulmonary diseases.

117. (C) Safety razor with extended handle. A safety razor with an extended handle is the appropriate component that allows this individual to overcome limited shoulder and elbow range of motion in order to reach his face. Attaching a safety razor or electric razor to a universal cuff (answers A and D) would benefit an individual who is unable to grasp a razor, but would not enable this individual to reach his face to shave. A safety razor with a built-up handle (answer B) would benefit an individual with limited finger flexion or strength, but it also would be ineffective in enabling this individual to reach his face. See Reference: Crepeau, Cohn, and Schell (eds). Holm, MB, Rogers, JC and James, AB: Activities of daily living.

118. (A) videofluoroscopy. A videofluoroscopy should be performed when it is suspected that the individual is aspirating. An individual who suddenly has a wet voice when there was no prior difficulty may have had a sudden change in medical status causing aspiration. He or she should be reevaluated to determine if there is aspiration into the larynx or trachea. Answers B, a change to thin liquids, and D, a regular diet, would be inappropriate for an individual who does not have a normal swallow or who may be

aspirating, because they are too difficult to control. Answer C, a tracheostomy tube, is usually in place prior to the initiation of a feeding program, because the individual was having difficulty with breathing, not swallowing or wet voice qualities. See Reference: Pedretti and Early (eds). Jenks, KN: Dysphagia.

119. (B) environmental adaptations and assistance for ADL. A patient who exhibits no capacity for new learning will be unable to benefit from therapy interventions that require the ability to transfer learning (answers A, C, and D). A compensatory approach of adapting the environment and recommending assistance for safe performance of daily activities is the most appropriate intervention. See Reference: Crepeau, Cohn, and Schell (eds). Giuffrida, CG and Neistadt, ME: Overview of learning theory.

120. (C) Oversized tee shirts and elastic top pants. For a child who experiences difficulty in self-dressing due to incoordination (as seen with athetoid CP), clothing should be loose fitting with simple or no fasteners. Oversized clothing is preferred to tight fitting garments (answers A and B). Garments with elasticized waist bands are better than those using zippers (answer B), or snaps and buttons (answer D). See Reference: Case-Smith (ed). Shepherd, J: Self-care and adaptations for independent living.

121. (D) set personal boundaries appropriate to the therapist-patient relationship. It is important to acknowledge the individual's need for sexual expression while supporting the sense of self and identifying acceptable relationships and behaviors. Setting boundaries while accepting the individual is the most appropriate therapeutic response. Outright rejection (answer A) may cause an individual to believe he or she is sexually undesirable or unlovable. Flirting back (answer B) may imply that a sexual relationship between the therapist and the patient is acceptable. Although the individual may need to know how SCI affects sexual functioning (answer C), the behavior that requires a response is not about a lack of knowledge, but rather about how to appropriately express sexual interest and the need for reinforcement of a sexual identity. See Reference: Pedretti and Early (eds). Burton, GU: Sexuality and physical dysfunction.

122. (C) state simple, concrete directions allowing time for delayed responses. Answer C is correct because, "many patients with TBI exhibit concrete thinking, in which they are able to interpret information only at the most literal level" (p. 681). Since processing of information is also an area of difficulty, allowing time for delayed responses is frequently necessary. Answer A, telling such people what is expected and asking them to begin would require abstract thinking and initiation of activities–both areas that are likely to be impaired. Answers B and C, relying on gestures, and providing written directions with pictures, may not be effective if visual perception is impaired. See Reference: Pedretti and Early (eds). Gutman, SA: Traumatic brain injury.

123. (A) shoulder flexion and protraction.
Answer A is correct because the infant changes from extensor influences on posture to development of flexion in the supine position. This requires the ability to flex and protract the shoulders against gravity in order to reach forward and upward to grasp toys. Answer B is not correct because shoulder extension and retraction would not be encouraged during supine activities when the toys are placed overhead. Answers C and D are not correct because most activities that involve looking and reaching can be accomplished without using head or trunk control against gravity in the supine position. See Reference: Mulligan. Typical child development.

124. (C) "The patient will perform lower extremity dressing with verbal cueing for energy conservation techniques 50% of the time."
Goals should be functional, measurable, and objective. Answer C meets those criteria. Answer B does not provide measurable criteria. Answer D describes what the practitioner will do. Short-term goals must relate to the long-term goal being addressed. Because the long-term goal being addressed is independence in dressing, the short-term goal must relate to dressing, not all activities of daily living (answer A). See Reference: Borcherding. Writing functional and measurable goals.

125. (C) have the individual predict his performance before an activity, then have him self-evaluate the performance. Having the individual predict his performance before an activity (self-estimation) and comparing his predicted performance with a self-evaluation of the actual performance can provide meaningful self-initiated feedback and would be the best way to increase awareness. Simply discussing the individual's perceptions (answer A) would not provide concrete immediate feedback about performance. Reviewing a checklist of necessary skills, answer B, would probably not be effective in increasing awareness since the patient feels he already possesses these skills. Answer D, ignoring the patient's perceptions, would not address the patient's therapeutic need to increase awareness and could lead to increased resistance. See

Reference: Pedretti and Early (eds). Wheatley, CJ: Evaluation and treatment of cognitive dysfunction.

126. (C) extension to promote finger flexion, and flexion to facilitate finger extension. The method used to maintain tenodesis in the hand of a person with quadriplegia is to keep the wrist extended to facilitate finger flexion, and flexed to promote finger extension. The other methods would stretch the tendons too much, which would not allow a tenodesis grasp. See Reference: Trombly and Radomski. Atkins, MS: Spinal cord injury.

127. (B) aerobic exercise. Gross motor activities, involving either aerobic exercise or stretching and relaxation, can help to reduce the physical symptoms associated with anxiety. Although line dancing (answer C) involves all of the elements of gross motor activities, it requires the individual to follow specific steps and movements, which could cause the patient to become more anxious. Sewing and handcrafts (answer A) and woodworking (answer D) would not be the best recommendation for reducing physical symptoms of muscle tension, because they are primarily fine motor activities that require sustained attention. See Reference: Creek (ed). Bracegirdle, H: Developing physical fitness to promote mental health.

128. (D) a long, thin nipple. According to Case-Smith (2001) "a variety of nipples are designed for use with children who have structural problems. These nipples compensate for lack of negative pressure and for limitations in tongue position and movement" (p. 477). Answer D, a long, thin nipple, works best for children with a recessed tongue and can assist with bringing the tongue forward while feeding. Answer A, a wide nipple, is typically indicated for the child with a cleft palate, while answer B, a nipple with a single hole, is most effective for children who perform better with a steady flow of liquid versus a burst of fluid typically provided via nipples with several holes. Answer C, a broad-based nipple, is most effective for children with a cleft lip since it tends to create suction. See Reference: Case-Smith (ed). Case-Smith, J, and Humphrey, R: Feeding intervention.

129. (C) Toothbrush with built-up handle. An individual with C7-C8 quadriplegia has the hand strength to hold a toothbrush with a built-up handle, answer C. An alternate method can be to position the toothbrush between the fingers. An individual with a C5 injury may require a mobile arm support for brushing teeth (answer A). Other individuals with injuries at the C5-C6 level may be able to use a universal cuff (answer B), or a wrist support with a utensil holder (answer D) to hold the toothbrush. See Reference: Christiansen and Matuska (eds). Garber, SL, Gregorio-Torres, TL: Adaptive strategies following spinal cord injury.

130. (A) observe, set the climate, and model desired behaviors. Answer A reflects typical leadership involvement in OT groups. Answer B is incorrect because it reflects minimal direction from the leader which is uncharacteristic of OT groups. Answer C is incorrect because the group leader performs these functions at the termination stage, rather than the initial stages of group development. Working individually with group members (answer D) is incongruous with current OT group treatment formats that use properties of the group to achieve therapeutic goals. See Reference: Crepeau, Cohn, and Schell (eds). Schwartzberg, SL: Group process.

131. (D) a raised-bed garden. The individual with back pain must avoid activities that stress the lumbar spine, such as prolonged bending/flexing of the spine. A raised-bed garden would allow gardening without bending. A wheelbarrow with elongated handles (answer B) would be more difficult to control while pushing than a wheelbarrow with normal handles, and therefore, would place undue stress on the low back. A 12-inch-high seat with tool holders (answer C) could benefit an individual with low endurance, but working on the ground from that position would be very difficult for an individual with back pain. Answer A, ergonomically correct hand tools, would assist individuals requiring joint protection of the hands and upper extremities as opposed to those with back pain. See Reference: Pedretti and Early (eds). Smithline, J and Dunlop, LE: Low back pain.

132. (C) Role-playing of social situations. Social skills training is accomplished in four progressive steps: instruction, demonstration of desired behaviors by the group leader, guided practice, and independent activities. The first step in this process, teaching about social skills and breaking down skills into smaller components, such as nonverbal behavior and listening skills, has been addressed in the group. The second step, directly demonstrating how the skills are performed also has been accomplished. The group members are now ready for guided practice, which "involves having the client perform an actual social skill under the watchful eye of the therapist and other members of the group" (p. 485). Role-playing of social situations is a technique used in guided practice. Answers A and B would occur after guided practice. Answer D, providing feedback on hygiene and appearance, may have some impact on social functioning, but would relate

more to ADL competence than social skill development. See Reference: Stein and Cutler. Leisure-time occupations, self-care, and social skills training.

133. (A) "jaw opening and closing are controlled with your index and middle fingers; place your thumb on the child's cheek." The correct position of the adult's hand for jaw control when the child is fed from the side is described in answer A. Answers B and D are incorrect because the thumb should be placed on the child's cheek to provide joint stability. Answer C is incorrect because controlling the child's jaw movement with the adult's whole hand provides less control of the child's jaw than the recommended method. Placing the adult's thumb on the child's ear (answer D) is also incorrect because of discomfort for the child, and because thumb placement should be near the fulcrum of jaw movement (at the temporomandibular joint). If the child is fed from the front, the adult's thumb is placed on the chin, with middle finger under the chin to control opening and closing of the jaw. The index finger then rests on the side of the child's face to provide stability. See Reference: Case-Smith (ed). Case-Smith, J and Humphry, R: Feeding intervention.

134. (D) provide wrist extension, MCP extension, and thumb extension. A low-level radial nerve injury results in decreased extension of the MP joints of the thumb and fingers. The purpose of this splint is to prevent the extensor tendons from overstretching as well as provide proper positioning of the hand for functional use. Answers A, B, and C are inappropriate functions for a dorsal dynamic splint. See Reference: Pedretti and Early (eds). Kasch, MC and Nickerson, E: Hand and upper extremity injuries.

135. (C) use of leisure time. How to deal with leisure time is a key occupational problem area for people with substance abuse problems because "...leisure activities and contexts are where alcohol and drugs are most commonly used" (p. 524). Use of leisure time is a very important area for the OT practitioner to address with a newly sober client who has been counseled to avoid situations and people associated with drinking alcohol. Identifying leisure interests and establishing plans for structuring large amounts of time without drinking can help support attempts to remain substance free. Answer A, work performance, also would be an area to explore, but would probably not be an area of skill development introduced early in the OT intervention process. Answer B, self-care skills, may need to be addressed as part of daily living skills performance, but would not impact as directly on avoiding substance abuse. Medication is not typically a feature of treatment for substance abuse so answer D also is incorrect. See Reference: Creek (ed). Chacksfield, J and Lancaster, J: Substance misuse.

136. (A) Within 6 months, the client will participate in classroom activities for 1 hour without disruptive outbursts, twice a day. A functional goal relates the skill to be developed to a child's environment or life tasks, therefore, making it more meaningful to the child and the family. Answers B, C, and D are measurable, but not functional goals, because they do not address the context in which the skill is applied. See Reference: Case-Smith (ed). Richardson, PK and Schultz-Krohn, W: Planning and implementing services.

137. (B) hyperextension of the PIP joint and flexion of the DIP joint. Answer B is the only answer provided that describes a swan-neck deformity. The pattern of hyperextension of the PIP and DIP joints (answer A) may be seen in lower motorneuron palsies. Flexion of the PIP joint and hyperextension of the DIP joint (answer C) is descriptive of a boutonniere deformity. An individual who has overstretched the volar plates at the PIP and DIP joints would have hyperextension of the MP joint and flexion of the DIP joint (answer D). See Reference: Pedretti and Early (eds). Buckner, WS: Arthritis.

138. (D) Ask the employer to provide an isolated cubical as the work space. An isolated cubical is a reasonable accommodation to request for an individual who is highly distractible. The Americans with Disabilities Act (ADA) requires employers to provide reasonable accommodations for individuals with documented disabilities that will enable them to work despite the disability. A job coach (answer A) is more appropriate for an individual who needs frequent cueing or assistance to perform their job. Frequent breaks (answer B) are a reasonable accommodation suitable for individuals with anxiety who need to manage stress. Although explaining the problem of distractibility to the employer (answer C) may open the lines of communication with the employer, it does not offer a solution. See Reference: Stein and Cutler. Tryssenaar, J: Vocational exploration and employment and psychosocial disabilities.

139. (A) Drawing a picture entitled "This is me." Children who have trouble expressing their emotions verbally are sometimes able to express their feelings in open-ended drawing activities. Among the answers given, answer A is the only projective activity. Answers B, C, and D are highly structured activities with minimal potential for open-ended expression. See Reference: Case-Smith (ed). Cronin, AS: Psychosocial and emotional domains.

140. (B) identify the individual's abilities, needs, and goals. Identifying the individual's abilities, needs, and goals should occur before any other steps in the process in order to make a match between the individual's abilities, environmental demands, and the appropriate technology to carry out desired daily occupations. Answers A, C, and D are steps which would come later in the process. See Reference: Christiansen and Baum (eds). Trefler, E and Hobson, D: Assistive technology.

141. (B) Handing out trays and utensils in a food service group. This individual demonstrates limitations in the area of interpersonal skills. Adequate interpersonal and social skills are necessary for successful employment. In order to develop these skills, the individual should be provided with opportunities to practice them in a structured environment. Handing out trays and utensils requires minimal interaction, and would provide an opportunity for this individual to practice interacting with others at a limited level. None of the other options provides the opportunity to develop interpersonal skills. See Reference: Stein and Cutler. Tryssenaar, J: Vocational exploration and employment and psychosocial disabilities.

142. (D) Alternate tasks that require standing with those that can be performed sitting. The performance component at issue in this question is fatigue. When fatigue impedes occupational performance, energy conservation techniques should be considered. Alternating sitting and standing activities is one method that can be applied to conserve energy; others include avoiding bending and stooping, avoiding unnecessary trips, using an appropriate work height, and relaxing homemaking standards. Convincing the individual to do something she can't afford (answer A) may not be in her best interest, and it is not an example consistent with the OT concept of collaborative decision making. Although increasing strength (answer B) may ultimately be useful, endurance is typically a more pressing issue for individuals with MS. Using the largest joints available for the task (answer C) is a joint protection technique more appropriate for an individual with arthritis. See Reference: Pedretti and Early (eds). Buckner, WS: Arthritis.

143. (B) Approach the individual briefly several times throughout the session without making any demands on him. This approach indicates to the individual that you accept his feelings and that you will not neglect him regardless of his withdrawn behavior. After several visits, the individual will be more likely to respond. In addition, the OT practitioner should match the individual's pace, and be careful not to make more demands of the individual than he is ready to handle. Depressed individuals may try to avoid contact with staff, and the OT practitioner must be careful not to reinforce this behavior by ignoring the client (answer A). Answers C and D both have a threatening or manipulative tone to them, and are unlikely to help establish a therapeutic relationship. See Reference: Early. Responding to symptoms and behaviors.

144. (B) Gently touch the infant's lips to encourage her to open her mouth and begin sucking motions. Answer B, gently touching the infant's lips, would most likely facilitate the suck-swallow reflex. "When the infant's lips are touched, the infant's mouth opens and sucking movements begin" (p. 91). Answer A, touching the infant's cheek before feeding, would most likely facilitate the rooting reflex. Answer C would most likely facilitate the phasic-bite reflex, while answer D, rubbing the infant's lips and cheeks simultaneously, would most likely frustrate the infant, because several different reflexes are being encouraged at the same time (e.g., the rooting reflex and phasic-bite reflex). See Reference: Solomon (ed). O'Brien, JC, Koontz Lowman, D, and Solomon, JW: Development of occupational performance areas.

145. (C) Ulnar styloid, distal head of radius, and thumb CMC joint. The ulnar styloid, distal head of the radius, and thumb CMC joints are the most common sites for pressure because of their overt bony prominences. Answers A, B, and D also are areas that could potentially be susceptible to skin breakdown, but are not primary sites of pressure when fabricating a resting pan splint. See Reference: Pedretti and Early (eds). Belkin, J and Yasada, L: Orthotics.

146. (C) give simple directions and patiently wait for responses. Severe depression can result in slowing of cognitive and motor functions, known as psychomotor retardation. The OT practitioner must not rush the individual (answer A), but should give him or her time to process information and respond. Too much stimulation (answers B and D) may cause the individual to withdraw even further. See Reference: Crepeau, Cohn, and Schell (eds). Ward, J: Adults with mental illness.

147. (B) a local wheelchair equipment vendor. Although any community resource may be helpful to a child and family with a severe physical disability, answer B is correct because of the possible breakdown of this already purchased piece of equipment. The OT practitioner needs to consider this possible

problem and provide local support for a solution. Therefore, although answers A, C, and D may serve as resources for other needs of the child, only a specialist in wheelchair equipment would be able to solve mechanical problems that arise. See Reference: Case-Smith (ed). Wright-Ott, C and Egilson, S: Mobility.

148. (D) has good UE range of motion, but difficulty accessing small targets. A large keyboard would be best for someone who has good range of motion, but difficulty accessing small targets (answer D). A person with limited range of motion, but adequate fine coordination (answer A) would benefit from a smaller or contracted keyboard. If someone fatigues rapidly when reaching for the keys (answer B), having to reach further on a large keyboard would cause more fatigue. A large keyboard would be more difficult for a person using one hand (answer C), because the hand would have to move farther to complete typing, adding more work to the process. See Reference: Pedretti and Early (eds). Anson, D: Assistive technology.

149. (B) Decreased arousal and drowsiness. Medication side effects are typically observed and reported by OT practitioners. Antianxiety medications reduce anxiety, but also may produce sleep, relax muscles, and impair memory (p. 317). Akathisia, extrapyramidal syndrome, and tardive dyskinesia (answers A, C, and D, respectively) are adverse effects commonly linked to antipsychotic medications. See Reference: Stein and Cutler. Medications related to psychosocial issues.

150. (A) macramé with short cords. Longer cords require more shoulder abduction with external rotation. Therefore, short cords (answer A) would be easiest for this type of individual. Fine cords (answer C) would be challenging for individuals with limited finger function. Thick cords (answer D) could be used to downgrade the activity for those individuals. However, the thickness of the cord would have no bearing on shoulder range of motion requirements. See Reference: Breines. Folkcraft.

151. (C) Change to a power wheelchair to reduce effort. Considering the progressive nature of the child's disease, as well as strength and endurance, the best recommendation would be to change to a power wheelchair. The child would be better able to participate in the cognitive tasks of school if less effort was required for mobility. Answer A, retaining the manual chair, would be counterproductive to functioning well at school, and strength will not improve with this child's condition. Answer B might make mobility slightly easier, but will not solve the long-term problem of decreasing strength and endurance. Answer D would still make demands on strength and energy that would appear inappropriate considering the nature of Duchenne's muscular dystrophy. The team's recommendation also should be integrated with the family's needs and resources. See Reference: Case-Smith (ed). Case-Smith, J, Rogers, J and Johnson, JH: School-based occupational therapy.

152. (D) Burn hand splints prevent stress on the tendons and ligaments, while decreasing edema. Burn hand splints prevent stress on the superficial tendons and ligaments, decreasing edema secondary to the avoidance of dependent positioning. Answer A, decreasing pain and allowing for active range of motion, is not correct because of the immobilizing nature of the static splint. Answers B and C, preventing scarring and skin grafting, are not primary reasons for utilizing burn hand splints upon admission to the intensive care unit. See Reference: Crepeau, Cohn, and Schell (eds). Rivers, EA: Skin system dysfunction: Burns.

153. (B) avoid use of power tools and sharp instruments. Individuals experiencing extrapyramidal syndrome, which may cause muscular rigidity, tremors, and/or sudden muscle spasms, should avoid using power tools or sharp instruments. Photosensitivity, an increased sensitivity to the sun, is another side effect often associated with neuroleptic medications that can be addressed by limiting sun exposure (answer A). Answer C is a strategy that can be used to avoid postural hypotension, a sudden drop in blood pressure resulting in feeling faint, or loss of consciousness when moving from lying or sitting to standing. Dry mouth is a common side effect of many drugs, and can be intensified by the dehydrating effects of caffeinated drinks and alcohol (answer D). Of all the above possible side effects of neuroleptic medications, answer B is most important precaution because it relates to the only side effect the client has experienced. See Reference: Creek (ed). Snowden, K, Molden, G, and Dudley, S: Long-term illness.

154. (A) provide gentle human touch to enable the infant to slowly respond to intervention. Although all answers are possible examples of applied calming techniques, the tactile system is the first to develop, and the most sophisticated, in the young NICU patient. Therefore, answer A is the most suitable for initial interaction contact. Answers B and C could be overstimulating because they involve the auditory and vestibular systems, which are fully operational during the youngest possible gestation viable for life, but are still immature. The visual system is the last to develop. Answer D is an optimal visual strategy for early infancy after 30 weeks' ges-

tation, when the infant's visual sensory system for visual interaction is maturing. See Reference: Case-Smith (ed). Hunter, JG: Neonatal Intensive Care Unit.

155. (D) "Recommend the use of lumbar support and regular performance of home program." The plan section of a discharge summary contains the patient's discharge disposition (e.g., to a nursing home or to outpatient therapy), recommendations for additional therapy or actions on the part of the patient (e.g., outpatient therapy, home health, or performing a home program), equipment needs or equipment provided to the patient, and plans for discharge, answer D. Answer A is a subjective report. Answer B is an example of a statement that belongs in the objective section of a discharge summary. Answer C belongs in the assessment section. See Reference: Borcherding. Documenting different stages of treatment.

156. (C) National Alliance for the Mentally Ill. This is a support group that is open to clients and families and focuses on education and support related to all mental illnesses. Al-Anon (answer A) is a support group for alcohol use among family members. Family therapy (answer B) is not a support group. Recovery, Inc. (answer D) is a self-help support group for clients with mental disorders. See Reference: Cara and MacRae (eds). Roth, S and McCune, CC: The client and family experience of mental illness.

157. (C) divide the laundry into several small loads for carrying. Dividing the laundry into several small loads (answer C) will decrease low back strain, as opposed to one or two large loads (answer D). Folding laundry from a basket on the floor next to the chair (answer A) would require bending and twisting, two movements that people with low back pain should avoid. Pain should be avoided when possible (answer B), and therefore preventive strategies should be urged to help the person avoid getting to the point of severe pain. See Reference: Pedretti and Early (eds). Smithline, J and Dunlop, LE: Low back pain.

158. (C) Word prediction software. Word prediction software anticipates the word desired and increases the speed of input by decreasing the number of keystrokes required. A larger monitor (answer A) may be useful when a child has difficulty seeing a screen or details on the screen. Voice output systems (answer B), which read text and provide cues, can be useful for children with autism, learning disabilities, cognitive delays and visual impairments. Masking inappropriate keys (answer D) reduces the number of options, and can help children who have difficulty finding the correct key. See Reference: Cook and Hussey. Augmentative and alternative communication systems.

159. (B) Raise the toilet. The minimum doorway width that allows a standard wheelchair to pass through easily is 32 inches. A standard toilet is 15 inches, which is 3 inches lower than the standard wheelchair seat. Raising the toilet to 18 inches would make transfers easier for this individual.

See Reference: Crepeau, Cohn, and Schell (eds). Holm, MB, Rogers, JC, and Stone, RG: Person-task-environment interventions: A decision-making guide.

160. (C) Can the child's feet reach the floor? A relaxed position during toilet use is essential to success in elimination training. The seat should be low enough so the child's feet can be used to help with postural stability. In addition, a seat design featuring a wide base, back support, and placement at a height that enables the child to place their feet firmly on the ground or on foot supports, will give the child a sense of comfort and security. Answers A, B, and D describe other useful considerations that should be addressed after the issue of support has been resolved. See Reference: Case-Smith (ed). Shepherd, J: Self-care and adaptations for independent living.

161. (B) An individual who cannot bear weight on the lower extremities. When an individual requires assistance due to decreased strength or balance, the sliding board is an appropriate device to include during transfer training. Answers A and C, the inability to follow commands and fatigue, are issues unrelated to the use of a sliding board. Answer D, when the individual is strong enough or demonstrates sufficient balance to perform a stand pivot transfer, a sliding board would not be indicated. See Reference: Pedretti and Early (eds). Creel, TA, Adler, C, and Tipton-Burton, M, and Lillie, SM: Mobility.

162. (C) use a diary to record each dosage after it is taken. Using a diary to record each dosage (answer C) would be most effective because it would provide the patient with a written record of when the medication was taken. Answer A, establishing a routine, and answer B, keeping the medications in a special location, could be helpful in reminding the patient to take the medication, but would not be as effective as a diary for remembering whether the medications were taken. Answer D, arranging to have a caregiver remind the patient, would not facilitate independence to medication management. See Reference: Early. Activities of daily living.

163. (A) Replace the spoon with a blunt-ended fork. For a child with incoordination and tremors, stabbing food with a blunt-ended fork is often more effective for feeding than using a spoon (answer A.) The food will not fall off the fork, and the blunt tines will prevent any injury to the child. Building up the spoon handle (answer B) is more appropriate for a child with a weak grasp. A swivel spoon (answer C), and bending the handle 45 degrees (answer D), are more appropriate for a child with limited forearm and wrist motion. See Reference: Case-Smith (ed). Case-Smith, J and Humphry, R: Feeding and oral motor skills.

164. (B) sip and puff switch. A sip and puff switch allows control through respiration (i.e., blowing air into and sucking air out of a straw positioned in front of the mouth activates the switch). This method would be particularly appropriate for a client with no functional movements. Answers A and C, joysticks and single digital switches, require mechanical activation through movement of some part of the body (e.g., hand, foot, head, chin). Mouth sticks, answer D, are usually used for direct access on keyboards or on environmental control unit (ECU) control panels. See Reference: Christiansen and Matuska (eds). Garber, SL and Gregorio-Torres, TL: Adaptive strategies following spinal cord injury.

165. (B) verbal and gestural cues only. The next least intrusive level of cues consists of the combination of verbal and gestural cues (answer B). Physical cues (answers C and D) are the most intrusive, and only verbal cues (answer A) are the least intrusive. See Reference: Case-Smith (ed). Shepherd, J: Self-care and adaptations for independent living.

166. (C) slight anterior tilt. According to Dudgeon and Deitz, "pelvic positioning with slight anterior tilt helps to distribute tissue pressure throughout the buttock and thigh...and for some individuals, this position inhibits abnormal reflexive responses" (p. 374). Answers A, B, and D would not be conducive to maximal postural positioning. See Reference: Trombly and Radomski. Dudgeon, B and Deitz, J: Wheelchair selection.

167. (D) Continuous reinforcement of correct responses. Continuous reinforcement is helpful with training of new behaviors and should be provided every time the correct behavior occurs. Intermittent reinforcement (answer A) and fixed interval reinforcement (answers B and C) are best for maintaining behaviors. See Reference: Bruce and Borg. Behavioral frame of reference—objective perspective.

168. (D) picking up raisins with pair of tweezers. While all answers describe methods to promote some aspect of handwriting skills, this activity is the only one that targets isolated finger use. Drawing on sandpaper (answer A) can be used to increase kinesthetic awareness and finger strength. Copying shapes (answer B) is primarily a perceptual motor task. Rolling out "Play Doh" (answer C) is an activity that can promote bilateral hand use and the development of palmar arches. See Reference: Case-Smith (ed). Amundsen, SJ and Weil, M: Pre-writing and hand-writing skills.

169. (B) to routinely inspect the skin closely for signs of skin breakdown. Teaching a patient with a residual limb to compensate for the lack of sensation with visual inspection is essential to prevent injury from skin breakdown. Answer A is incorrect because tapping, rubbing, and application of textures are used when a residual limb is hypersensitive. Answer C, deep massage, is a technique used to loosen and prevent scar adhesions. Answer D, teaching procedures of skin hygiene, is important, but would not, by itself, prevent skin breakdown, which is the primary concern when the residual limb lacks sensation. See Reference: Pedretti and Early (eds). Keenan, DD and Rock, LM: Upper extremity amputations.

170. (C) supervision. At this level, the child performs the task on his own, but cannot be safely left alone, or he may need verbal cueing or physical prompts for 1% to 24% of the task. At the independent level (answer A), the child performs the complete task, including the set-up. At the independent with setup level (answer B), the child performs the task after someone sets it up. Minimal assist (answer D) signifies that the child performs 50% to 75% of the task independently, but needs physical assistance, or other cueing, for the remainder of the task. See Reference: Case-Smith (ed). Shepherd, J: Self-care and adaptations for independent living.

171. (A) isometric exercises. Isometric exercises involve contracting the muscles without joint movement or a change in muscle length. Isotonic exercises (answer B) shorten muscle length, which results in joint movement. Progressive resistive exercises (answer C) are a type of isotonic exercise in which resistance is increased during exercise repetitions. With the arm immobilized, the individual would be unable to perform isotonic exercises. Passive exercises (answer D) are performed by an outside force. Passive range of motion (PROM) exercise, for instance, results in joint motion, but does not involve any active muscle contraction. Passive exercises could not be performed by an individual whose joint is immobilized. See Reference: Pedretti and Early (eds). Breines, EB: Therapeutic occupations and modalities.

172. (D) perform slow push-ups against the wall. Having the child perform push-ups against the wall (answer D) is an activity which provides joint compression of the upper extremities with motor activity—a combination which will have a normalizing effect on the nervous system. Answers A and C are not correct because they emphasize additional tactile input. Answer B is not correct because it emphasizes slow vestibular input. See Reference: Kramer and Hinojosa (eds). Kimball, JG: Sensory integration frame of reference: Theoretical base, function/dysfunction continua, and guide to evaluation.

173. (C) Swing-away footrests and removable armrests. After swinging away footrests and removing armrests, the individual can perform a sliding board transfer without being blocked by the wheelchair. Answers A and B include nothing that would facilitate a sliding board transfer. One-arm drive (answer A) is useful for individuals with the use of only one upper extremity. A low backrest (answer A) is useful for those who require minimal trunk support, because it allows greater freedom of movement for the arms and shoulders. A reclining backrest (answer B) benefits individuals who are unable to sit upright for prolonged periods of time, or who need to recline for weight shifts. Elevating footrests (answer D) are desirable for individuals with lower extremity edema. Answer D is incorrect because although removable armrests may make transfers easier, elevating footrests would not. A footrest would need to be a detachable or swing-away type for it to be moved out of the way. See Reference: Pedretti and Early (eds). Creel, TA, Adler, C, Tipton-Burton, M, and Lillie, SM: Mobility.

174. (B) providing a method for guided self-assessment. Guided self-assessment of each individual's stressors and stress reactions is the first step in designing a stress management program. Time management techniques (answer A), which help individuals schedule, prioritize, and develop appropriate attitudes about daily task requirements, may comprise one of the following sessions. Aerobic exercise (answer C) is an appropriate method for reducing stress in individuals with MS, but care should be taken in designing a program that will not lead to overheating. Progressive relaxation exercises (answer D) involve systematic tensing and relaxing of muscles, and are not appropriate for individuals with hypertension, cardiac disease, upper motor neuron lesions, or spasticity. See Reference: Crepeau, Cohn, and Schell (eds). Giles, GM: Interventions to improve personal skills and abilities Section VIII: Stress management.

175. (B) Cooperative partnership between two disciplines. According to Case-Smith: "In consultation, the therapist and teacher (or other professional) form a cooperative partnership and engage in a reciprocal, problem solving process" (p. 769)(answer B). Answer A, following up within the home environment, would typically be carried out via a home care OT practitioner, while answers C and D would not be conducive to the school-based consultative process. See Reference: Case-Smith (ed). Case-Smith, J, Rogers, J. and Johnson, J.H.: School-based occupational therapy.

176. (A) Stocking the shelves at a local grocery. OT interventions for the transition from school to adult life should focus on real-life functional activities in actual work settings. Working in a natural setting affords students opportunities to develop skills necessary for success in community jobs. Working in a sheltered workshop or in their own school environment does not provide real-life settings for job training. Reading help wanted ads and role playing interviews (answer D) are not considered vocational training. See Reference: Case-Smith (ed). Spencer, K: Transition services: From school to adult life.

177. (D) Group meeting in formats such as community forum or focus groups. Each method of data gathering has both advantages and disadvantages; however, answer D, group meeting formats such as community forum or focus groups, holds the greatest potential for gaining the opinions of a number of people in the targeted population. Answer A, reviewing of records about the target population, may provide useful information about diagnoses and types of disabilities, but nothing about groups members' perceived needs. Answer B, written questionnaires, will get input from the population, but takes time and may result in low return rates and therefore not be as representative as desired. Answer C, individual interviews, could provide useful information, but also could be too time consuming in terms of both giving the interviews and analyzing the data. See Reference: Scaffa, ME (ed). Brownson, CA: Program development for community health: planning, implementation, and evaluation strategies.

178. (A) repetition, high force, and awkward joint postures. Repetition, high force, and awkward joint postures are work-related risk factors that are frequently associated with cumulative trauma disorders. Answer B, progressive resistive exercises, joint mobilization, and weight bearing, are interventions OT practitioners may use with a variety of conditions. Answers C and D, inflammation, swelling, pain, fatigue, cramps, and paresthesias, are all considered to be potential symptoms of cumulative trauma disorders, not factors that contribute to the condition. See Reference: Pedretti and Early (eds).

Kasch, MC and Nickerson, E: Hand and upper extremity injuries.

179. (C) Attempt to provide meaningful activities that will engage attention. Answer C, providing activities, is the best approach because activities can help people with hallucinations to "...divert attention from their symptoms" (p. 157). Answer A, leaving people experiencing hallucinations alone would have no benefit in reducing attention to the hallucination. Answer B, completely isolating the person from others, is not recommended because interpersonal contact can be beneficial for reinforcing reality and reducing hallucinations. Answer D, moving the person to a more stimulating environment, can have the effect of increasing hallucinations if they find the environmental stimuli too stressful. See Reference: Cara and MacRae (eds). MacRae, A: Schizophrenia.

180. (C) produce a flyer identifying risk factors for cumulative trauma disorders. Cumulative trauma disorders are viewed as a mechanism of injury for tendonitis, nerve compression syndromes, and myofascial pain. Associated risk factors include repetition, high force, awkward joint posture, direct pressure, vibration, and prolonged static positioning. Answer A, osteoarthritis disorders, frequently present with stiffness, redness, and edema, and are not caused by cumulative trauma. Answer B, peripheral vascular disease, is unrelated to the diagnoses mentioned in the question and is more commonly associated with the vascularity of the client. A neuroma (answer D) is specifically related to an amputation, nerve injury or suture. See Reference: Pedretti and Early (eds). Kasch, MC and Nickerson, E: Hand and upper extremity injuries.

181. (B) fall prevention. All of the answers are important to the quality of life and independence for individuals living in an ALF. However, falls are the leading cause of accidental death in people over 65 and are a major reason for nursing home placement. See Reference: Bonder and Wagner (eds). Tideiksaar, R: Falls.

182. (B) educate employees about ergonomic adaptations including correct typing techniques, posture, hand positioning, and equipment modification. Educating employees on correct positioning and equipment modification would be an effective way to introduce this population to a change in task methods related to keyboarding which may prevent CTD. Answers A, C, and D are incorrect because they represent interventions that might occur at some point following the onset of CTD. See Reference: Pedretti and Early (eds). Kasch, MC and Nickerson, E: Hand and upper extremity injuries.

183. (C) environmental modification. Environmental modification is the area of intervention that can best assist in maintaining safety and supporting function at home by providing the physical and sensory environments to compensate for deficits. Strength and endurance activities (answer A) will have no direct effect on safety in the home. Cognitive rehabilitation techniques (answer B) are not indicated for conditions with progressive cognitive deterioration. Use of assertiveness skills (answer D) would be inappropriate for dealing with the kinds of communication problems encountered with persons who have Alzheimer's disease. See Reference: Pedretti and Early (eds). Glogoski, C: Alzheimer's disease.

184. (C) Provide a screen to reduce peripheral visual stimuli. Although all the answers given describe techniques that could assist the student, the use of a screen is most appropriate in a mainstream classroom, because the other methods or adaptations (answers A, B, and D) could have a negative impact on the other childrens' ability to learn. See Reference: Case-Smith (ed). Schneck, CM: Visual perception.

185. (A) Pain management techniques. Work hardening programs focus on returning individuals to work in physically appropriate settings, as quickly as is feasible, through reconditioning. As part of that program, pain management techniques (answer A) are included to assist the person with managing and coping with pain during work-related activities. A work hardening program would teach proper body mechanics to prevent further injury rather than focus on energy conservation (answer C), which is emphasized with individuals who need to minimize or avoid fatigue. Vocational counseling (answer D) helps individuals enhance their vocational potential and addresses skills necessary for job seeking and job acquisition. While balancing work and leisure (answer B) is important for maintaining overall health, it is not the emphasis of a work-hardening program. See Reference: Pedretti and Early (eds). Burt, CM: Work evaluation and work hardening.

186. (A) Work environment, structure of work tasks, rules, and supervision. Answer A, assessment of the work environment, tasks and supervision, would be key to making recommendations concerning accommodations for those with psychiatric problems, such as ways to "eliminate distraction, provide frequent supervision, flexible work hours and breaks, etc." (p. 308). Assessment of the architectural barriers would be irrelevant unless the population had physical disabilities as well. Answers C and D, assessment of work aptitudes, interests, and capacities of the individuals, would be relevant for placement recommendations of individuals, but not accommodation recommendations for the worksite regarding the population. See Reference: Scaffa, ME (ed). Scheinholz, MK: Community-based mental health services.

187. (B) is medically necessary. Medicare defines medical necessity as "that which can withstand repeated use, is primarily and customarily used to serve a medical purpose, and is generally not useful to a person in the absence of illness or injury" (p. 394). Medicare part B does not typically cover items such as elevated toilet seats, grab bars, or adaptive equipment because they are not considered to be medically necessary. Answers A, C, and D may all be a part of the broader statement of medical necessity not pertaining to Medicare part B. See Reference: McCormack, Jaffe, and Goodman-Lavey (eds). Thomas, VJ: Reimbursement.

188. (D) is no longer homebound. In order to receive home care services, "the service recipient must be confined to home, a condition referred to as homebound...the patient may not be bedridden, but leaving the residence must require a considerable or taxing effort" (p. 22). Most insurance carriers cover home care only when the individual is unable to leave his or her residence without assistance. After the individual is able to leave the residence, the individual cannot continue to receive home care services (answer A) and would be referred to outpatient services. Without knowing the individual's specific goals, it is not possible to say whether she has achieved them (answers B and C). See Reference: Piersol and Ehrlich (eds). Zahoransky, M: The system and its players.

189. (D) call 911. The OT practitioner should be knowledgeable about situations that may be potentially dangerous for patients. This question requires that the practitioner be knowledgeable about the appropriate ranges for heart rate and blood pressure. Both of the measures are above safe ranges and indicate that the patient is medically unstable. Therefore, immediate medical services would be necessary. Answers A, B, and C do not recognize the seriousness of the situation and could delay the necessary medical attention. See Reference: Crepeau, Cohn, and Schell (eds). Doherty, RF: Cardiopulmonary dysfunction in adults.

190. (D) the title of the job, employer's expectations, how much productivity is expected, and how the employee's performance will be measured. Job descriptions usually contain the title of the job, the employer's expectations, how much productivity is expected, and how the employee's performance will be measured. Items that are not required but may complement an individualized job description are personality characteristics, past experience requirements, and accomplishments. Previously established mutual goals, quality of patient care, achievement of predicted outcomes, and evidence of relationship building (answer A) are components of a performance review. Answers B and C include items such as references and accomplishments of the candidate that are not typically found in a job description, but are more appropriately located on a resume. See Reference: McCormack, Jaffe and Goodman-Lavey (Eds). MacDonell, CM: Personnel management: measuring performance, creating success.

191. (D) sheltered workshops. Sheltered workshops are designed to help individuals master basic work skills. Working with supported employment or in a fast food setting with a job coach (answers B and C) are similar in that they incorporate actual job sites for developing work skills. Adult activity centers (answer A) focus on work-related and leisure activities. See Reference: Early. Work, homemaking, and child care.

192. (A) selected tasks in which aides have been trained, with close supervision. To maximize efficiency and cost-effectiveness of therapy services, there has been an increased use of OT aides. Such aides must be very closely supervised, and are expected to receive site specific training in selected activities determined by the supervising OT practitioner, and must be utilized in accordance with state regulations. Activities and levels of supervision in answers B, C, and D are all beyond the scope of the OT aide. See Reference: Crepeau, Cohn, and Schell (eds). Cohn, ES: Interdisciplinary Communication and Supervision of Personnel.

193. (B) fidelity. Fidelity is defined as remaining faithful to the patient's best interest. This includes statements regarding the confidentiality of patient information. Answer A, informed consent, is in reference to the rights of individuals to be provided information regarding their health care as well as to make choices about their own health care. Answer C, beneficence, is the concept of striving to bring about the best possible outcome for patients served through treatment modalities. Answer D, nonmaleficence, is defined as "the obligation to avoid doing harm to another or to avoid creating a circumstance in which harm could occur to another" (p. 954). See Reference: Crepeau, Cohn, and Schell (eds). Hansen, RA: Ethics in occupational therapy.

194. (C) A COTA contributes to the process, but does not complete the task independently. The COTA participates in this process by providing factual information to the OTR and collaboratively identifying discharge needs (answer C). However, because of the analytical nature of provision of discharge recommendations, the COTA does not complete this activity independently. Answers A and B are incorrect because they do not take into account the analytical nature of the task. Answer D is incorrect because it does not allow for the input of data from the COTA. See Reference: AOTA: Guidelines for supervision, roles, and responsibilities during the delivery of occupational therapy services.

195. (D) order only the lightweight wheelchair and hospital bed. Medicare defines medical necessity as "that which can withstand repeated use, is primarily and customarily used to serve a medical purpose, and is generally not useful to a person in the absence of illness or injury" (p. 394). Answers B and C are incorrect because they include items that are not considered "durable medical equipment" (e.g., reachers, a shower chair, or a hand-held shower). Depending on the patient's medical condition, a bedside commode may be covered. The family may have the option of paying for non-qualifying items out-of-pocket (answer A) if they choose to. See Reference: McCormack, Jaffe, and Goodman-Lavey (Eds). Thomas, VJ: Reimbursement.

196. (B) Sterilize it before using it again. OSHA has set out strategies to protect individuals from potential exposure to HIV and hepatitis B virus. This situation would be an example of an engineering control. These controls are to modify the work environment to reduce risk of exposure. Other examples are using sharps containers, eyewash stations, and biohazard waste containers. Answers A, C, and D would not meet guidelines set forth by OSHA regarding equipment that has come into contact with open wounds. See Reference: Pedretti and Early (eds). Buckner, WS: Infection control and safety issues in the clinic.

197. (A) Community newsletter. Community newsletters are examples of external marketing, commonly used to educate consumers about OT. Answers B, C, and D are all examples of internal marketing strategies. See Reference: Jacobs and Logigian (eds). Jacobs, K: Marketing occupational therapy services.

198. (D) A patient with the diagnosis of a CVA and left neglect caught his left arm in the wheel of the wheelchair, resulting in a cut and bruise. An incident report should be completed whenever a situation occurs that is harmful to the patient or practitioner. This includes, but is not limited to, falls, burns, cuts, and contact with hazardous materials. While the information in answers A, B, and C is worthy of report in the appropriate form of documentation, only answer D would result in an incident report. See Reference: AOTA: Enforcement procedures for occupational therapy code of ethics.

199. (C) Interpret the results based on data collected by the COTA. Once the OTR has assigned performance of an evaluation to a COTA, the OTR is responsible for analyzing and interpreting the results. Service competency (answer A) would need to be established prior to the COTA administering the evaluation. Collecting data (answer B) is the responsibility of the COTA in this scenario. Developing the treatment plan (answer D) would follow analysis of the data. See Reference: AOTA: Guidelines for super-

vision, roles, and responsibilities during the delivery of occupational therapy services.

200. (D) Cost-benefit analysis. "Program managers...need to be intimately aware of the resources necessary for various programs and the financial implications of providing these resources. Cost-benefit analysis must be done, including projected revenues" (p. 900). Outcomes measurements (answer A) are taken at the completion of service intervention and are used to evaluate the effectiveness of the intervention. Utilization reviews (answer B) assess the care that is provided to ensure that services were appropriate and not overutilized or underutilized. Program evaluation (answer C) is a method used to determine how well the program's goals have been achieved. See Reference: Crepeau, Cohn, and Schell (eds). Perinchief, JM: Documentation and management of occupational therapy services.

Simulation Examination 2

■ EVALUATION

1. An OT practitioner has received an order to evaluate an individual who is 2 days post total hip arthroplasty, and expected to be discharged to home in 2 days. The most important areas to focus on are:
    A. cognitive and perceptual functioning.
    B. work, self-care, and leisure performance.
    C. upper and lower extremity strength, ROM, and coordination.
    D. the need for adaptive equipment and assistance from others.

2. In assessing the dressing skills of a 5-year-old child, the OT observes that the child is able to put on a jacket, zip the zipper, and tie a knot in the draw string, but needs verbal cueing to tie a bow. The OT would MOST likely determine that the child's dressing skills are:
    A. age appropriate.
    B. delayed.
    C. advanced.
    D. limited.

3. An OT practitioner is performing a home management evaluation of an ambulatory individual with cerebral palsy who is cognitively intact, but exhibits an ataxic gait pattern. The PRIMARY focus of the evaluation should be:
    A. safety and stability.
    B. the individual's ability to reach and bend.
    C. whether the individual has adequate strength to perform homemaking tasks.
    D. fatigue and endurance levels.

4. An OT practitioner is assessing a school age child with cerebral palsy who absolutely refuses to cooperate with the initial evaluation. What should the OT do NEXT?
    A. Continue to gently coerce the child into completing the assessment.
    B. Switch assessment tools and encourage the child to partake in the Canadian Occupational Performance Measure.
    C. End the session and initiate a phone interview with the child's parents and teacher.
    D. Explain to the child that he will miss recess due to the inability to cooperate with therapy.

5. Which of the following methods is BEST for evaluating a hook grasp?
    A. Direct the individual to hold a sewing needle while it is being threaded.
    B. Observe the individual lift a tall glass half filled with water.
    C. Have the individual hold a heavy handbag by the handles.
    D. Hand the individual a key to place in a lock.

6. While standing and holding onto furniture, a 3-year-old boy with delayed motor development shifts his weight onto one leg and steps to the side with the other. This movement pattern is BEST described as:
    A. creeping.
    B. walking.
    C. cruising.
    D. clawing.

7. An OT practitioner is evaluating the sensation of an individual who recently sustained a cerebrovascular accident (CVA) and has adapted the method of response to include nodding and pointing to a card with a picture of the correct answer. This method of response would be MOST appropriate for an individual who has:
    A. expressive aphasia.
    B. receptive aphasia.
    C. agnosia.
    D. ataxia.

8. An OT practitioner is observing an individual who has had a stroke and notes that the person seems unable to correctly position slices of cheese and ham onto bread or to then place another piece of bread on top to assemble a sandwich. This behavior would MOST likely be reported as:

   A. constructional apraxia.
   B. ideomotor apraxia.
   C. visual agnosia.
   D. unilateral neglect.

9. An OT practitioner is assessing an individual with dysphagia. Which of the following should the OT address FIRST?

   A. Jaw pain and tooth grinding habits
   B. Cranial nerve function
   C. Mental status, oral structures, and motor control of head
   D. Muscle length control via finger-to-nose tests

10. When performing a "naturalistic observation" of dressing skills with a young child diagnosed with developmental delay, an OT practitioner should FIRST:

   A. provide oversized clothing to ensure success.
   B. have the child dress and undress in a distraction-free corner of the clinic.
   C. provide assistance as needed to minimize frustration.
   D. observe the child entering the clinic and taking off his coat and shoes.

11. Many individuals who participate in outpatient cardiac rehabilitation programs take beta blockers. The best method for evaluating tolerance for exercise with these individuals is to:

   A. perform isometric testing.
   B. use a perceived exertion scale.
   C. monitor heart rate and blood pressure.
   D. calculate maximum age-adjusted heart rate (MAHR).

12. An individual with mental illness wants to travel to the library independently, but keeps getting lost. Which of the following actions should the OT practitioner take FIRST in the evaluation process?

   A. Take the individual to the library and obtain a library card.
   B. Assess the individual's ability to read.
   C. Identify the bus that goes to the library and obtain a bus schedule.
   D. Assess the individual's topographical orientation skills.

13. The OT practitioner is observing dressing skills in an individual with COPD. While putting on his shirt, the individual becomes short of breath and stops to rest before finishing with the shirt and going on to his trousers. This behavior MOST likely indicates a deficit in:

   A. postural control.
   B. muscle tone.
   C. strength.
   D. endurance.

14. Which of the following assessment methods would an OT practitioner MOST likely choose in order to learn about a family's values and priorities?

   A. Interview
   B. Skilled observation
   C. Inventory
   D. Standardized test

15. Evaluation results for a person with arthritis will MOST accurately reflect true functional abilities if scheduled:

   A. early morning (8 to 10 a.m.).
   B. afternoon.
   C. late morning (10 to 11 a.m.).
   D. early morning and again in the afternoon.

16. A child running in the playground trips and falls forward, landing on outstretched arms. This behavior is BEST described as a(n):

   A. primitive reflex.
   B. righting reaction.
   C. equilibrium reaction.
   D. protective extension response.

17. In order to screen an individual referred for a work-hardening program, the OT practitioner needs to locate background information about the individual's work history. The BEST method for obtaining detailed information about the individual's job requirements is to:

   A. interview the individual.
   B. examine the results of an analysis of the individual's job.
   C. look up the individual's job in the Dictionary of Occupational Titles.
   D. request information from the referring physician.

18. A teenager is hospitalized with anorexia nervosa. When collecting data on the individual's life history, values, and self-confidence level, the OT practitioner will MOST likely obtain this information through a(n):

A. overall physical assessment.
B. occupational performance history interview.
C. activity configuration.
D. psychoeducational session.

19. An individual requires 40% to 50% assistance from the OT to transfer from his wheelchair to a sliding board and to lift his legs from the wheelchair into and out of a bathtub. According to Functional Independence Measure (FIM) Levels, the individual will require which level of assistance to complete the transfer?

A. Total assistance
B. Minimal assistance
C. Moderate assistance
D. Maximal assistance

20. The primary evaluation skill used by an OT practitioner who is evaluating a severely developmentally disabled adult is:

A. administering standardized cognitive assessments.
B. observing and interpreting patterns of behavior.
C. classifying levels of disability.
D. administering functional performance tests.

21. An OT practitioner is performing an environmental assessment to determine accessibility for an individual who will be returning home. The FIRST step in this process is to:

A. identify the barriers to movement and function in the home environment.
B. identify and analyze the tasks and occupations that the individual will be performing in the home.
C. identify the aspects of the environment that support movement and function in the home.
D. determine the social environment of the individual.

22. A 4-month-old infant being seen for an OT assessment shows a strong preference for the left hand when reaching for a rattle at midline. Considering the development of dominance in normal children, the OT practitioner is MOST likely to conclude that:

A. further observation and evaluation of right-sided dysfunction is indicated.
B. development of hand dominance is proceeding in a typical manner.
C. hand dominance will not develop until the child is 1 year old.
D. unilaterality precedes bilaterality in typical development.

23. An individual who had a stroke is copying a picture of a clock. The drawing appears as a lopsided circle with a flat side on the left. The numbers one through eight are written in numerical order around the right side of the clock. The hands are correctly drawn on the clock to represent three o'clock. The individual's performance appears to demonstrate:

A. right hemianopsia.
B. left unilateral neglect.
C. cataracts in the left eye.
D. bitemporal hemianopia.

24. An OT practitioner measures an individual's elbow PROM three times, and gets three different measurements, varying by up to 10 degrees. The BEST action for the therapist to take is to:

A. check the alignment of the goniometer.
B. use a larger goniometer.
C. use a smaller goniometer.
D. attempt to force the individual's arm further into flexion.

25. The OT practitioner is making recommendations to a community living site for a 13-year-old child who has mental retardation. Which of the following statements most accurately describes the functional ability of this child who is in the moderate (trainable) range of intellectual ability?

A. The client requires nursing care for basic survival skills.
B. The client can usually handle routine daily functions.
C. The client requires supervision to accomplish most tasks.
D. The client is able to learn academic skills at the third to seventh grade level.

26. During a perceptual evaluation, an OT practitioner determines that an individual exhibits constructional apraxia, body scheme disturbances, and unilateral neglect. During the functional part of the evaluation, these deficits are MOST likely to be exhibited as self-care difficulties related to:

    A. spatial relations.

    B. dressing apraxia.

    C. anosognosia.

    D. figure-ground discrimination.

27. An individual diagnosed with substance abuse exhibits difficulty gluing two pieces of a birdhouse together, becomes increasingly agitated, and finally storms out of the room to get a cigarette. This behavior would provide most information about the person's:

    A. eye-hand coordination.

    B. stress management.

    C. visual perception.

    D. fine motor skills.

28. When working with a child who exhibits tactile defensiveness, which of the following areas should be evaluated FIRST?

    A. Reading skills

    B. Dressing habits

    C. Social skills

    D. Leisure interests

29. An adolescent with a history of shoplifting and gang violence has been hospitalized with a diagnosis of conduct disorder. During a task group, the OT practitioner should carefully observe the individual's:

    A. perceptual-motor performance.

    B. leisure and vocational interests.

    C. attention span and social interaction skills.

    D. interest in and ability to perform multiple roles.

30. A homecare OT is evaluating a child with autism. Which of the following environmental factors might interfere with the child's performance in the home?

    A. How the child's affect and use of language is used within the home setting

    B. How the child reacts to the OT upon arrival to the home

    C. Cluttered spaces in the rooms with apparent limited access to toys

    D. Observation of the child experiencing difficulties while riding his bike outside

31. A supermarket employee with obsessive-compulsive disorder takes an hour to stock 24 soup cans on the shelf because once he has placed the cans on the shelf, he removes them and starts over because "all the labels were not lined up exactly in the same direction." Which of the following methods would MOST effectively evaluate this individual's work performance?

    A. Functional assessment of work-related skills, such as carrying and opening cartons and shelving items

    B. Cognitive assessment using the Allen's Cognitive Levels evaluation

    C. Verbal interview focusing on the requirements of the individual's job

    D. Task evaluation using a "clean" medium like a puzzle

32. An OT is assessing process performance skills in a 10-year-old child with a pervasive developmental disorder. The OTR would MOST likely attempt to determine if the child can do which of the following:

    A. demonstrate appropriate use of sandpaper and hammer while constructing a birdhouse.

    B. engage in an activity without demonstrating self-stimulation behaviors.

    C. consistently place a backpack in a designated cubby when entering the classroom.

    D. perform in the role of "student" within the classroom setting.

33. An OT practitioner is evaluating two-point discrimination in an individual with a median nerve injury. The MOST appropriate procedure is to:

    A. apply the stimuli beginning at the little finger and progress toward the thumb.

    B. test the thumb area first, then progress toward the little finger.

    C. present test stimuli in an organized pattern to improve reliability during retesting.

    D. allow the individual unlimited time to respond.

34. An OT practitioner is preparing to evaluate a preschool child who has upper extremity orthopedic issues. The OT will MOST likely obtain the majority of informal assessment data through:

    A. measurement tools that assess overall hand function.

    B. dynamometer and pinch meter function.

    C. observation of play and upper extremity/hand function.

    D. functional independence measures.

35. A newly referred patient complains of frequently dropping lightweight items and reports a numb feeling in both hands. Which of the following instruments is MOST important for evaluating this individual?
- A. Goniometer
- B. Dynamometer
- C. Pinch meter
- D. Aesthesiometer

36. When measuring elbow range of motion with a goniometer, the axis of the goniometer must be positioned:
- A. at the lateral epicondyle of the humerus.
- B. at the medial epicondyle of the humerus.
- C. parallel to the longitudinal axis of the humerus on the lateral aspect.
- D. parallel to the longitudinal axis of the radius on the lateral aspect.

37. The OT practitioner working with an infant observes the presence of the first stage of voluntary grasp. Which of the following would be the MOST appropriate statement for documenting this behavior?
- A. The infant is exhibiting radial palmar grasp.
- B. The infant is exhibiting pincer grasp.
- C. The infant is exhibiting ulnar palmar grasp.
- D. The infant is exhibiting palmar grasp.

38. An individual demonstrates the ability to pick up a penny from a flat surface. The OT practitioner would document this as which type of prehension?
- A. Lateral
- B. Palmar
- C. Tip
- D. Spherical

39. An OT practitioner is evaluating an individual diagnosed with early-stage Alzheimer's disease who lives with her husband, though the husband works during the day. Which of the following is the MOST important area to address in the initial evaluation?
- A. Ability to chew and swallow
- B. Kitchen safety
- C. Anger management
- D. Recognition of family members

40. An individual recovering from a peripheral nerve injury demonstrates weakness in thumb opposition. Which of the following instruments most effectively evaluates strength in the affected area?
- A. Aesthesiometer
- B. Pinch dynamometer
- C. Dynamometer
- D. Volumeter

41. An OT practitioner observes a 5-year-old child with Down syndrome and low muscle tone sitting on the floor exclusively using a "W" sitting position. This observation MOST likely indicates that the child is:
- A. developing atypically.
- B. using a noncompensatory position to achieve stability.
- C. demonstrating typical development for a child with Down syndrome.
- D. using a position normal for a younger child, not for a 5-year-old child.

42. During a mealtime feeding evaluation of an individual who has sustained a brain injury, the OT practitioner observes that the client does not attempt to eat, though the food is accessible and he has expressed that he is hungry. The practitioner documents that the individual is MOST likely exhibiting problems with:
- A. attention.
- B. concentration.
- C. initiation.
- D. apraxia.

43. A preschool child with spastic cerebral palsy uses "bunny-hopping" for functional mobility during an OT evaluation. This indicates that a primitive pattern is being used for mobility. Which of the following reflexes is MOST likely being used by the child?
- A. Symmetrical tonic neck reflex
- B. Asymmetrical tonic neck reflex
- C. Tonic labyrinthine reflex
- D. Neck righting reflex

44. A 6-month-old child, when pulled into sitting with several trials, demonstrates a head lag. This movement MOST likely indicates that head control is:
- A. developing in a typical manner.
- B. slightly delayed by 1 month.
- C. significantly delayed by several months.
- D. advanced.

45. An individual who alternately laughs and cries without apparent provocation throughout an evaluation would be identified as exhibiting:

A. mania.
B. emotional lability.
C. paranoia.
D. denial.

46. In using an assessment that is "norm referenced" for children, the OT practitioner assumes that the test:

A. measures normal behavior of children.
B. compares performance with a normative sample.
C. is valid and reliable.
D. should be used with a normal population.

47. The MOST important items to assess when evaluating motor control after a traumatic injury include:

A. developmental factors.
B. muscle tone, postural tone, pain, and coordination.
C. blood pressure, heart rate, endurance, and confusion.
D. self-concept and self-awareness.

48. An OT practitioner is conducting a pre-discharge interview with a patient who has been treated on the psychiatric unit for schizophrenia. The question which the therapist asks, "Are you ready to go home today?" is an example of a(n):

A. open question.
B. closed question.
C. directed or leading question.
D. double question.

49. An individual has been referred to OT following an upper extremity injury resulting in partial paralysis. Which of the following assessments would be MOST important for an OT practitioner guided by a biomechanical frame of reference?

A. Adaptive equipment needs
B. Tone, reflex development, automatic reactions
C. Strength, range of motion, coordination
D. Habits, values, roles

50. An OT practitioner witnesses a seizure in a child with hydrocephalus. The MOST relevant information to document is:

A. the child's positioning during the seizure.
B. objective signs and duration of the seizure.
C. responsiveness during the seizure.
D. facial expression during and after the seizure.

■ INTERVENTION PLANNING

51. An individual has been referred to OT following open heart surgery and a period of prolonged bed rest. After the individual is able to tolerate sitting unsupported at the edge of the bed, the NEXT activity the OT practitioner should introduce is:

A. peeling potatoes while seated.
B. wheelchair propulsion at 1.2 mph.
C. taking a shower.
D. walking at 1 mph.

52. A two-and-a-half-year-old child can locate visually and understand directions about the spatial concept of "in," the NEXT spatial concept to develop would MOST likely be the concept of:

A. behind.
B. first.
C. on.
D. last.

53. A middle-aged individual with a diagnosis of major depressive disorder is admitted to the hospital following an overdose of sleeping pills. What activity would the OT practitioner recommend FIRST to achieve the present goals of increasing his sense of competence and development of enjoyable leisure activities?

A. Pouring and glazing chess pieces
B. Designing and building a doll house
C. Copper tooling using a template
D. Learning how to play bridge

54. The MOST appropriate goal for an individual who sustained a C7-C8 spinal cord injury is to be able to perform wheelchair-to-commode transfers at which of the following levels?

A. Independent with a transfer board
B. Minimal to moderate assistance with a transfer board
C. Dependent in all transfers
D. Assisted, using a stand-pivot transfer

55. An OT is treating a child with autism. To maximize the child's benefit from therapy, the therapist would present activities in a therapeutic environment that:

A. is lively and colorful, facilitating active involvement.
B. provides many options, encouraging decision making.
C. involves many toys and activities, promoting exploratory learning.
D. is highly structured, facilitating step by step learning.

56. After administering an interest checklist, the OT practitioner documents that an individual has identified a few vague, solitary leisure interests. Based on this information, what is the BEST activity to use in the next session of a leisure counseling group?

   A. A leisure inventory assessment

   B. An activity exploring leisure opportunities and problems

   C. An activity which encourages the individual to sign up for social activities

   D. A calendar of community leisure activities for the next few weeks

57. A mother of four who was diagnosed with a right CVA is receiving home care OT services to improve left upper extremity function and sitting and standing balance. The MOST appropriate activity for the OT to recommend would be:

   A. stacking cones.

   B. door pulley.

   C. folding laundry.

   D. throwing a ball.

58. When fabricating a splint for an individual with rheumatoid arthritis, which one of the following is MOST appropriate for the purpose of resting the joints, decreasing pain, and preventing contractures?

   A. A protective MP joint splint

   B. A wrist stabilization splint

   C. An ulnar drift positioning splint

   D. A volar pan splint for hand and wrist

59. In the comfortable, but crowded OT clinic of a mental health partial hospitalization program, a client is having difficulty concentrating on problem-solving tasks. Which of the following environmental strategies would be MOST likely to enhance the client's ability to perform the problem-solving tasks in this clinic setting?

   A. Play pleasant background music.

   B. Decrease the intensity of lighting in the clinic.

   C. Allow the person to perform tasks in a quiet, separate area.

   D. Adjust the temperature and ventilation in the clinic.

60. An individual is participating in an assertiveness training group within a psychiatric rehabilitation program. The expected outcome of this intervention is that the individual will MOST likely improve the ability to:

   A. engage in relevant conversations with coworkers.

   B. use appropriate facial expressions when disagreeing with coworkers.

   C. express disagreement with coworkers in a productive manner.

   D. use courteous behavior when disagreeing with coworkers.

61. A child with behavioral problems has difficulty with peer interactions. Which of the following aspects of the treatment plan is MOST important?

   A. Provide activities in an authoritarian environment.

   B. Allow the child the opportunity to develop basic social skills on his own.

   C. Provide enjoyable activities in a safe and accepting environment.

   D. Strictly enforce rules for group play.

62. An OT practitioner is planning to review kitchen activities with an individual who underwent a total hip replacement and is to return home tomorrow. Since the chart says that this person is touch-down weight-bearing (TDWB), how will the weight-bearing restriction impact the way she practices the kitchen activities?

   A. The person should perform all kitchen activities from a sitting position.

   B. Standing kitchen activities can be performed by placing about 50% of the person's body weight on the affected leg.

   C. Standing kitchen activities can be performed by placing the majority of weight through both arms, using toes for balance (about 10% of weight).

   D. The person will be able to perform all standing activities without weight-bearing restriction.

63. An individual has been referred to OT for instruction in stress management techniques prior to discharge the next day. Which of the following methods is MOST appropriate?

   A. Autogenic training

   B. Meditation

   C. Deep breathing and verbalization

   D. Work simplification and energy conservation

64. A child with learning disabilities resulting in low frustration tolerance and poor self-esteem is learning how to tie shoelaces. Which of the following methods would be MOST appropriate for the OT to introduce to this child?

    A. Physical guidance

    B. Verbal cues

    C. Backward chaining

    D. Forward chaining

65. An OT practitioner who works in an outpatient facility recommends that individual's with Parkinson's disease be treated in a therapeutic group. The PRIMARY reason for selecting group treatment is:

    A. it is more effective in preventing motor problems associated with Parkinson's disease.

    B. it provides social interaction and support, as well as activity.

    C. it is an effective way to present therapeutic exercise activities.

    D. it requires less therapist time because the therapist can leave once the group has started.

66. An OT practitioner is working with a client experiencing anxiety who would benefit by having an outlet for emotional turmoil associated with past emotional and physical abuse. The type of activity that would offer the BEST opportunity for expression would be:

    A. meditation and yoga exercises.

    B. journal and diary writing.

    C. personal hygiene and grooming classes.

    D. aerobics and fitness program.

67. An individual with amyotrophic lateral sclerosis is no longer able to ambulate for kitchen or home management activities. Which of the following interventions BEST addresses the goals of independence in meal preparation for this individual?

    A. Meal preparation techniques using a wheelchair

    B. Training in the use of adapted cooking equipment

    C. Simple cooking activities while standing at the counter for gradually increasing amounts of time

    D. Beginning with cold meals and progressing to hot meals

68. An OT practitioner has performed a pre-employment assessment on a person with a history of mental illness to prepare for the client's entry into "supported employment" in a warehouse. Which of the following reflects the MOST important use of the assessment results for the OT and the mental health team?

    A. Anticipating challenges the client may face to plan strategies that will support performance

    B. Determining prevocational OT groups that would be most appropriate for the client

    C. Providing the employer with information about the client's abilities and skills

    D. Helping to predict if the client will be successful in this type of work

69. An OT practitioner is working with an individual following an UE amputation to determine whether a hook terminal device or a functional prosthetic hand would be most appropriate. The individual's primary concern is his ability to return to work and function as a carpenter. The MOST important factor in the therapist's recommendation would be that a:

    A. functional prosthetic hand has a better cosmetic appearance.

    B. hook provides better prehensile function and allows greater visibility of objects.

    C. hook weighs less than a hand.

    D. functional hand is covered by a rubber glove that stains easily.

70. To promote play skills and self-expression in a child who is withdrawn, the OT practitioner should FIRST select activities that:

    A. promote open-ended symbolic play, such as using action figures, puppets, and dolls.

    B. provide a defined structure, such as simple craft activities with instructions.

    C. promote social interaction, such as a game of tag with peers.

    D. provide a means of tension release, such as leather tooling or wedging clay.

71. An OT practitioner is selecting foods for an initial treatment session with an individual with dysphagia. In general, which of the following foods would be MOST appropriate?

    A. Vegetable soup

    B. Salad

    C. Watermelon

    D. Eggs

72. An OT practitioner is selecting treatment activities to use with a young adult diagnosed with schizophrenia that would help to increase her ability to receive, process, and respond to sensory information. The MOST suitable type activities to address this area would include:

A. social skills training.
B. vestibular stimulation and gross motor exercise.
C. life skills.
D. expressive projects.

73. The OT practitioner is selecting activities for a school age child with postural control deficits. Which activity would BEST promote postural control?

A. Sliding down a playground slide
B. Playing "Simon Says"
C. Swimming
D. Playing on a trampoline

74. An OT practitioner is planning treatment for an individual who recently experienced a left CVA resulting in right-sided hemiplegia and motor apraxia. To BEST facilitate the individual's attempts to perform morning ADL, the therapist should plan to:

A. provide the individual with detailed, step-by-step commands for each task throughout the ADL process.
B. make the environment as simple and uncluttered as possible and use sharp contrast to make objects clearly stand out.
C. have the individual visualize the task first and then provide general statements such as "Let's get ready."
D. teach the individual to move slowly through the environment and encourage touching of objects during the task.

75. A child demonstrates aggressive and disruptive behavior in school as a result of a low sensory threshold. Which of the following suggestions would be MOST useful to discuss with the teacher regarding an upcoming class bus trip to the zoo?

A. Review the bus rules with the child and apply consequences consistently.
B. Let the child sit at the front of the bus and use a tape player with earphones.
C. Give the child the responsibility of monitoring classmates as "bus patrol."
D. Let the child set the criteria for a successful trip, and provide a reward if the criteria are met.

76. A physical education teacher is being treated for osteoarthritis of the upper and lower extremities. Using a client-centered approach to prevent further complications, the OT practitioner should recommend:

A. lifting weights three times a week for 1 hour.
B. listening to relaxation tapes three times a week before bedtime.
C. vocational retraining.
D. low-impact aerobics three times a week for 1 hour.

77. A child with poor anticipatory postural control demonstrates inadequate playground skills, losing her balance when trying to anticipate movement. Which of the following activities will BEST promote the development of these skills?

A. Ballet
B. Soccer
C. Basketball
D. Ping-pong

78. An OT practitioner is working on sequencing skills with a young person who has had a TBI. Which of the following is the MOST effective activity to promote development of these skills?

A. Leather stamping using tools in a random design
B. Stringing beads for a necklace, following a pattern
C. Putting together a 20-piece puzzle
D. Playing "Concentration"

79. An OT practitioner is planning a program for an individual who needs to increase shoulder strength, range of motion, and endurance. Which of the following activities is MOST suitable for periodic upgrading?

A. Blowing up and tying balloons of various sizes
B. Playing a game of balloon darts
C. Painting faces on balloons
D. Playing balloon volleyball

80. An OT practitioner receives a consult for an infant in the NICU whose mother has a history of drug abuse during pregnancy. Using a sensory integrative approach, what is the FIRST action the therapist should take?

 A. Determine the mother's current medical status, parental involvement, and support systems.

 B. Recommend a social work referral to address social concerns, provide emotional support and community program information, and make a referral to the Department of Human Services.

 C. Modify the environment to protect the infant from excessive and/or inappropriate sensory stimulation prior to direct intervention.

 D. Assess motor and behavioral skills to identify areas of developmental delay in order to educate family and medical staff of necessary positional and environmental strategies for skill acquisition.

81. The MOST appropriate overall intervention approach that an OT practitioner would use for an individual diagnosed with a severe and progressive form of dementia would focus on:

 A. improving their social skills in relating to others.

 B. creating new habits of time use.

 C. implementing compensatory environmental strategies to maximize safety and function.

 D. facilitating resumption of previous life roles and independence.

82. When providing occupational therapy for children who have been diagnosed with a terminal illness, the PRIMARY focus for OT intervention would be:

 A. educational activities.

 B. play and self-care activities.

 C. socialization activities.

 D. motor activities.

83. Which scar management technique is MOST appropriate to utilize during the rehabilitative phase of treatment with an individual who sustained a partial thickness burn 6 months ago?

 A. Preventing scar development through static splinting

 B. Controlling edema to prevent loss of range of motion

 C. Minimizing scar hypertrophy through compression garments and proper skin care

 D. Promoting self-care skills in order to resume the role of homemaker

84. A preschooler is having difficulty performing tasks requiring eye-hand coordination as a result of poor visual tracking skills. The FIRST activity the OTR uses to promote visual tracking skill is:

 A. tossing and catching a water balloon.

 B. catching and bursting soap bubbles.

 C. throwing and catching a beach ball.

 D. playing softball.

85. An OT practitioner wants to provide functional activities as part of an individual's hand rehabilitation program. Which of the following activities is appropriate?

 A. Active and self range of motion techniques

 B. Crafts, games, and self-care tasks

 C. Cone stacking, pegs, and pulleys

 D. Mild, moderate, and resistive theraband exercises

86. An OT practitioner is working with an individual who was admitted to an inpatient psychiatric program with diagnoses of major depressive disorder and Stage 4 AIDS. The BEST general focus of treatment at this point would be to:

 A. restore and maintain performance of self-chosen occupations that support performance of valued occupational roles.

 B. increase physical endurance and maintain desired self-care tasks.

 C. facilitate resolution of current and anticipated losses through the grieving process.

 D. restore and maintain functional performance of the individual's primary work role.

87. Which of the following will MOST effectively decrease edema in the hand once a wrist fracture has healed?

 A. Contrast baths and retrograde massage

 B. Hot pack applications

 C. Paraffin treatments

 D. Sensory re-education and pendulum exercises

88. An individual with underreactive sensory processing has been referred to OT. Based on a sensory integration frame of reference, activities for this individual should have which of the following facilitory characteristics?

 A. Arrhythmic and unexpected

 B. Arrhythmic and slow

 C. Sustained and slow

 D. Unexpected and rhythmic

89. A flight attendant with a back injury is participating in a work-hardening program. The individual can successfully simulate distributing magazines to all passengers in a plane using proper body mechanics. To upgrade the program gradually, the OT practitioner should NEXT request that the individual simulate:

    A. serving from the beverage cart.

    B. distributing blankets and pillows.

    C. distributing magazines to half of the passengers in the plane.

    D. putting luggage in the overhead compartments.

90. An OT practitioner in the school system is developing transition activities for a group of developmentally disabled 16-year-old students. Which of the following activities would be BEST for addressing goals related to transition?

    A. Role-play ordering food in the classroom.

    B. Go out for lunch at a fast-food restaurant.

    C. Order a takeout lunch by phone.

    D. Select lunch items from a picture menu in the classroom.

91. The goal for providing hand splints to a child with active juvenile rheumatoid arthritis is to:

    A. inhibit hypertonus.

    B. increase range of motion.

    C. prevent deformity.

    D. correct deformity.

92. An OT is working with a child who has mild spastic cerebral palsy. The evaluation has shown that the child has poor in-hand manipulation skills. What type of the following would MOST likely improve the development of this skill?

    A. Grasping blocks to build a building

    B. Placing pegs from one pegboard to another

    C. Carrying a bag of Lego blocks with a handle

    D. Removing a nut from a bolt

■ IMPLEMENTING INTERVENTION

93. A patient diagnosed with Parkinson's disease is being seen by an OT practitioner to develop a routine for performing self-care activities. The OT should instruct the patient that self-care activities:

    A. are more easily performed if coordinated with consistent timing of medications.

    B. should be performed before medications are taken.

    C. should be attempted only with the assistance of others.

    D. should be performed at intervals throughout the day until completed.

94. The OT practitioner is working on handwriting skills with a school-age child with decreased proprioception in the hand and wrist. Which of the following would the OT recommend for writing?

    A. A wide pen

    B. Attach rubber bands to the eraser and the child's wrist.

    C. A soft triangle grip

    D. A pediatric weighted utensil holder

95. An OT practitioner is working with an elderly individual who has diabetes, poor vision, and peripheral neuropathies, resulting in difficulty discriminating between medications. The BEST adaptation for the therapist to provide is:

    A. Braille labels.

    B. labels with white print on a black background.

    C. a pill organizer box.

    D. brightly colored pills with each type of medication a different color.

96. A child with a diagnosis of ADHD also exhibits perceptual deficits. The activity the OT practitioner would MOST likely recommend for this child to train visual attention is:

    A. playing a game of "Memory" where images are matched by memory.

    B. assembling a 200-piece puzzle.

    C. finding "Waldo" against a complex visual background.

    D. blowing cotton balls into a target.

97. An OT practitioner is addressing concerns about sexual activity with a person who has left-sided hemiplegia with spasticity. The BEST recommendation for positioning during sexual intercourse for this person would be:
   A. lying on the left side, propped up with pillows.
   B. lying on the right side, propped up with pillows.
   C. lying in a supine position.
   D. lying in a prone position.

98. The OT practitioner is treating a child with a standard above-elbow amputation who is experiencing hypersensitivity of the residual limb. The therapist would MOST likely perform which of the following interventions in the preprosthetic phase of treatment?
   A. Play activities to strengthen the residual limb
   B. Activities to increase the range of motion of the residual limb
   C. Play activities that incorporate tapping, application of textures, and weight-bearing to the residual limb
   D. Dressing activities for practicing putting on and taking off the UE prosthesis

99. An OT practitioner is assisting an individual with mild hemiparesis in transferring from the wheelchair to a mat table using a stand pivot transfer technique. After locking the brakes, the FIRST verbal cue the OT gives to the individual is:
   A. "stand up."
   B. "scoot forward to the edge of the wheelchair."
   C. "unfasten the wheelchair brakes."
   D. "position the wheelchair so that it directly faces the mat table."

100. A young child has just learned to sit independently on the floor. To facilitate the NEXT step toward refining postural reactions in sitting, the OT should encourage the child to:
   A. Sit straddling a bolster with both feet on the floor.
   B. Maintain sitting balance on a scooter while being pulled.
   C. Ride a "hippity-hop" without falling off.
   D. Maintain floor-sitting position with the therapist providing pelvic support.

101. An individual with left upper extremity flaccidity is observed sitting in a wheelchair with his left arm dangling over the side. The FIRST positioning device the OT should introduce to the individual is a(n):
   A. lap tray.
   B. wheelchair armrest.
   C. arm sling.
   D. arm trough.

102. An OT practitioner is ordering a wheelchair for an individual with progressive MS. The MOST important consideration the practitioner can make is the adaptability of the wheelchair in anticipation of:
   A. gradual gains in strength.
   B. growth of the individual.
   C. further decline.
   D. improved wheelchair mobility.

103. An OT practitioner working in a sheltered workshop with adults with developmental disabilities is preparing for a group of individuals functioning at Allen's Cognitive Level 4. Which of the following is the BEST method for introducing an assembly activity?
   A. Provide repetitive, one-step activities.
   B. Demonstrate a three-step assembly process.
   C. Provide project samples for individuals to duplicate.
   D. Provide written directions for the individuals to follow.

104. The OT is teaching the parents of a child with spastic quadriplegia how to effectively position the child in sitting so that participation in family games can be facilitated. What is the OT MOST likely to recommend?
   A. Make sure the child's head is upright.
   B. Make sure the child's arms are on the armrests.
   C. Make sure the child's back is straight.
   D. Make sure the child's pelvis is secured in seat.

105. An elderly individual who ambulates with a walker in the home states he does not like sponge baths and would like to resume taking showers, but is afraid of falling. Which of the following should the therapist do FIRST?
   A. Suggest bathtub bathing instead of showering.
   B. Encourage the client to purchase a shower chair.
   C. Demonstrate how using a shower chair improves safety.
   D. Explain that therapy will boost his confidence level when showering.

106. An individual who demonstrates compulsive behaviors is unable to complete a cookie baking activity because he spends so much time measuring and remeasuring ingredients. Upon observing this, how should the OT practitioner respond?

    A. Tell him that measuring so many times is unnecessary.

    B. Encourage him to talk about his fears.

    C. Acknowledge that he uses rituals to cope with anxiety.

    D. Discontinue group work and treat him individually.

107. Which of the following is the MOST important adaptation to recommend to an individual returning home following a total hip replacement?

    A. Move items from high cabinets to lower locations.

    B. Obtain a raised toilet seat.

    C. Place high contrast tape at the edge of each step.

    D. Install a handheld shower head.

108. An OT is adapting a chair for a student with extensor tone. Which of the following should the therapist recommend to the teacher in order to inhibit the child's extensor tone, while maintaining a functional seated position in the classroom?

    A. Provide lateral trunk supports to the seat.

    B. Place a seat belt at a 45-degree angle at the hips.

    C. Insert a wedge-shaped seat that is higher in the front.

    D. Install a lapboard.

109. A resident of a long-term care facility is receiving OT because of difficulties with eating. The FIRST step the OT practitioner should perform at mealtime is to:

    A. provide skid-proof placemats, plate guard, and utensils with built-up handles.

    B. observe for swallowing after each bite of food.

    C. instruct the caregivers about a special eating setup for the resident.

    D. position the person in an upright posture, making sure head is flexed slightly and in midline.

110. Several individuals recovering from substance use disorders are about to be discharged from an inpatient psychiatric unit to a variety of community programs. Which of the following areas is MOST important to address in a discharge planning group?

    A. Developing ADL and IADL routines

    B. Learning how to use leisure time

    C. Relapse prevention

    D. Enhancing social participation skills

111. An individual is learning how to perform transfers into a bathtub 2 weeks after a total knee replacement, but is still unable to extend or flex the knee more than 20 degrees. Which of the following would MOST likely allow for safe tub transfers?

    A. Wait another 2 to 4 weeks, because tub transfers are contraindicated until 4 to 6 weeks after surgery.

    B. Use a hand rail attached to the side of the tub.

    C. Use a tub transfer bench and leg lifter.

    D. Use a low kitchen stool with rubber tips.

112. The OT practitioner is attempting to increase playfulness with a 7-year-old girl with sensory integrative dysfunction. The child experiences difficulties with motor tasks and often complains that no one likes her. After establishing rapport with the child, the OT would MOST likely introduce which of the following?

    A. Playing a game of "Go Fish"

    B. Playing a game of checkers

    C. Jumping rope

    D. Role playing a tea party with "Barbie" dolls

113. Which of the following is the MOST effective way for an OT practitioner to structure the intervention environment for a patient who exhibits seductive or sexual acting out behavior?

    A. Provide a stimulating environment that offers options for engagement in real life activities.

    B. Provide a large area of personal space, where the person is protected from physical contact with others.

    C. Provide a quiet, relaxed environment, but not isolated from other people.

    D. Provide an environment where all possible distractions have been removed or reduced.

114. The OT practitioner is instructing an individual with COPD in energy conservation techniques. Which of the following should the practitioner recommend in order to limit the amount of work needed during bathing?

    A. A reacher
    B. A shower chair and terry bath robe
    C. A bath mitt
    D. Proper body mechanics

115. An individual diagnosed with chronic obstructive pulmonary disease is participating in a pulmonary rehabilitation program. Which of the following will the OT practitioner MOST likely recommend?

    A. Perform pursed-lip breathing when doing activities.
    B. Use a long-handled sponge while in the shower.
    C. Take hot showers to reduce congestion.
    D. Avoid air conditioned rooms during warm months.

116. In carrying out inpatient treatment groups for individuals with schizophrenia, the OT practitioner would be MOST likely to use which of the following intervention methods initially?

    A. Projective media, such as clay, to facilitate expression of feelings
    B. Allowing an individual group member to work in an isolated area away from the group
    C. Simple and highly structured activities
    D. Discussions about the individuals' delusions

117. An OT practitioner is instructing an individual with arthritis how to maintain range of motion while performing household activities. Which of the following activities MOST effectively accomplishes this?

    A. Use short strokes with the vacuum cleaner.
    B. Keep elbow flexed when ironing.
    C. Keep lightweight objects on low shelves.
    D. Use a dust mitt to keep fingers fully extended.

118. An OT practitioner is working with a child with a significant developmental disability who frequently bites his siblings and parents. Which of the following would the OT MOST likely recommend?

    A. Encourage the parents to use verbal feedback, and explain to the child that biting is inappropriate.
    B. Tell the parents to enforce time-out periods for each biting incident.
    C. Encourage the child to wear a necklace with chewable objects attached.
    D. Tell the parents that the child will eventually stop biting when one of his siblings bites him back.

119. An individual with an anxiety disorder feels so overwhelmed he cannot get himself from his room to OT group each morning. Which of the following strategies will be MOST helpful?

    A. Reduce distractions and keep the lights low.
    B. Provide a stimulating environment with real life opportunities.
    C. Give him a tour of the OT department and a schedule of activities.
    D. Leave doors open and avoid being alone with the individual.

120. Following a hip replacement, a patient is limited to "toe touch" weight-bearing on the operated extremity. The OT practitioner should instruct the patient to do which of the following during performance of ADLs?

    A. Transfer on and off a commode seat while using a walker.
    B. Work on bed mobility by rolling and pushing with both heels.
    C. Eat all meals in bed independently.
    D. Try to perform distal lower extremity dressing without assistive devices.

121. An OT practitioner is evaluating a 2-year-old child who demonstrates decreased protective reactions. In which of the following positions would the therapist MOST likely place the child in order to elicit protective reactions?

    A. Supine on a mat
    B. In the therapist's lap
    C. On a tiltboard or bolster
    D. Prone on a mat

122. A male patient with an indwelling catheter asks the OT practitioner for advice concerning sexual activity. Which of the following responses is MOST appropriate?

    A. Refer the patient to his physician.

    B. Discuss precautions necessary for sex when an indwelling catheter is present.

    C. Teach the individual how to remove and replace the indwelling catheter.

    D. Explain that it is dangerous and difficult to have sex when an indwelling catheter is present.

123. An individual is experiencing headaches at work due to increased neck and shoulder tension resulting from computer keyboarding. The BEST stress management approach for the OT practitioner to suggest in this situation is:

    A. assertiveness training focusing on increasing the individual's assertiveness with his or her supervisor.

    B. relaxation exercises while incorporating breaks into the day if using the keyboard frequently.

    C. cognitive reappraisal training to decrease the individual's tendency to focus on the negative side of work events.

    D. teaching the individual more effective problem-solving strategies.

124. An OT practitioner provides a leather-working activity to an individual with C7 quadriplegia in order to increase grip strength. Which component of this activity would be MOST effective in promoting this goal?

    A. Holding the hammer

    B. Holding the stamping tools

    C. Squeezing the sponge to wet the leather

    D. Lacing with the needle

125. The OT practitioner is observing a 3-year-old child during tooth brushing. The child demonstrates good bilateral upper extremity/ hand strength, but decreased dexterity. Which piece of equipment would the OT MOST likely encourage the child to use during brushing?

    A. A small soft bristle toothbrush

    B. A Velcro strap attached to a toothbrush

    C. An electric toothbrush

    D. A soft sponge-tipped toothette

126. An individual with a C6 spinal cord injury is unable to button his shirt. The OT would be MOST likely to select which type of adaptive equipment to assist this individual with buttoning?

    A. A buttonhook with an extra long, flexible handle

    B. A buttonhook with a knob handle

    C. A buttonhook on a 0.5 inch diameter, 5 inch long wooden handle

    D. A buttonhook attached to a cuff that fits around the palm

127. A very confused nursing home resident is frequently found in the rooms of other residents in the middle of the night. Which of the following environmental adaptations would MOST effectively prevent wandering?

    A. Apply wrist restraints after the client has fallen asleep.

    B. Keep hallways clear of obstructions to prevent injury.

    C. Install an alarm on the client's door.

    D. Suggest the night shift staff provide closer supervision.

128. An individual with a high level spinal cord injury is returning home. Which type of adaptive technology would the individual MOST likely require to ensure safety in the home?

    A. A simple electronic aid to daily living (EADL)

    B. A dedicated device with 911 auto-dial backup

    C. A remote control power door opener

    D. An electric page turner

129. The OT is working with a 6-year-old child who occasionally drops his utensils when eating because of a slight decrease in hand range of motion/grasp limitation. Which piece of equipment would the OT MOST likely recommend FIRST?

    A. Swivel utensils

    B. Pediatric universal holders

    C. Foam tubing around the utensils

    D. Weighted utensils

130. An OT practitioner is treating an individual who has been refusing to wear his splint, and now reports it is lost. Prior to fabricating another splint, the therapist should FIRST:

A. give the individual 48 hours to locate the splint, then fabricate a new one if the first cannot be found.

B. determine if there are any motivational or cultural issues interfering with splint-wear compliance.

C. ask the individual to find the splint and demand that he begin wearing it or you will call his physician.

D. discharge the individual because he has no interest in regaining function.

131. An individual who has MS is standing at a table folding laundry and begins to complain of fatigue. The BEST way to adapt the activity would be to:

A. suggest the individual complete the activity in a seated position.

B. recommend the individual upgrade the activity by ironing all of the shirts prior to folding.

C. stop the activity and break the task into components to determine where the activity went wrong.

D. suggest that the individual stop the activity so a more effective task can be introduced.

132. A preteen with a diagnosis of spastic cerebral palsy is enjoying independent use of his computer-assisted technology, but complains of general fatigue. The OT should assist the student by:

A. decreasing the amount of energy expended while working with the computer through an alternative keyboard.

B. increasing the size of the computer screen

C. encouraging the student to request assistance when feeling fatigued.

D. taking turns with the student while typing homework assignments

133. An OT practitioner is fabricating a splint for an individual who has carpal tunnel syndrome. Which of the following splint fabrication techniques should be adhered to in order to allow for adequate digit motion?

A. Trim lines of the splint should extend distal to the MCP crease.

B. Trim lines of the splint should extend proximal to the DIP joint.

C. Trim lines of the splint should extend proximal to the MCP crease.

D. Trim lines of the splint should extend distal to the ulnar fifth MCP crease.

134. An OT practitioner is working with an individual who has severe cognitive deficits. Using a functional skill training approach, the MOST appropriate method to teach the individual to brush his or her teeth is based on:

A. rote repetition of the task sub-steps with gradually fading cues.

B. practice of fine-motor activities that incorporate motions needed in tooth brushing.

C. teaching a caregiver how to set up the task and guide the client's performance.

D. use of instructional cards, which the individual will learn to use as a reminder of how to perform the task.

135. A 3-year-old child with a severe physical disability and no cognitive delays does not have a form of functional mobility. What is the MOST APPROPRIATE age that a powered wheelchair should be considered for this child?

A. 3 years

B. 4 years

C. 6 years

D. 8 years

136. Which of the following would the OT practitioner recommend to a 12-year-old child with mild visual impairments who desires independent use of the telephone within his home?

A. A speaker phone

B. A hands-free phone

C. A phone with extra large buttons

D. A phone with a receiver holder

137. Specific recommendations have been made for electronic assistive technology for an adult with muscular dystrophy. After the devices are ordered and modified as necessary, the NEXT step in the process of implementation is for the OT practitioner to:

A. evaluate how well the whole system works.

B. evaluate if the assistive technology devices match the needs of the client.

C. train the client in the operation of the assistive technology system and in strategies for its use.

D. determine if funding is available for the recommended assistive technology.

138. An individual has demonstrated competence in heating canned soup. The OT practitioner recommends modifying the treatment plan and upgrading the cooking activity to:

    A. baking brownies.
    B. making an apple pie.
    C. making toast.
    D. making a fresh fruit salad.

139. A child with quadriplegia complains of frequently slumping to the side when sitting in a wheelchair. The OT practitioner would MOST likely recommend which of the following to enable the child to maintain optimal wheelchair positioning?

    A. A reclining wheelchair
    B. An arm trough
    C. Lateral trunk supports
    D. Lateral pelvic supports

140. An OT practitioner is working with a 17-year-old girl with impaired mobility, dexterity, and communication skills. The teenager is within functional limits cognitively. Which of the following would the OT MOST likely recommend to the family regarding emergency alert systems in the event of a fire?

    A. Position a wireless cell phone within the girl's reach.
    B. Establish an exit routine in order to get out of the house quickly in the event of a fire.
    C. Review "fire prevention within the home" literature.
    D. Recommend that the girl wear an emergency alert system pendant around her neck.

141. A resident of a long-term care facility who is in a weakened condition and has mild cognitive deficits is being seen by the OT practitioner in the mornings to help re-establish dressing routines. The BEST way to structure the task is to:

    A. have the resident select the clothing they prefer, then have the OT dress the client.
    B. have the resident dress in bed with garments that are stretchy and one size larger than usual, and then preview each step of the process with the resident.
    C. have the resident walk to retrieve clothing garments and encourage independent performance.
    D. place clothing within close reach of the resident, encourage the resident to proceed with dressing as you provide distant supervision.

142. An OT is working with a fifth grade child with spina bifida who will need to self-catheterize twice a day. The OT will MOST likely communicate to the child's teacher that in order to perform independently the child will need:

    A. assistance with awareness and sequencing.
    B. good hand strength, range of motion, and perceptual awareness.
    C. a powered bidet.
    D. reducer rings.

143. When teaching deep breathing techniques to manage stress, the OT practitioner should instruct the individual to:

    A. make a fist, and then gradually relax it.
    B. focus on a rhythmic, repetitive word.
    C. walk rapidly until an increased heart rate is achieved.
    D. deeply inhale and slowly exhale.

144. While participating in activities to improve strength, an individual with multiple sclerosis who was recently admitted to the hospital complains of fatigue. Which of the following actions is the MOST appropriate for the OT practitioner to take?

    A. Instruct the individual to work through the fatigue to complete the session.
    B. Instruct the individual to work through the fatigue for another 5 to 10 minutes.
    C. Discontinue strengthening activities.
    D. Give the individual a rest break.

145. An OT practitioner making a bedside visit finds the patient poorly positioned with an edematous upper extremity caught between the mattress and the bed rail. The MOST appropriate intervention to address the edema in the upper extremity is to:

    A. elevate the arm on pillows so it rests higher than the heart.
    B. massage the arm gently, stroking toward the fingers.
    C. instruct the patient to avoid active range of motion.
    D. instruct the patient to avoid PROM.

146. An OT practitioner is fabricating a static splint that will assist with the maintenance of a functional hand and finger position while keeping the soft tissues of the hand in a mid-range position. Which splint would the OT MOST likely select to address these needs?

    A. Bivalve cast
    B. Resting pan splint
    C. Dynamic extension splint
    D. Wrist cock-up splint

147. An individual is about to be discharged from outpatient OT after rehabilitation for a hand injury. The individual has not been able to work for 3 months and is unable to perform all of the job requirements as a truck driver. Which of the following should the OT practitioner recommend at discharge?

    A. A home exercise program

    B. Home health OT

    C. Work hardening

    D. No further OT services

148. A young boy with hemiplegia has difficulty putting on his socks each morning before school. Which of the following should the OT practitioner recommend?

    A. Encourage the child to wear tight fitting socks.

    B. Teach the child to sit in a chair with a back support, lift the affected leg onto a stool, and use socks with a wide opening.

    C. Encourage the child to request assistance from his mother when putting on socks.

    D. Teach the child to sit in a chair and lift and place the unaffected foot up on a small stool, and use socks with a wide opening.

149. An individual in an OT group has a history of monopolizing the group without giving others an opportunity to participate in the group process. What is the most effective approach for working on the individual's social conduct and group skills during a gardening activity?

    A. Give the individual a specific task such as filling up the water containers.

    B. Have the individual assign tasks to various group members.

    C. Have the individual observe the group.

    D. Pair the individual with another group member for a specific task.

150. An individual with Guillain-Barré syndrome was recently admitted to a rehabilitation unit and is expected to remain for 3 to 4 weeks. At what point in the rehabilitative process should the OT practitioner order adaptive equipment for this individual?

    A. After the patient and family have accepted the individual's disability

    B. As soon as the insurance provider approves it

    C. Within the first week of therapy

    D. Just before discharge

151. An OT practitioner is treating a restaurant worker with carpal tunnel syndrome. The MOST important instruction for the practitioner to give this individual is to avoid or modify activities that encourage:

    A. increased wrist extension, such as carrying dishes on a tray at shoulder height.

    B. pressure on the wrist in neutral position, such as scrubbing pots and pans.

    C. tasks that increase ulnar deviation, such as wiping tables.

    D. increased radial deviation, such as screwing and unscrewing and filling sugar, salt, and pepper containers.

152. An individual's weight has changed during the course of hospitalization, and there is now a space of 2.5 inches between the individual's hips and the sides of the wheelchair. Which is the BEST recommendation regarding proper wheelchair fit?

    A. Obtain a wider wheelchair because this one is now too narrow.

    B. Encourage the individual to lose weight.

    C. Pad the sides of the wheelchair to improve the fit.

    D. Obtain a narrower wheelchair because this one is now too wide.

153. An individual who sustained severe burns is ready for the rehabilitative phase of treatment after 3 weeks in intensive care. Prior to performing ADL training, the MOST important action for the OT practitioner to take would be to:

    A. debride the wound.

    B. remove compression garments.

    C. perform UE strengthening activities.

    D. perform skin conditioning techniques.

154. An OT practitioner is leading an assertiveness group with clients demonstrating low self-esteem. The MOST important curative factor to regularly include in an assertiveness group is a:

    A. leader who provides the group members with definitions of assertion, passivity, and aggression.

    B. group leader who allows and encourages all group members to physically and verbally release their aggressive feelings toward inanimate objects.

    C. practitioner who demonstrates common assertiveness techniques to the group members.

    D. practitioner who encourages group members to share similar situations and reactions with one another.

155. A child with a diagnosis of moderate mental retardation is currently performing at the second grade level. The child can MOST likely:

A. write a grocery list.

B. understand basic concepts related to money.

C. perform simple division.

D. write an accurate short story about his summer vacation.

156. An OT practitioner documenting the progress of a client using the SOAP note format would include which of the following in the "subjective information" section?

A. "The OT practitioner will establish a daily self-feeding routine using verbal and physical cues to encourage the client to open containers on the lunch tray."

B. "The client has been able to identify closed liquid beverage containers on the meal tray for four of six presentations."

C. "The client is able to identify and drink liquids presented in cups without lids but leaves beverages in closed containers untouched."

D. "The client asks for more beverages during meals and appears surprised when the OT practitioner indicates beverages in closed containers are on the meal tray."

157. An OT practitioner is preparing to do a parachute activity as part of a sensory integration program. Since several of the patients in the group are taking antipsychotic medications, the OT should be alert for which possible side effect that could occur as a result of this activity?

A. Postural hypotension

B. Photosensitivity

C. Excessive thirst

D. Blurred vision

158. An individual reports that back pain during sexual activity is so severe that it prevents any enjoyment. The BEST strategy to recommend is:

A. use a side lying position.

B. time sexual activity for periods of high energy.

C. avoid discussing pain with the sexual partner because it may be a "turn off."

D. identify alternative methods for meeting sexual needs that do not cause pain.

159. An OT practitioner is working with an individual who is experiencing a manic episode and demonstrating expansive behaviors in the clinic. Given that this individual has expressed interest in all kinds of craft activities, which type of craft activity would the OT be MOST likely to select to provide external structure for the client?

A. Detailed needlepoint project requiring fine stitches

B. Using clay to shape an object of one's choice

C. A watercolor painting project

D. Finishing a prefabricated wood birdhouse from a kit

160. The mother of an 18-month-old child with hypertonia reports that dressing is extremely difficult. When teaching the parent how to put shoes and socks on the child, the OT should suggest that the mother FIRST:

A. flex the child's hips.

B. flex the child's knees.

C. flex the child's ankles.

D. flex the child's toes.

161. An OT is explaining to a teacher the kind of high technology aid that can be used to help a multiple handicapped student who has speech and writing deficits in the classroom. Which intervention would the OT MOST likely recommend for this child?

A. An environmental control unit

B. A Wanchik writer

C. A head pointer

D. An electronic augmentative communication device

162. An OT practitioner is leading a discussion with a group of individuals who are diagnosed with major depressive disorder. The MOST helpful therapeutic communication approach for the practitioner to take is to:

A. be upbeat, positive, and cheerful when encouraging the individuals to discuss their feelings.

B. offer even-tempered acceptance, reflecting back what is heard without agreeing that the situation is hopeless.

C. remain silent and still while the individuals are describing their feelings.

D. allow the individuals to structure and lead the group discussion.

163. To practice transfers using a transfer board, the OT practitioner must have the individual use a wheelchair that has:

    A. detachable footrests.

    B. detachable armrests.

    C. anti-tip bars.

    D. brake handle extensions.

164. A third-grader's readiness for discharge from direct OT, as a related service, has been determined on the basis of:

    A. whether the areas of concern to the OT interfere with the child's education.

    B. the degree of functional skills possessed by the child.

    C. the level of independence in ADL.

    D. the degree of accessibility of the learning environment.

165. An individual's family wants to build a ramp to the primary entrance of the home. The OT practitioner advises the family that the ramp should be graded with a maximum slope of:

    A. 1 inch of ramp for every foot of rise in height.

    B. 1 foot of ramp for every inch of rise in height.

    C. 10 inches of ramp for every 2 inches in height.

    D. 1 foot of ramp for every foot of rise in height.

166. An OT practitioner asks an individual in a manic state what he would like to do in craft group. The individual answers, "I'm a really good carpenter so I'm going to build my kids a club house." The BEST response is to:

    A. support him in this choice.

    B. tell him he doesn't have the necessary attention span at this time.

    C. redirect him toward an activity that doesn't require sharp tools.

    D. suggest a more realistic activity.

167. The OT practitioner is working with a child who has upper extremity weakness and incoordination. The child wishes to put on and take off her pants independently. Which of the following would the OT MOST likely recommend?

    A. Pants with Velcro inserts placed in the zipper area

    B. Pants with an elastic waistband

    C. Cotton pants with large buttons inserted where the zipper area is located

    D. Pants with an enlarged zipper pull attachment

168. A school-age child with visual perceptual deficits is being discharged from OT. Which compensatory technique for dealing with visual figure-ground problems should the OT practitioner recommend to the child's teacher?

    A. Place a red line on the left side of the page.

    B. Use a timer for certain activities.

    C. Teach the child to use lists and color coding of books and folders.

    D. Block out all areas of a page except important words.

169. When preparing to discharge a child with juvenile rheumatoid arthritis, what is the MOST important information to share with the child's school teacher?

    A. A summary of the child's cognitive and visual perceptual skills

    B. Adaptive equipment/ADL needs in the classroom

    C. Information on the child's range of motion status

    D. A summary of the child's progress in OT

170. In the middle of a wheelchair to bed transfer, an obese patient begins to slip from the grasp of an average size OT practitioner. The BEST action for the OT to take is to:

    A. ease the patient onto the floor.

    B. reverse the transfer, getting the patient back in the wheelchair.

    C. continue the transfer, getting the patient to the bed.

    D. call next door for assistance.

171. An OT practitioner is reviewing bathing skills with a 13-year-old child when the client suddenly asks questions regarding his sexuality. What should the OT do FIRST?

    A. Refer the teenager to someone who has increased knowledge regarding the subject of sexuality, such as a psychologist.

    B. Tell the client that you don't mind appropriately discussing sexuality-related questions as long as his parents are comfortable with the idea.

    C. Attempt to change the subject because the child is too young to be educated on this topic.

    D. Try to openly and honestly address the client's questions to the best of your knowledge.

172. An OT practitioner is conducting an ongoing assertiveness training group. Which of the following strategies would be MOST helpful in facilitating group cohesion and exchange of feedback among group members?

    A. Define assertiveness, passivity, and aggression for the group members.

    B. Allow and encourage all group members to release their aggressive feelings physically and verbally toward inanimate objects.

    C. Demonstrate commonly used assertiveness techniques to the group members.

    D. Encourage group members to share similar experiences and reactions with each other.

173. An OT practitioner is educating a caregiver regarding manual wheelchair mobility. Which of the following is the BEST way to teach the caregiver to propel a wheelchair down a steep ramp?

    A. Tip the wheelchair backward and guide it down the ramp backward.

    B. Tip the wheelchair backward and guide it down the ramp forward.

    C. Allow the patient to propel the wheelchair independently.

    D. Obtain the assistance of a second individual.

174. An OT practitioner is working with an individual who is confused and having difficulty placing both feet into his pants legs. Which is the MOST appropriate preparatory method for the OT to use to prepare the individual to progress to actual dressing training?

    A. Pulling up pants during toileting activities

    B. Teaching the individual to use a reacher to pull up his pants to knee level

    C. Pulling off socks using a dressing stick

    D. Having him place his feet through loops of therapeutic band

■ OCCUPATIONAL THERAPY FOR POPULATIONS

175. An occupational therapy manager is developing a proposal for OT services in the Neonatal Intensive Care Unit. Using the Developmental Support Care approach as the basis for services, how would the occupational therapist BEST describe OT's scope of practice in the NICU?

    A. Modifying the environment to protect the infant from overstimulation and inappropriate stimuli

    B. Providing PROM, positioning and handling, fabrication of splints, and referral to early intervention

    C. Educating parents and hospital staff

    D. Implementing motor and behavioral skill acquisition through developmental milestone positioning

176. An OT practitioner has been employed as a consultant to reduce the application of restraints for the population of several long-term care facilities operated by a large company. The MOST appropriate service for the OT practitioner to provide is:

    A. identifying legal issues related to restraint reduction.

    B. providing staff education, recommendations, and support for restraint alternatives.

    C. investigating incidents of resident abuse related to restraint reduction.

    D. assessing the level of risk and liability involved with restraint use.

177. An OT practitioner working for the school system as a consultant has identified a general need to enhance the fine coordination skills of elementary school students to facilitate better writing skills. The MOST appropriate action for the consultant to take to address the needs of this population would be to:

    A. screen students for writing problems, and provide in-depth assessment of those identified.

    B. provide remedial activities for those students identified as having fine coordination deficits.

    C. recommend activities to develop fine coordination that teachers can incorporate into classroom programming.

    D. recommend additional OT staff to provide direct services for students.

178. An OT practitioner has been asked to develop health promotion programs for adults with severe and multiple disabilities in a long-term care residential environment. What program focus would BEST address the overall health promotion and wellness needs of this population?

A. Physical fitness programs which emphasize increasing activity levels
B. Educational programs emphasizing safety education and prevention
C. Programs emphasizing engagement in social and productive activities
D. Programs emphasizing training in assistive technology options

179. The OT staff in an outpatient facility are developing goals for a new, multidisciplinary work hardening program. Which of the following goals is MOST appropriate for this program?

A. ADL retraining to increase the ability to perform household skills independently
B. Progressive resistive exercise to increase endurance for self-care skills
C. Work simulation to increase strength and endurance for necessary work-related skills
D. Vocational retraining to increase the ability to reenter the job market

180. An OT practitioner is attending a meeting with a community agency requesting consultation services. The NEXT step in this process would be to:

A. negotiate a contract.
B. establish a trusting relationship.
C. assess the problem.
D. develop goals.

181. An OT practitioner is consulting in a long-term care setting to recommend programs for residents who seem isolated and disengaged from the other residents. Which activity format would be BEST for enhancing self-esteem, providing opportunities for socialization, and assisting residents in integrating past experiences with present life?

A. Reminiscence groups
B. Meditation groups
C. Grooming activities groups
D. Movement activities and games groups

182. An occupational therapist has been hired by a community residence for women with mental health issues as a consultant to address the problem of low motivation and low activity levels in the areas of activities of daily living and instrumental activities of living. The consultant in this situation would:

A. provide occupational therapy treatment to increase occupational performance in the areas identified.
B. develop a plan with staff to change the social environment to one that will enhance motivation and activity levels.
C. design a range of living skills groups so that every resident will be included.
D. help the residents to achieve personal goals, make decisions or change behaviors.

183. An OT practitioner is advising the social workers in a residence for teenage mothers with HIV on how to help the young mothers develop parenting skills. Which of the following areas would be MOST important to focus on when working with the mothers of infants in terms of infant health and well-being?

A. Activities that promote mother-child communication and foster attachment
B. Modeling and discussing appropriate disciplinary techniques
C. Activities that promote language development and cognitive skills
D. Peer interaction for both mothers and babies

184. An older adult day care facility has contracted an OT practitioner to develop programming for its clients at risk for falls. The BEST type of program to provide regular group physical activity and enhance balance would be:

A. safe transfer training.
B. walking.
C. tai chi.
D. gardening.

185. An OT is part of a team developing a policy for discontinuation of services to students in school-based settings. The MOST appropriate time to terminate services is when a student:

A. fails to achieve long-term objectives after 1 month.
B. is unable to accomplish short-term goals identified at the time of the initial evaluation.
C. no longer makes substantial progress regardless of several adjustments made to intervention techniques.
D. transitions from elementary to middle school.

186. An OT practitioner is working as a consultant to a long-term care facility that is designing a dementia care unit. The OT practitioner would MOST likely recommend which type of environmental attributes as therapeutic?

A. Controlled stimulation with meaningful sensory cues
B. High sensory stimulation to encourage active engagement
C. Subdued, low sensory stimulation environment, to prevent agitation
D. Stimuli that are very similar to those found in the residents' home environments

■ SERVICE MANAGEMENT AND PROFESSIONAL PRACTICE

187. Which of the following is the BEST method for demonstrating service competency in a standardized evaluation?

A. Observe performance of the standardized test by a competent OT practitioner.
B. Observe a competent OT practitioner, then practice, then teach another individual how to administer the test.
C. Follow procedures exactly as outlined in the test manuals.
D. Obtain the same results as another OT practitioner who has demonstrated service competency.

188. An OTR and COTA share and coordinate therapy for a caseload. Which of the following jobs would be MOST appropriate for the COTA to perform:

A. completing the chart reviews.
B. completing the nonstandardized portions of the evaluation.
C. interpreting the results of the nonstandardized portion of the evaluation.
D. independently designing a treatment plan for the individual.

189. The MOST important goal for an OT practitioner to convey to a level I fieldwork student is to:

A. facilitate clinical reasoning.
B. achieve competence.
C. assist the student in developing a general comfort level with client needs.
D. encourage the student to partake in ethical and reflective practice.

190. "3-27-05: ADL evaluation and treatment for diagnosis of RCVA: Three times a week for 1 month. Signed, M. Johnson, MD." Upon reading this statement, the OTR would interpret this as a:

A. referral.
B. screening.
C. goal setting.
D. treatment planning.

191. An OTR and a COTA work in a collaborative relationship. The teamwork between the two professionals is BEST exemplified by which of the following?

A. The OTR completes the assessment and instructs the COTA to provide a specific intervention.
B. The COTA updates the OTR on the progress a patient has made in the past week, and both provide information to update the goals.
C. The COTA gives a progress note to the OTR and the OTR writes the discharge summary based on the progress note.
D. The OTR tells the COTA what type of equipment to order for a patient and the COTA orders the equipment from a medical equipment company.

192. A home health OT has received a referral for an individual with Medicare coverage. Which one of the following actions must occur before the therapist can initiate evaluation or treatment?

A. Identify the deficits that impair functional abilities.
B. Establish short- and long-term goals.
C. Obtain a physician's plan of care identifying services to be provided.
D. Obtain the individual's history of the current illness.

193. An OTR with expertise in hand rehabilitation is assessing a COTA's service competency in hand function assessment. At what point is service competency established?

A. When the COTA consistently obtains the same results as the OTR
B. After the COTA passes the NBCOT examination
C. When the COTA has obtained a specified number of continuing education credits in hand rehabilitation
D. After the COTA has practiced for a minimum number of years, as specified by state licensure

194. The trend toward health status and away from health care focuses on enhancing wellness through activities using various strategies, including education and behavioral change efforts. The OT practitioner's role in this trend is BEST described as:

    A. occupational behavior.

    B. intervention.

    C. self-efficacy.

    D. health promotion.

195. An OT practitioner violates the Occupational Code of Ethics and is censured by the NBCOT. The OT contacts a lawyer and learns that censure is:

    A. a formal written expression of disapproval against a practitioner's conduct that is issued and retained in the NBCOT's files.

    B. a formal, public disapproval of a practitioner's conduct.

    C. probation, in which a practitioner is given a period of time to retain the counseling or education required to remain certified.

    D. a permanent revocation of NBCOT certification.

196. An OT manager is preparing the outpatient OT staff for a visit from an accrediting agency. The accrediting agency that surveys inpatient and comprehensive outpatient rehabilitation programs is BEST represented by which of the following:

    A. AOTA.

    B. JCAHO.

    C. CARF.

    D. NBCOT.

197. An OTR/COTA team begins to provide occupational therapy services through a certified home health agency. What is the MOST critical component for establishing a successful collaborative relationship in this treatment setting?

    A. Determining reimbursement when completing joint visits

    B. Establishing a system for the OTR to countersign the COTA's documentation

    C. Creating effective communication via weekly staff meetings, voice mail, and faxes

    D. Developing a handout to educate future clients regarding how the OTR/COTA team will provide services

198. A manager of an OT department is attempting to increase the visibility of the OT department within the hospital setting. This type of promotion is commonly done through internal marketing. In order to market internally, the OT manager would MOST likely employ which of the following?

    A. A community newsletter

    B. A presentation to physicians

    C. A local community workshop

    D. A booth at a local health fair

199. After completing a chart review, the OT practitioner enters the room of a new patient who states that he does not want to be seen by any of the therapists because his insurance has run out and he cannot afford to pay for the treatment. Which of the following actions would be MOST appropriate for the OT practitioner to take?

    A. Treat the individual per the physician's order and notify the nurse about the patient's refusal.

    B. Based on his refusal, do not treat the individual and document the interaction in the chart.

    C. Treat the individual, but do not charge or document the services.

    D. Do not treat the individual and only charge for the time spent completing the chart review.

200. An OT practitioner wishes to assess the results of a life skills training program provided to individuals at a shelter for abused women. Which of the following methods would be the MOST comprehensive method for obtaining this information?

    A. Final evaluation of each client involved

    B. Client satisfaction survey

    C. Program evaluation

    D. Utilization review

Answers for Simulation Examination 2

1. (D) the need for adaptive equipment and assistance from others. The hospital stay following total hip arthroplasty is usually less than a week, and the OT practitioner must prioritize what can reasonably be accomplished in that time. Determining an individual's need for adaptive equipment and how much assistance is required for ADLs (answer D) are the highest priority for occupational therapy evaluation and are reasonable goals for such a short length of stay. While work and leisure performance (answer B) are important aspects of occupational performance, they may need to be addressed later by the OT practitioner working with the individual in home health, as an outpatient, or in an extended care facility. Addressing deficits in strength, ROM, or coordination (answer C) also may be necessary to enhance occupational performance, but the need for intervention would likely extend beyond acute care as well. While cognitive/perceptual functioning (answer A) is critical to safe ADL and IADL performance, these areas are more thoroughly assessed prior to surgery in order to determine the client's ability to adhere to the prescribed precautions post-surgery. See Reference: Trombly and Radomski. Bear-Lehman, J: Orthopaedic conditions.

2. (A) age appropriate. The child being observed is performing a dressing activity which is age appropriate for a 5-year-old child. A typical child at this age can dress unsupervised and is able to tie and untie knots, but generally does not know how to tie a bow independently. See Reference: Case-Smith (ed). Shepherd, J: Self-care and adaptations for independent living.

3. (A) safety and stability. Incoordination, tremors, ataxia, and athetoid movements may result from conditions that affect the central nervous system, such as Parkinson's disease, CP, multiple sclerosis, and head injuries. "The major problems encountered in ADL performance [for people with incoordination] are safety and adequate stability of gait, body parts, and objects to complete the tasks" (p. 148). Strength (answer C) was not identified as an area of concern for this individual. The ability to reach and bend (answer B) is of primary concern for those with limitations in range of motion. Endurance level (answer D) is a primary concern for individuals with MS, Guillain-Barré syndrome, ALS, and other neurological conditions that cause them to fatigue quickly. See Reference: Pedretti and Early (eds). Foti, D: Activities of daily living.

4. (C) End the session and initiate a phone interview with the child's parents and teacher. When a child refuses to participate in therapy, the OT should attempt to contact the child's parents and/or teacher (answer C). According to Mulligan, "informal interviews with the child and his or her parents are helpful to gain information about the child's interests, strengths, and challenges and will help you uncover child and family priorities...they also give you an opportunity to establish rapport with your clients and for you to explain what you hope to accomplish throughout the evaluation process" (p. 37). Answer (A), continuing to force the child to participate in therapy, may have detrimental effects on the child, causing them to never participate in the therapeutic process, while answer (B), encouraging the child to partake in the COPM evaluation, would not be appropriate at this time since the child refuses to participate in the evaluation process. However, it may be an alternative in the future since the COPM can be used to "measure the child's (or the parents') perception of the child's performance" (p. 42). While answer (D), threatening the child to take away something of significance (such as recess time), will most likely have detrimental effects on the child's perception of both occupational therapy and the therapist treating him. See Reference: Mulligan. Mulligan, S: A Guide to Evaluation.

5. (C) Have the individual hold a heavy handbag by the handles. The hook grasp is strongly based on the use of digits two to five. The thumb is not always required for the hook grasp and can remain inactive. A needle would be held with a two-point pinch while being threaded (answer A). A glass would be held with a cylindrical grasp (answer B). Finally, a key being placed in a lock would be held by a lateral pinch (answer D). See Reference: Pedretti and Early (eds). Belkin, J and Yasuda, L: Orthotics.

6. (C) cruising. The described pattern is cruising (answer C). Cruising occurs at approximately 12 months of age and directly precedes walking (answer B). Creeping (answer A) refers to four-point mobility in a prone position with only hands and knees on the floor, a pattern that occurs between the ages of 7 and 12 months. Clawing (answer D), also called "fanning," is the ability to spread the toes to maintain balance in standing. See Reference: Case-Smith (ed). Wright-Ott, C and Egilson, S: Mobility.

7. (A) expressive aphasia. Expressive aphasia (answer A) interferes with an individual's verbal or written expression, but not comprehension of verbal or written information. An individual with expressive aphasia would be able to indicate the correct response by nodding or pointing to the stimulus used or a card marked with the correct response. Individuals with receptive aphasia (answer B) cannot comprehend spoken or written words and symbols; therefore, they cannot understand verbal directions or consistently respond to stimuli. Individuals with receptive aphasia may be able to imitate or follow a demonstration, but these techniques do not work for sensory evaluation. An individual who has agnosia or ataxia (answers C and D) would be able to understand directions, but be unable to accurately indicate an area because of impaired recognition of the body part or impaired coordination. The method of response may be adapted by using verbal description of an area or cue cards. See Reference: Trombly and Radomski. Woodson, AM: Stroke.

8. (A) constructional apraxia. An individual with constructional apraxia exhibits difficulty performing the construction of one or more objects onto each other as needed in making a sandwich or putting on clothing in the proper sequence or position. Ideomotor apraxia (answer B) is the inability to imitate gestures or perform a purposeful motor task on command even though the person understands the idea or concept of the task. Visual agnosia (answer C) is an inability to recognize familiar objects. Unilateral neglect (answer D) occurs when the individual neglects the affected side of the body and performs activities toward or with the unaffected side. See Reference: Trombly and Radomski. Quintana, LA: Assessing abilities and capacities: vision, visual perception, and praxis.

9. (C) Mental status, oral structures, and motor control of head. A dysphagia evaluation usually consists of assessing a client's mental status, oral motor structure, and head, trunk, and extremity motor functions (answer C). Answer A is most related to an evaluation of TMJ. Answer B, a cranial nerve assessment, would typically be performed by a physiatrist and/or neurologist. Answer D, muscle length control or dysmetria (a result of overshooting or pointing past an object) is typically not included in the assessment of dysphagia. See Reference: Pedretti and Early (eds). Jenks, KN: Dysphagia

10. (D) observe the child entering the clinic and taking off his coat and shoes. "In a naturalistic observation, the therapist gathers information in the typical or natural setting [in which] the activity occurs" (p. 494). The most reliable information can be gained by observing the child as he or she normally does the activity; this is especially true of children with developmental delay, who may have difficulty generalizing learning from one situation to another. Therefore, answer B may not provide a sample of the child's true skill level. Answers A and C describe situations in which the practitioner is providing assistance, therefore not allowing the child to demonstrate his skill in independent dressing. See

Reference: Case-Smith (ed). Shepherd, J: Self care and adaptations for independent living.

11. (B) use a perceived exertion scale. Beta blockers blunt heart rate response, and can result in inaccurate heart rate (answer C) calculations. Determination of MAHR (answer D) is commonly used in cardiac rehabilitation to determine appropriate exercise intensity, but relies on accurate heart rate calculation. A perceived exertion scale (answer B), such as the Borg Scale of Perceived Exertion asks the individual to describe how much they feel they are exerting, ranging from "no work at all" to "very, very heavy work." Isometric testing (answer A) is one way of measuring neuromuscular endurance, but isometric contraction is often contraindicated for individuals with cardiac conditions. See Reference: Trombly and Radomski. Huntley, N: Cardiac and pulmonary diseases.

12. (D) Assess the individual's topographical orientation skills. To plan an appropriate intervention, the individual's community mobility skills must first be assessed. Constantly getting lost is a strong indicator that the individual may be impaired in the area of topographical orientation. Learning to take the bus and obtaining a library card (answers A and C) are important steps toward independent library use, but should occur after evaluation has been completed. Individuals may enjoy using a library whether they can read or not so the ability to read is not essential to this goal and does not need to be evaluated (answer B). See Reference: Creek (ed). Lewis, P and Miller, T: Community.

13. (D) endurance. A deficit in endurance (answer D) is demonstrated by the individual's inability to sustain cardiac, pulmonary, and musculoskeletal exertion for the duration of the activity. Answer A, a deficit in postural control, would be correct if the client had been unable to maintain his balance while putting on the shirt. A deficit in muscle tone (answer B) would have been evident if the client had demonstrated spasticity while putting on the shirt. Inability to push his arms through the resistance created by the shirt sleeve would demonstrate a deficit in strength (answer C). See Reference: Crepeau, Cohn, and Schell (eds). Kohlmeyer, K: Sensory and neuromuscular function.

14. (A) Interview. Interviews provide "an opportunity for the parents to identify their values and priorities about the skills being evaluated by the therapist" (p. 207). Open-ended questions are best for eliciting information regarding the family's feelings about the intervention. Answers B, C, and D are structured observation methods, through which information on specific skills or functional levels is collected. See Reference: Case-Smith (ed). Stewart, KB: Purposes, processes, and methods of evaluation.

15. (D) early morning and again in the afternoon. Individuals with arthritis should be evaluated in the morning and afternoon to assess the functional abilities of the individual during and after morning stiffness. Evaluating the individual only in the morning (answers A and C) or only in the afternoon (answer B) accurately reveals the individual's functional level at only one time of day. Individuals with arthritis have many changes in functional status after morning stiffness has disappeared. See Reference: Pedretti and Early (eds). Buckner, WS: Arthritis.

16. (D) protective extension response. "Protective extension responses are postural reactions that are used to stop a fall or to prevent injury when equilibrium reactions fail to do so" (p. 74). Equilibrium reactions (answer C) involve "automatic, compensatory movements...used to maintain the center of gravity over the base of support" (p. 74). Righting reactions (answer B) "bring the head and trunk back into an upright position" (p. 74). Primitive reflexes (answer A) are automatic movements that occur involuntarily and disappear as the infant matures. See Reference: Solomon (ed). Lowman, DK: Development of occupational performance components.

17. (B) examine the results of an analysis of the individual's job. The job analysis is a detailed description of the physical, sensory, and psychological demands of a job. The job analysis may be performed by an occupational therapist or other professional involved in the case. Examples of performance requirements include tasks such as lifting, walking, sitting, standing, and reaching, as well as seeing, hearing, and interpersonal skills. Interviewing the individual (answer A) is useful to obtain information about his or her perception of the injury, motivation for returning to work, and sense of responsibility for rehabilitation. However, the worker may not be able to give an objective, detailed, and concise analysis of the job. The Dictionary of Occupational Titles (answer C) provides generic job descriptions, but does not contain as much specific information as a job analysis. A physician (answer D) is unlikely to have the depth of information necessary or the time available to provide the necessary information. See Reference: Pedretti and Early (eds). Burt, CM: Work evaluation and work hardening.

18. (B) occupational performance history interview. According to Henry (2003), "the occupational performance history interview gathers information about a client's occupational adaptation over time and can be used with adolescents...it consists of three parts: a semi-structured interview concerning the client's occupational life history, three rating scales, and a life history narrative" (p. 293). Answer A, a physical assessment, would be used to determine the individual's baseline regarding strength, endurance, and balance, while answers C and D would most likely be used by the OT to gain additional insight into the individual's struggle with anorexia nervosa after the occupational performance history interview was conducted. See Reference: Crepeau, Cohn, and Schell (eds). Cohn, ES, Boyt Schell, BA, and Neistadt, ME: Overview of evaluation.

19. (C) Moderate assistance. Moderate assistance is defined as having the ability to complete the task with supervision and cueing, while requiring physical assistance for approximately 50% of the task. The individual who requires minimal assistance (answer B) is able to complete a task with supervision and cueing, while requiring physical assistance for less than 20% of the task. An individual who needs supervision, cueing, and physical assistance for 50% to 80% of the task is performing at the maximal assistance level (answer D). An individual is rated total assist (answer A) when he or she is able to perform less than 20%, or a few steps, of the activity independently. See Reference: Pedretti and Early (eds). Adler, C: Spinal cord injury.

20. (B) observing and interpreting patterns of behavior. The correct answer is observing and interpreting patterns of behavior, answer B, because to plan intervention, the therapist must be first able to identify the level of the individual's functioning in certain key areas, such as the ability to initiate and follow simple directions through observation of what may appear as "meaningless and aimless behaviors" (p. 51). Answer A, administering standardized cognitive assessments and answer D, administering functional performance tests, are inappropriate evaluation methods for severely developmentally disabled adults because of the limited behavioral skills of these individuals. The ability to classify levels of developmental disability (answer C) is not the responsibility of the occupational therapist. See Reference: Ross and Bachner (eds). Kellogg, HA: Clinical issues characterizing adults.

21. (B) identify and analyze the tasks and occupations that the individual will be performing in the home. The first step in the process is to analyze the tasks and occupations that the individual will be performing at home because this forms the basis of the entire assessment and recommendations that will be offered. This also will provide a framework for determining how well the individual can perform the tasks within the particular environment being surveyed. Answers A, C, and D are also important aspects of the process, but occur after the first step. See Reference: Pedretti and Early (eds). Smith, P: Americans with Disabilities Act: Accommodating persons with disabilities.

22. (A) further observation and evaluation of right-sided dysfunction is indicated. Answer A is correct because infants usually use a bilateral approach at this age. Although unilaterality occurs several months later, most children alternate hands in many activities until age 6 years. This means that this infant should be observed for possible right-sided dysfunction. Answer B is incorrect because unilaterality at age 4 months is not typical development. Answer C is incorrect because hand dominance begins to develop at age 3 to 6 months, and answer D is incorrect because bilaterality precedes unilaterality in the course of infant development. See Reference: Case-Smith (ed). Exner, CE: Development of hand skills.

23. (B) left unilateral neglect. The correct answer is left unilateral neglect (answer B) which is the inability to respond or orient to perceptions from the left side of the body. This deficit also is apparent when an individual eats only half the food on his plate or shaves only half of his face. Unilateral neglect is contralateral to the side of a brain lesion; therefore, left unilateral neglect would result from right-sided brain damage. Left neglect occurs most commonly in right hemisphere lesions. A cataract (answer C) would cause a visual impairment with detail on both sides of a page. Bitemporal hemianopia (hemianopia also is referred to as hemianopsia), also known as "tunnel vision," occurs when the individual's peripheral vision is lost (answer D). The individual would still be able to cross midline with cataracts or bitemporal hemianopsia (answer D). A right hemianopsia would not see the right side, and this type of patient would draw all the figures on the left side of the page. Visuospatial deficits are an important factor influencing functional independence outcomes. Visuospatial ability should be taken into account when establishing treatment goals as well as during discharge planning. See Reference: Trombly and Radomski. Quintana, LA: Assessing abilities and capacities: vision, visual perception, and praxis.

24. (A) check the alignment of the goniometer. If the goniometer is not aligned correctly, any joint measurements will demonstrate a discrepancy. A variability of 5 degrees is normal between two different evaluators, and may be that much less on a retest by the same therapist. Changing the size of the goniometer to larger (answer B) or smaller (answer C) during measurements could make the discrepancy greater, because it could make aligning the arms of the goniometer with the landmarks

more difficult. It is much faster to check the alignment of the goniometer first when using one of the proper length for the job. Forcing the individual's arm further into flexion (answer D) would be painful to the individual because measurements are taken at the end of the individual's full range of motion and the joint would be unable to go further. See Reference: Trombly and Radomski. Trombly, CA and Podolski, CR: Assessing abilities and capacities: Range of motion, strength, and endurance.

25. (B) The client can usually handle routine daily functions. Answer B is correct because it describes the skills of an individual with moderate or trainable mental retardation. This child would most likely be able to complete ADLs, live in a group home setting, and do unskilled work in a sheltered workshop. Answer A describes a child with profound mental retardation, answer C describes a child with severe mental retardation, and answer D describes a child who is mildly mentally retarded and educable. See Reference: Case-Smith (ed). Rogers, SL, Gordon, CY, Schanzenbacher, KE, and Case-Smith, J: Common diagnoses in pediatric occupational therapy.

26. (B) dressing apraxia. To some extent, dressing apraxia is a result of impaired awareness of the affected side and the relation of body parts to the clothing, as well as difficulty with assembly of the clothing onto the body and "...treatment is aimed at ameliorating those deficits." (p. 607). Difficulty with spatial relations (answer A) is a problem with awareness of the relationship of one's self to another object. A person with anosognosia (answer C) is unaware of any deficits. Figure-ground discrimination (answer D) is the ability to distinguish an object from its background. See Reference: Trombly and Radomski. Quintana, LA: Optimizing vision, visual perception, and praxis abilities.

27. (B) stress management. Many addicts use drugs and alcohol as a way to fill leisure time and to manage stress or boredom. When this individual experienced frustration with the birdhouse project, he was unable to manage this stress, became agitated, escaped the challenge, and sought out an addictive substance (the cigarette). Individuals with problems related to eye-hand coordination, visual perception, or fine motor performance (answers A, C, and D) also may have difficulty gluing pieces of a birdhouse together. However, the behaviors described above, in combination with the diagnosis of substance abuse, make answer B the most likely answer. See Reference: Crepeau, Cohn, and Schell (eds). Ward, JD: Adults with Mental Illness.

28. (B) Dressing habits. Certain dressing habits (answer B) may indicate tactile defensiveness, e.g., the child may show poor tolerance of certain textures or avoid wearing turtlenecks, socks, or shoes. Conversely, some children may never take off their shoes in order to avoid tactile overstimulation. Reading skills (answer A), social skills (answer C), and the choice of hobbies (answer D), could be affected secondarily, as a result of intolerance to certain textures or human touch or the inability to concentrate. However, because of the close connection between dressing and tactile tolerance, knowledge of the child's dressing habits will give the OT practitioner the most reliable information. See Reference: Case-Smith (ed). Parham, LD and Mailloux, Z: Sensory integration.

29. (C) attention span and social interaction skills. Conduct disorders often involve aggression toward people or animals and destruction of property. When working with this population, OT typically addresses the areas of attention span, impulse control, age appropriate social role performance, and social skills. Children with developmental delays typically require intervention for perceptual-motor skills (answer A). Multiple role performance (answer D) is more developmentally relevant to adulthood than to adolescence. Although leisure and vocational interests (answer B) may be relevant to the adolescent population, the issues of attention span and social interaction would be more significant for an individual with conduct disorder. See Reference: Early. Understanding psychiatric diagnosis: The DSM-IV.

30. (C) Cluttered spaces in the rooms with apparent limited access to toys. According to Mulligan (2003), "from the moment you enter the child's space or environment (e.g., home or classroom) take note of any specific characteristics that may have potential to enhance or hinder the child's performance. For example, are spaces cluttered or do they appear to allow children to move freely?" (p. 36). Answers A and B are primarily related to behavioral characteristics rather than environmental, while answer (D), observing the child riding his bike, is not considered to be part of the child's household environment. See Reference: Mulligan. Mulligan, S: A guide to evaluation.

31. (A) Functional assessment of work-related skills, such as carrying and opening cartons and shelving items. Observation of the individual performing actual job responsibilities (answer A) will provide more objective and measurable information about the individual's strengths and weaknesses in the area of job performance than a verbal interview (answer C) or task evaluation (answer D). Although a "dirty" medium may be contraindicated when initially working with an individual with OCD of the washing type, it would not be an issue

for this individual because his OCD is of the checking type. There is nothing to indicate the individual has cognitive deficits; therefore, a cognitive evaluation (answer B) would not be indicated. See Reference: Early. Data collection and evaluation.

32. (A) demonstrate appropriate use of sandpaper and hammer while constructing a birdhouse. Assessing if the child can use tools in accordance with their intended purpose, while constructing a birdhouse is most representative of a process performance skill. Process performance skills typically look at the child's ability to modulate his or her energy, temporal, spatial, and object organizational skills. Answers B, C, and D are most representative of performance patterns, such as engaging in self-stimulation behaviors, daily routines, and role performance. In Miller-Kuhaneck, H: Autism: A Comprehensive Occupational Therapy Approach, ed. 2, AOTA Press, Bethesda, MD. 2004. See Reference: Miller-Kuhaneck. Clark, G, Miller-Kuhaneck, H, and Watling, R: Evaluation of the child with an autism spectrum disorder.

33. (A) apply the stimuli beginning at the little finger and progress toward the thumb. The general guidelines for sensation testing are that an individual's vision should be occluded, the stimuli should be randomly applied with intermingled false stimuli (opposite of answer C), a practice trial should be performed before the test, and the unaffected side or area should be tested before the affected side or area (opposite of answer B). With a median nerve injury, the ulnar side of the hand is the uninvolved side, and should be tested first. Also, the tested individual should be given a specified amount of time in which to respond; therefore, answer D is incorrect. See Reference: Trombly and Radomski. Bentzel, K: Assessing abilities and capacities: Sensation.

34. (C) observation of play and upper extremity/hand function. The observation of play and hand function is the most appropriate way to obtain assessment information during infancy and preschool ages. "Much of the assessment, during infancy and preschool, centers around observation of play and hand function" (p. 609). Answers A, B, and D are all appropriate choices after the child is old enough for formal assessment. See Reference: Case-Smith (ed). Gartland, S and DuBois, SA: Occupational therapy in preschool and childcare settings.

35. (D) Aesthesiometer. People with sensory loss in the hand often drop things because they are not receiving adequate sensory input. An aesthesiometer measures two-point discrimination with a movable point attached to a ruler that has a stationary point at one end. The dynamometer (answer B) and pinch meter (answer C) are both used to measure strength.

An individual with a loss of strength would drop heavy, not lightweight items. A goniometer (answer A) is a tool with two arms used to measure movement at a joint. One arm is held stationary while the other arm moves around an axis of 360 degrees. See Reference: Pedretti and Early (eds). Kasch, MC and Nickerson, E: Hand and upper extremity injuries.

36. (A) at the lateral epicondyle of the humerus. The lateral epicondyle of the humerus is the bony prominence on the lateral side of the elbow. The medial epicondyle (answer B) is the bony prominence on the medial side of the elbow. The stationary arm of the goniometer should be positioned parallel to the longitudinal axis of the humerus on the lateral aspect (answer C). The movable arm of the goniometer should be positioned parallel to the longitudinal axis of the radius on the lateral aspect (answer D). See Reference: Trombly and Radomski. Trombly, CA and Podolski, CR: Assessing abilities and capacities: Range of motion, strength, and endurance.

37. (C) The infant is exhibiting ulnar palmar grasp. Ulnar palmar grasp precedes the other types of grasp. The infant first grasps on the ulnar side of the hand against the palm, then with all four fingers against the palm (palmar grasp), and finally the grasp moves to the radial side of the hand (radial grasp). The highest level of grasp is pincer grasp, in which the pad of the index finger meets the opposed thumb. See Reference: Case-Smith (ed). Exner, CE: Development of hand skills.

38. (C) Tip. Tip prehension is accomplished by flexing the IP joint of the thumb, and the PIP and DIP joints of the finger, and bringing the tips of the thumb and finger together. This type of prehension is used to pick up objects such as a pin, nail, or coin. Lateral prehension (answer A) is formed by positioning the pad of the thumb against the radial side of the finger. This prehension pattern is used for holding a pen, utensil, or key. Palmar prehension (answer B), also known as three-jaw chuck, is formed by positioning the thumb in opposition to the tips of the index and middle fingers, forming a pad-to-pad opposition. This form of prehension is commonly used to lift objects from a flat surface and to tie a shoelace. A spherical grasp (answer D) is typically used for holding a ball or other round objects. See Reference: Pedretti and Early (eds). Belkin, J and Yasuda L: Orthotics.

39. (B) Kitchen safety. Short-term memory loss is one of the earliest symptoms of Alzheimer's disease. Because her husband is still working, this individual may want to continue preparing meals. Kitchen safety issues, such as remembering to turn off the stove, would be the most important of the options

listed to evaluate. The awareness of declining abilities may be very frustrating for some individuals, leading to anger, social withdrawal, and depression. There may be a need for anger management strategies (answer C), but this issue is a secondary concern to safety. Difficulty with motor abilities develop as the disease progresses, and the ability to chew and swallow (answer A) may need to be evaluated in the later stages. Severe memory loss (answer D), inability to process information, and loss of communication skills also may develop in the later stages of the disease. See Reference: Crepeau, Cohn, and Schell (eds). Ward, J: Adults with mental illness.

40. (B) Pinch dynamometer. A pinch dynamometer is used to measure the strength of a three-jaw chuck grasp pattern (also known as palmar pinch) as well as key (lateral) pinch and tip pinch. All of these pinch patterns require thumb opposition. For each of these tests, the individual performs three trials, which the evaluator averages together; the result is compared to a standardized norm. An aesthesiometer (answer A) measures two-point discrimination. A dynamometer (answer C) measures grip strength, but is not particularly sensitive to thumb opposition. A volumeter (answer D) measures edema in the hand. See Reference: Crepeau, Cohn, and Schell (eds). Kohlmeyer, K: Sensory and neuromuscular function.

41. (C) demonstrating typical development for a child with Down syndrome. Answer C is correct because exclusive "W" sitting is commonly seen in children with low muscle tone. The child is compensating for an inability to achieve stability in a variety of positions that require dynamic postural control, depending on skeletal rather than neuromuscular structures for stability. Answers A and D are not correct because exclusive "W" sitting would be considered both typical and age appropriate for a 5-year-old child with Down syndrome. Answer B is not correct because exclusive "W" sitting is considered to be a compensatory position. See Reference: Kramer and Hinojosa (eds). Schoen, SA and Anderson, J: Neurodevelopmental treatment frame of reference.

42. (C) initiation. Initiation, or the ability to begin a task, affects a person's spontaneity in performing activities and how much he or she is able to perform. An individual with initiation problems may be able to plan or carry out activities, but may be unable to begin until prompted by another person. Problems with attention (answer A), concentration (answer B), or apraxia (answer D) would be evidenced if the eating activity were performed incorrectly or incompletely. See Reference: Gillen and Burkardt (eds). Arnadottir, G: Impact of neurobehavioral deficits on activities of daily living.

43. (A) Symmetrical tonic neck reflex. The correct answer is A because the symmetrical tonic neck reflex, when present, provides the child with bilateral arm extension and hip flexion with the head raised (and bilateral arm flexion and hip extension with the head lowered), which can be used to move forward. Answers B, C, and D are not correct because these primitive patterns do not assist the child into a quadruped position; rather they primarily affect prone and supine positioning. See Reference: Crepeau, Cohn, and Schell (eds). Kohlmeyer, K: Sensory and neuromuscular function.

44. (C) significantly delayed by several months. Answer C is correct because at 6 to 7 months of age, a child should initiate mature head flexion (head positioned slightly forward) when pulled into a sitting position. The child assists with pulling of the arms and some trunk flexion or use of the abdominals at this age. Usually by 2 months of age, an infant is beginning to assist with being pulled to sit with some head flexion. By 3 to 4 months of age, a child should demonstrate partial head flexion, where the head is in line with the trunk. Answers A, B, and D are not correct because they do not address the significance of the child's delay in head control. See Reference: Case-Smith (ed). Nichols, DS: Development of postural control.

45. (B) emotional lability. Emotional lability is the rapid shifting of moods. Emotional lability may be one of the symptoms observed in individuals experiencing mania (answer A). Paranoia (answer C) describes enduring beliefs about being harmed. Denial (answer D) is not acknowledging the presence of information. See Reference: Cara and MacRae (eds). MacRae, A: Psychopathology and the diagnostic process.

46. (B) compares performance with a normative sample. Norm referencing is a term applied to standardized or formal tests that have been given to a large number of persons in a specific population called the normative sample. When a child is tested with a norm-referenced test, the scores are compared with those of the normative sample; this provides information on how a child performs compared with the average performance of the normative sample. Answers A and D are incorrect. Being "norm referenced" does not guarantee that the test is valid and reliable unless evidence for these characteristics is provided, so answer C also is incorrect. See Reference: Case-Smith (ed). Richardson, PK: Use of standardized tests in pediatric practice.

47. (B) muscle tone, postural tone, pain, and coordination. Muscle tone, postural tone, pain, and coordination are evaluated both through the involved and uninvolved extremity to determine motor control after injury. Answer C, evaluation of vital signs, endurance, and confusion, is associated with evaluation of cardiopulmonary function. Answer D, assessment of self-concept and self-awareness, is related to the psychological impact of trauma. Answer A, developmental factors, pertains to an individual's life experiences and how those experiences relate to coping with the musculoskeletal disorder. See Reference: Pedretti and Early (eds). Preston, LA: Motor control.

48. (B) closed question. Closed questions can be answered with one-word responses such as "yes" or "no." Open questions (answer A) are very broad and can be answered many different ways. Leading questions (answer C) suggest the desired response. A double question (answer D) asks two questions at once or forces a choice. See Reference: Early. Medical and psychological models of mental health and illness.

49. (C) Strength, range of motion, coordination. The biomechanical approach is based on enhancing strength, range of motion, and endurance (answer C). The biomechanical approach is typically used when impairment does not affect the intact central nervous system. This approach is primarily used for individuals who have had a traumatic injury or illness that has affected the musculoskeletal system. The rehabilitative approach (answer A) emphasizes making an individual as independent as possible, compensates for limitations, and incorporates the use of adaptive equipment (answer A). The neurodevelopmental approach (answer B) is used for individuals who are born with a central nervous system dysfunction, have experienced an illness, or have had an injury to the neural system. The neurodevelopmental approach is based on using sensory input and developmental sequences to promote function. Evaluation focuses on tone, reflex development, and automatic reactions. The Model of Human Occupation recognizes that human performance is organized and directed by volition, habituation, and mind-brain-body subsystems. This model emphasizes the importance of habits, values, roles (answer D), interests, and personal causation. See Reference: Trombly and Radomski. Trombly, CA: Conceptual foundations for practice.

50. (B) objective signs and duration of the seizure. In order to assess the efficacy of antileptic medication or during periods of gradual withdrawal, staff members are often asked to monitor the child for seizure activity. Type and duration of seizures should be documented carefully. Observations about the child's position (answer A), responsiveness (answer C), and facial expression (answer D) are important observations, but not as significant as documenting the objective signs and duration of the seizure. See Reference: Case-Smith (ed). Rogers, SL, Gordon, CY, Schanzenbacher, KE, and Case-Smith, J: Common diagnosis in pediatric occupational therapy practice.

51. (D) walking at 1 mph. The MET value for sitting at the edge of the bed is 1.3, and the MET value for walking 1.2 mph is 2. The MET values for peeling potatoes (answer A), propelling a wheelchair at 1.2 mph (answer B), and taking a shower (answer C) are 2.5, 2, and 3.5, respectively. Although it is unrealistic to expect the entry-level practitioner to memorize a MET table, several factors can help the therapist assess the demand of any given task. For example, upper extremity activity work produces a greater cardiovascular response than lower extremity work. Because both peeling potatoes and propelling a wheelchair primarily use the upper extremities, one can deduce that the cardiac demand from those activities would be greater than walking very slowly. Taking a shower not only involves repeated UE use, but adds the environmental factor of heat, which also contributes to the demands on the cardiovascular system. See Reference: Dutton. Introduction to biomechanical frame of reference.

52. (C) on. According to Solomon (2000), "the ability to use the spatial and directional concepts of "in" and "off" usually develops by about 30 months. By about 36 months of age, the infants usually begin to understand the concept of "on" (p. 277), thus making answer C correct. Answers A, B, and D are incorrect, because basic concepts such as "behind," "first," and "last" do not typically develop until age five-and-a-half. See Reference: Solomon (ed). Jones, L. and Machover, P.: Occupational performance areas: Daily living and work and productive activities.

53. (C) Copper tooling using a template. When choosing activities to address self-competence and self-confidence, it is important first to choose activities that are relatively simple, structured, of short duration, and guaranteed to provide a successful experience to the patient. Answers A and B are fairly complex projects that require decision making, several sessions to complete, and have the potential for problems in any of the many stages of construction. Although they may be appropriate later in the treatment program, they are contraindicated at the beginning of treatment. Learning to play bridge (answer D) may be a good choice when addressing development of leisure activities, but it also involves learning a series of steps and interacting with others, requirements that are premature at this stage in treatment. See Reference: Early. Responding to symptoms and behaviors.

54. (A) Independent with a transfer board. An individual injured at the C7-C8 level should be able to perform transfers independently either with or without sliding board. They do not typically require minimal to moderate assistance (answer B). Stand-pivot transfers (answer D) are appropriate for individuals who can come to a standing position and bear some weight on the lower extremities. Individuals with injuries C4 or higher are unable to provide physical assistance during transfers, but may provide verbal direction (answer C). See Reference: Pedretti and Early (eds). Adler, C: Spinal cord injury.

55. (D) is highly structured, facilitating step by step learning. Therapeutic activities should be presented in an environment free from extraneous stimuli to help the child focus on a task. The activities should be carefully graded and presented in a sequence tailored to the sensory capacities and preferences of each child. Stimuli-laden therapeutic environments such as those described in answers A, B, and C can be more beneficial to the child who is better able to use imagination and self-direction than to the autistic child. See Reference: Case-Smith (ed). Rogers, SL, Gordon, CY, Schanzenbacker, KE and Case-Smith, J: Common diagnosis in pediatric occupational therapy practice.

56. (B) An activity exploring leisure opportunities and problems. The OT practitioner can assist individuals in developing self-knowledge of leisure and play preferences (p. 357), which is the first step in making choices about leisure and play participation. Answer B, an activity exploring leisure opportunities and problems, is the best answer because this type of activity could assist this individual in developing knowledge about other leisure opportunities and explore his feelings about engaging in these opportunities. This individual's previous leisure interests are already known, so answer A, a leisure inventory assessment, would be a duplication of information. Answer C, an activity which encourages the individual to sign up for social activities, may not be effective since the individual has indicated no interest in these activities so far. Answer D is premature at this point because the individual has not identified any goals around which to plan future leisure activities. See Reference: Crepeau, Cohn, and Schell (eds). Primeau, LA: Play and leisure.

57. (C) folding laundry. Folding laundry (answer C) challenges balance and upper extremity function in ways that are more functional than stacking cones or throwing a ball. Rather than seeking contrived activities (answers A, B, and D) that challenge single skill deficits, the focus of home care is to find ways for the patient to actually perform the daily activities that are presenting the challenges. Because this patient is the mother of four, it is presumed that her occupational role includes homemaking activities. See Reference: Piersol and Ehrlich (eds). Seibert, C: The clinic called home.

58. (D) A volar pan splint for hand and wrist. A volar pan splint is indicated for the wrist, fingers, and thumb joints during acute synovitis. A wrist stabilization splint (answer B) would be indicated for wrist pain and to protect the extensor tendons from rupture. An ulnar drift positioning splint (answer C) would be used to prevent ulnar drift, while maintaining joint alignment for grasp and pinch activities. A protective MP joint splint (answer A) would assist in keeping the MP joints in normal alignment, while preventing volar subluxation. See Reference: Pedretti and Early (eds). Buckner, WS: Arthritis.

59. (C) Allow the person to perform tasks in a quiet, separate area. An important aspect of intervention for the occupational therapist is the ability to change aspects of the environment to maximize the performance of a client. All of the answer choices are environmental strategies which can have an impact on the ability to become engaged in an activity and can affect performance, but answer C, allowing the person to perform tasks in a quiet area, is most likely allow concentration when a person is easily distracted (p. 32). Answer A, the use of music can be very effective to "shift a person's attention, soothe agitation, and as an aid with visualization techniques" (p. 32), but may provide too much sensory stimulation. Answer B, decreasing the lighting, may help decrease the level of stimulation in the room, but also could encourage relaxation, rather than focused concentration. Answer D, adjusting the temperature and ventilation in the clinic, could enhance the working environment if it were previously too hot and stuffy, but from the question, the human environment seems to be the most distracting feature in the clinic. See Reference: Cara and MacRae (eds). MacRae, A: Environmental and cultural considerations.

60. (C) express disagreement with coworkers in a productive manner. Assertiveness training focuses on developing the ability to "...articulate one's needs while respecting the rights of others" (p. 152) and express feelings in an appropriate and productive manner. Answers A, B, and D are examples of additional social interaction skills; however, they do not address an assertiveness component. Answers A and B are examples of actions taken when engaging in conversation, and answer D is an example of proper social conduct. See Reference:

Bruce and Borg. Behavioral frame of reference-objective perspective.

61. (C) Provide enjoyable activities in a safe and accepting environment. Children who learn to enjoy activities alone will be more likely to cooperate with peers in a group activity. It is unlikely that the child will initiate and develop social interaction in an environment that inhibits independence (answer A). Children with peer interaction problems need to be taught some basic social skills (unlike answer B) in order to increase successful peer interaction. Children will more likely learn and accept rules and limits established by their group than by an authority figure (answer D). See Reference: Kramer and Hinojosa (eds). Olson, LJ: Psychosocial frame of reference.

62. (C) Standing kitchen activities can be performed by placing the majority of weight through both arms, using toes for balance (about 10% of weight). Teaching strategies for weight-bearing restrictions for a person with a total hip replacement is very important when planning to address ADL activities with individuals who have had hip replacement surgery because weight-bearing can affect the healing of the hip joint. Placing the majority of weight through arms, using toes for balance (about 10% of weight), answer C, is the correct guideline for touch-down weight-bearing. Answer A, performing all activities from a sitting position, would reflect non-weight-bearing status. Placing 50% of the body weight on the affected leg during standing activities, answer B, would be the rule for partial weight-bearing. Performing all standing activities without restriction, answer D, is another way of saying the person may be full weight-bearing. See Reference: Crepeau, Cohn, and Schell (eds). Dolfi, Cm Leibold, ML and Schreiber, J: Adult Orthopedic Dysfunction.

63. (C) Deep breathing and verbalization. "Deep (diaphragmatic) breathing involves slowly inhaling and exhaling to reduce tension in the shoulders, trunk, and abdomen...deep breathing is relatively easy to learn, requires no equipment, and can be done anywhere" (p. 641). In addition to this, the act of verbalization, simply talking with friends regarding one's stress, can reduce stress levels. "Friends can offer different perspectives, new suggestions, and support, all of which are helpful in extricating a person from feeling stuck with a problem situation" (p. 641). Answers A and B, autogenic training and meditation, are useful stress management techniques, but both require a considerable amount of time and practice in order to successfully implement. Answer D, work simplification and energy conservation, typically impact endurance and the performance of an actual task. See Reference: Crepeau, Cohn, and Schell (eds). Giles, GM: Stress management.

64. (C) Backward chaining. In backward chaining (answer C) the OT completes all of the steps of a task except the last one. As the child becomes competent, the OT completes all, but the last two steps, and so on, until the child is able to perform the entire activity. This method provides immediate gratification, and is particularly useful for children with low frustration tolerance and poor self-esteem. Physical guidance (answer A) requires the least amount of cognitive ability, and provides the child the opportunity to learn through a sensory motor experience. Verbal cues (answer B) may be perceived as intrusive and critical by children with low self-esteem. Forward chaining (answer D) begins with the child completing the first step and the practitioner completing the rest. When competent, the child progressively takes on more of the steps. This method is beneficial for individuals who have difficulty with sequencing and generalizing skills. See Reference: Case-Smith (ed). Shepherd, J: Self-care and adaptations for independent living.

65. (B) it provides social interaction and support, as well as activity. Parkinson's disease frequently causes social isolation because of decreased mobility and communication; therefore, group treatment is particularly valuable for these clients. Answer A is incorrect because group treatment is not necessarily better for addressing motor problems. Presenting exercise activities (answer C) can be effective in groups, but it would not be the primary reason to select a therapeutic group for clients with Parkinson's. Answer D is incorrect because the therapist is responsible for leading a therapeutic group and would not leave until the group session has concluded. See Reference: Pedretti and Early (eds). Schultz-Krohn, W: Parkinson's disease.

66. (B) journal and diary writing. Although answers A, C, and D would benefit the self-confidence and stress management needs of women struggling with anxiety and other issues associated with emotional and physical abuse, they are not purely expressive activities. Keeping a journal would be most effective in assisting individuals in expressing their inner thoughts, feelings, anxieties, and beliefs. Another benefit of keeping a journal is that it can become the focus of distressing thoughts and may help the person to release the disturbing feelings when the book closed (p. 218). See Reference: Cara and MacRae (eds). Levitt, VB: Anxiety disorders.

67. (A) Meal preparation techniques using a wheelchair. As the disease progresses, individuals with ALS lose the strength required for ambulation, and therefore, begin to use wheelchairs. The development of meal preparation skills using a wheelchair, such as transportation of items, addressing work heights, using adaptive equipment (answer A encompasses answer B), and safety issues, is therefore the best answer. Gradually increasing standing tolerance (answer C) is not appropriate for this individual because motoric function will continue to deteriorate. Developing competence in preparing cold meals before advancing to hot meals (answer D) is more appropriate for individuals with cognitive or perceptual deficits. See Reference: Dutton. Rehabilitation postulates regarding intervention.

68. (A) Anticipating challenges the client may face to plan strategies that will support performance. The supported employment model of services focuses on placing a client in a job of choice and then providing on-the-job training, assessment, and support. Answer A, anticipating challenges the client may face and plan strategies to support performance, is the most useful aspect of pre-employment evaluation information for planning services within this model (p. 599). Participation in graduated or transitional work preparation programs such as prevocational groups (shown to be less effective than the supported employment approach) are not typically part of the supported employment approach; therefore, answer B is incorrect. Answers C and D reflect uses of the assessment data for predicting the client's possible success or failure within a particular job environment and would be less relevant to the OT or mental health team for the purpose of supportive services to client. See Reference: Cara and MacRae (eds). Auerback, ES and Jeong, G: Vocational programming.

69. (B) hook provides better prehensile function and allows greater visibility of objects. The fact that a hook TD provides better prehensile function and allows greater visibility of objects would be the most important consideration for a person whose primary concern is functioning as a carpenter. Answers A, C, and D are incorrect because although they can be important considerations for some people with UE amputations, they are not as relevant to this person's goals. See Reference: Pedretti and Early (eds). Keenan, DD and Rock, LM: Body-powered protheses.

70. (A) promote open-ended symbolic play, such as using action figures, puppets, and dolls. Toys that elicit feelings (answer A) and expression can be used to promote beginning play skills, beginning interaction, and communication skills. Inherent in open-ended play is the fact that there is no right or wrong way and failure is not possible. Structured craft activities (answer B) do not provide sufficient opportunity for self-expression and carry the possibility of failure, because there is a right and wrong way to do them. As an initial activity, a game of tag (answer C), especially one that involves peers, may be perceived as threatening and overwhelming by the child. Activities that promote tension release (answer D) do not directly address play skills, rather, they focus on the powerful motor action only. See Reference: Case-Smith (ed). Morrison, CD and Metzger, P: Play.

71. (D) Eggs. Eggs provide a uniform, "soufflé or semisolid" (p. 524) texture which is an easier consistency to control in the mouth. Answers A, B, and C are all foods that are contraindicated in those with dysphagia diets because vegetable soup and salad (answers A and B) have "mixed textures" (p. 524), and watermelon (answer C) has seeds, all of which require a higher degree of oral manipulation for chewing and swallowing. See Reference: Gillen and Burkardt (eds). Avery-Smith, W: Dysphagia management.

72. (B) vestibular stimulation and gross motor exercise. The sensory integration treatment approach, which aims to improve the reception and processing of sensory information within the central nervous system, uses both vestibular stimulation and gross motor exercises (answer B). Social skills training (answer A), also would be appropriate for an individual with schizophrenia, but for the purpose of developing interpersonal skills. Answer C, life skills would be used for addressing self-care skills and independent living goals, and expressive projects (answer D) might be used when an individual needs opportunities for nonverbal communication and outlets for emotion and creativity. Although these interventions may be a part of the overall treatment program, this type of individual would benefit from being able to receive and process sensory information before embarking on more complex treatment formats. See Reference: Early. Medical and psychological models of mental health and illness.

73. (D) Playing on a trampoline. Postural control refers to the ability to maintain balance during functional movements. Activities that require a child to respond by changing body position to maintain balance encourage the use of postural reactions. Playing on a trampoline would be the best activity, because it requires a child to continuously change body position to adapt to changes in gravity while jumping. Answer A, sliding down a sliding board, would stimulate vestibular processing. Imitating gestures, as in answer B, playing "Simon Says," would facilitate perceptual processing. Swimming, answer C, would be a

good activity to improve a child's endurance. See Reference: Solomon (ed). O'Brien, JC: Play.

74. (C) have the individual visualize the task first and then provide general statements such as "Let's get ready." Answer C is correct because visualizing a task and its movement sequences helps the individual with motor apraxia by giving a visual model to refer to during the activity. Using general comments such as "Let's get ready," rather than specific step-by-step directions, is more effective because individuals with motor apraxia have difficulty imitating or initiating motor tasks on command, though they understand the concept of the task. Answer A, step-by-step commands, would add to the confusion for an individual with motor apraxia, but would be helpful for the individual with ideational apraxia who may not understand the concept of the task, but may be able to perform individual steps of the task on command. Removing visual distractions and enhancing the visual environment, as in answer B, is useful for individuals with visual perceptual deficits, rather than motor apraxia. Answer D, having the individual move slowly and touch objects during the task, is a method aimed at improving spatial relations' perception. See Reference: Gillen and Burkardt (eds). Rubio, K and Gillen, G: Treatment of cognitive-perceptual deficits: a function-based approach.

75. (B) Let the child sit at the front of the bus and use a tape player with earphones. A child who is seated in the front of the bus will experience less jostling by peers, resulting in less tactile and visual stimulation. Also, the earphones will reduce auditory overload. The method described in answer B addresses the underlying problem of the child's low tolerance for sensory stimulation. Answers A, C, and D are behavioral management techniques that do not take the child's hypersensitivity into account. See Reference: Case-Smith (ed). Cronin, AF: Psychosocial and emotional domains.

76. (D) low-impact aerobics three times a week for 1 hour. Based on the information provided, the low-impact aerobics activity is the most client-centered of the choices. Answer A, lifting weights, is considered to be an activity that promotes hyperextension and resistance, possibly leading to increased pain, immobility, and further damage to the joints, in addition to joint pain and fatigue. Answer B, the use of relaxation tapes, would be an appropriate selection for assisting an individual to cope with the potential psychosocial aspects of arthritis. Answer C, vocational retraining, is not indicated based on the information provided. See Reference: Pedretti and Early (eds). Buckner, WS: Arthritis.

77. (A) Ballet. To promote the development of anticipatory control, movement should be slow, predictable, and controlled from a stable base. Participation in a dance class would involve controlled movement from a stable base. Answers B, C, and D are activities that feature faster moving objects whose speed and direction of movement cannot be controlled by the player, and require quick reactions to unpredictable stimuli. See Reference: Case-Smith (ed). Nichols, DS: The development of postural control.

78. (B) Stringing beads for a necklace, following a pattern. This is the only activity of those listed that requires the individual to follow a sequence to achieve the desired outcome. Leather stamping in a random design (answer A) does not require sequencing skills, but does require coordination, visual-motor integration, and strength. Putting together a puzzle (answer C) requires perception of spatial relations. Playing "Concentration" (answer D) requires memory and attention span. See Reference: AOTA: Practice Framework. Table 2. Performance skills—process skills.

79. (D) Playing balloon volleyball. An activity such as balloon volleyball may be graded for improving strength by adding resistance to the arm in the form of weights. Endurance may be improved by adding more repetitions of the movement. Raising the height of the net can increase the range of motion required. Blowing up and tying balloons (answer A) and painting faces on balloons (answer C) are primarily fine motor activities. An individual who throws darts at balloons (answer B) would be able to increase the resistance needed for shoulder strengthening by adding weight to the arms or using balloons with thicker rubber. However, this activity is less suitable to increase the number of repetitions, because the repeated loud noise associated with bursting the balloons would be annoying. See Reference: Pedretti and Early (eds). Breines, E: Therapeutic occupations and modalities.

80. (C) Modify the environment to protect the infant from excessive and/or inappropriate sensory stimulation prior to direct intervention. Preterm infants with histories of maternal drug abuse have multiple sensory needs often resulting in poor self-regulation and behavioral organization. Answers C and D both incorporate sensory integration approaches. However, answer C best demonstrates an initial intervention to promote the neurobehavioral organization required to tolerate direct handling. Answers A and B are important in determining appropriate treatment plans for the infant and family. However, a social work referral should be made after initial assessments are completed to make the most appropriate recommendations for social service involvement, if needed. Although identifying maternal medical status and treatment compliance issues are of great importance to best determine eventual educational and disposition recommendations, it is not the primary sensory intervention focus of the OT team. See Reference: Case-Smith (ed). Hunter, JG: Neonatal intensive care unit.

81. (C) implementing compensatory environmental strategies to maximize safety and function. Interventions directed toward improvement are typically unrealistic when working with individuals diagnosed with progressive cognitive disorders. "Since improvement is not generally expected, therapy seeks to maintain maximum functioning as long as possible through the teaching of compensatory strategies and by careful environmental management." These disorders are characterized by deteriorating courses. A social skills emphasis (answer A) is more appropriate for individuals with schizophrenia. Habit restructuring (answer B) is more appropriate for those with substance abuse disorders. Role resumption (answer D) is more appropriate for those with mood disorders. See Reference: Early. Understanding psychiatric diagnosis: The DSM-IV.

82. (B) play and self-care activities. "When providing OT care for children with terminal illness, the underlying principle is to add quality to their remaining days. There are two performance areas that occupational therapists should address in children with terminal illness: (1) play activities and (2) activities of daily living" (p. 838). Educational activities (answer A) would not address the emphasis of adding quality of life. Play activities help the child to focus interest and express feelings, and may incorporate socialization and motor activities (answers C and D), but neither of these types of activities alone would be the primary goal. Self-care activities allow the child to maintain independence and purposefulness. See Reference: Case-Smith (ed). Barnstorff, MJ: The dying child.

83. (C) Minimizing scar hypertrophy through compression garments and proper skin care. Minimizing scar hypertrophy through compression garments and proper skin care is imperative upon wound closure. Answer A, preventing scar formation via static splinting, is typically performed during the surgical or postoperative phase of treatment. Controlling edema (answer B) and promoting self-care skills (answer D) are not goals directly related to scar management and are more commonly initiated during acute care intervention. See Reference: Pedretti and Early (eds). Utley-Reeves, S: Burns and burn rehabilitation.

84. (B) catching and bursting soap bubbles. This activity involves visually tracking a slow moving target and requires minimal fine motor precision to accomplish a successful "hit." Answers A, C, and D also require visual tracking and eye-hand coordination, but they involve faster moving targets that require immediate, more precise movement. These activities can be used to promote advanced skills as the child's visual tracking ability improves. See Reference: Case-Smith (ed). Dubois, SA: Preschool services.

85. (B) Crafts, games, and self-care tasks. Crafts, games, and self-care tasks can best be described as functional activities that should be a component of hand rehabilitation. Answers A, C, and D are all considered to be adjunct activities that may be implemented as a precursor to functional activities. See Reference: Pedretti and Early (eds). Kasch, MC and Nickerson, E: Hand and upper extremity injuries.

86. (A) restore and maintain performance of self-chosen occupations that support performance of valued occupational roles. The individual's depression is likely to be in reaction to the AIDS disease and major loss of functioning at Stage 4. Stage 4 of AIDS generally means severe physical and neurological changes. Because the change of function can be broad, answer A is the most comprehensive approach. Answers B and C are too restrictive to be a "major focus." Answer D, restoration of work, is typically unrealistic at Stage 4 of AIDS. See Reference: Crepeau, Cohn, and Schell (eds). Pizzi, M and Burkhardt, A: Occupational therapy for adults with immunological diseases: AIDS and cancer.

87. (A) Contrast baths and retrograde massage. Contrast baths cause vasodilation and vasoconstriction, which facilitate a pumping out of the edema. Retrograde massage assists with the facilitation of blood and lymph movement. Answers B and C, hot packs and paraffin, can assist with soft tissue and joint mobility as well as pain, but are often contraindicated in cases where edema is present because the direct heat source increases blood flow to the area, and subsequently increases edema. Answer D, sensory re-education, would address the client's limitations with sensation, not edema, and pendulum exercises are typically performed in a dependent position to increase shoulder ROM, thus potentially increasing edema in the hand. See Reference: Pedretti and Early (eds). Kasch, MC and Nickerson, E: Hand and upper extremity injuries.

88. (A) Arrhythmic and unexpected. Sensory integration treatment is complex and highly individualized, and must be monitored carefully to observe the effects of sensory input of varying types on the individual. Sensory modulation dysfunction characteristics requiring facilitatory sensory input should be unexpected, arrhythmic, uneven, or rapid input (answer A). Answer B is not correct because, although arrhythmic input is excitatory, slow sensory input is inhibitory. Sustained and slow sensory input (answer C) is inhibitory, not facilitatory. Answer D is incorrect because, although facilitatory input is unexpected, rhythmic input is inhibitory. See Reference: Bundy, Lane, and Murray (eds). Lane, S: Sensory modulation.

89. (A) serving from the beverage cart. When distributing magazines, the flight attendant uses negligible reaching, bending, pushing, or pulling movements. Serving from the beverage cart involves pushing and pulling on a horizontal plane, and somewhat more resistive reaching and bending than that required to distribute magazines. Blankets and pillows (answer B) are lightweight like magazines, and would not be considered an upgrade. Putting luggage into the overhead compartments (answer D) would be the final step in the work-hardening process, because it involves the most weight and the riskiest back position. Distributing magazines to half of the passengers (answer C) would be downgrading the activity. See Reference: Pedretti and Early (eds). Smithline, J and Dunlop, LE: Low back pain.

90. (B) Go out for lunch at a fast-food restaurant. Answer B, go out for lunch at fast-food restaurant, is correct because a key principle in intervention for effective transition includes using natural environments and cues, and increasing community-based instruction as the student gets older Classroom-based activities and simulated activities (answers A, C, and D) are not as effective in promoting development of the community member role as activities that actually take place in the community. See Reference: Case-Smith (ed). Spencer, K: Transition services: From school to adult life.

91. (C) prevent deformity. A child with juvenile rheumatoid arthritis will need splinting to prevent deformity (answer C) and maintain range of motion. Hypertonus (answer A) is not a characteristic of this condition. Due to the active nature of the child's condition, increasing range of motion (answer B) may be contraindicated. The correction of deformity (answer D) also may be contraindicated with this child due to the active nature of the disease. See Reference: Case-Smith (ed). Rogers, SL, Gordon, CY, Schanzenbacher, KE, and Case-Smith, J: Common diagnoses in pediatric occupational therapy practice.

92. (D) Removing a nut from a bolt. Answer D describes one type of in-hand manipulation called rotation. Rotation is the movement of an object around one or more of its axes, where objects may be turned horizontally or end over end, with the pads of the fingers, as when one would unscrew a nut from a bolt. Answers A, B, and C are incorrect because they describe activities with no in-hand manipulation that essentially keep an object in a certain position as it is grasped, released, or carried. See Reference: Case-Smith (ed). Exner, CE: Development of hand skills.

93. (A) are more easily performed if coordinated with consistent timing of medications. An individual with Parkinson's disease should learn to effectively utilize the time period of reduced symptoms resulting from medication use to efficiently engage in ADLs. Medications taken regularly and consistently aid the establishment of routines for self-care. Performance of self-care activities before medications (answer B) and stretched out throughout the day (answer D) would not make best use of the medication's positive effects. Answer C is incorrect because it discourages attempts for independent functioning. See Reference: Pedretti and Early (eds). Schultz-Krohn, W, Foti, D, and Glogoski, C: Degenerative diseases of the central nervous system.

94. (D) A pediatric weighted utensil holder. "Children who lack sensory discrimination skills in the hands...use the weighted holder. The weight increases proprioceptive (deep-pressure) feedback to the joints and muscles in the hand and wrist, adding to children's awareness of the position and movement of the hand, fingers, and wrist in relation to the pencil and paper" (p. 264). Answers A and C, a wide pen and soft triangle grip, would assist a child with decreased grip, while answer B, rubber bands, would assist a child who has difficulty opposing their thumb into the web space. See Reference: Solomon (ed). Jones, LMW and Machover, PZ: Occupational performance areas: Daily living and work and productive activities.

95. (B) labels with white print on a black background. White print on a black background is easier to see for individuals with poor vision. Using Braille labels (answer A) is not appropriate for individuals with peripheral neuropathy because they have decreased tactile sensation in their fingertips. A pill organizer box (answer C) is useful for taking pills on schedule and is particularly helpful for individuals who have memory deficits or complex medication regimens. If the pills were presorted in the box, the individual could safely take them without actually identifying them. However, using the pill organizer does not address the issue of medication differentiation. Brightly colored pills (answer D) would make it easier to identify different medications; however,

the therapist has no control over how pills are manufactured and what colors are used. See Reference: Sladyk, K and Ryan, SE (eds). Jamison, PW: A retired librarian with sensory deficits.

96. (D) blowing cotton balls into a target. Children with ADHD have difficulty with sustained attention and effort. Answers A, B, and C require sustained visual vigilance and involve delayed gratification. In contrast, blowing cotton balls into a target is a short-term activity with immediate reward for successful completion; therefore, it responds to the child's dual needs. See Reference: Crepeau, Cohn, and Schell (eds). Florey, L: Psychosocial dysfunction in childhood and adolescence.

97. (A) lying on the left side, propped up with pillows. Using activity analysis, one can deduce that (answer A) lying on the left side, propped up with pillows, is the correct answer. This allows the unaffected right extremities to remain free, and provides weight-bearing to the affected side to assist with tone reduction. The pillows behind the individual allow support, and the individual may lean against the pillows also to provide pressure relief as needed to the affected side, because sensation may be reduced on that side along with movement. Lying on the right side (answer B) would not provide any tone reduction, which is needed during a stressful activity such as sexual intercourse. This position also would impair the movement of the unaffected extremities, which would be needed for activities involving foreplay or applying contraceptive devices. Lying in a supine (answer C) or prone (answer D) position would not provide tone reduction to an individual with spasticity, and could be uncomfortable without many pillows to assist with positioning comfortably. Also, an individual lying prone has less mobility than when he or she is lying on the right side. See Reference: Pedretti and Early (eds). Burton, GU: Sexuality and physical dysfunction.

98. (C) Play activities that incorporate tapping, application of textures, and weight-bearing to the residual limb. Massage, tapping, use of textures, and weight-bearing on the distal end of a residual limb are techniques used to develop tolerance to touch and pressure in the hypersensitive limb. Answers A and B will not affect hypersensitivity, and answer D is incorrect because the child is in the preprosthetic phase and does not yet have access to the prosthesis. See Reference: Trombly and Radomski. Celikyol, F: Amputations and prosthetics.

99. (B) "scoot forward to the edge of the wheelchair." When the OT has the individual scoot forward to the edge of the wheelchair, this helps the individual position the body over the feet and causes the weight to shift forward during a transfer. The individual is much easier to transfer when the weight is shifted forward. If the person attempts to stand up (answer A) from a regular seated position, and the weight is shifted back during a transfer, it may require more than one person to assist with the transfer. Answer C, unfasten the wheelchair brakes, is incorrect because the wheelchair needs to be stabilized in a locked position before standing. Positioning the wheelchair facing the mat table (answer D) allows no room for the OT to stand and assist with the pivot. See Reference: Pedretti and Early (eds). Creel, TA, Adler, C, Tipton-Burton, M. and Lillie, SM: Mobility.

100. (A) Sit straddling a bolster with both feet on the floor. Once the child has learned to sit independently on the floor, an external stabilizing support is no longer necessary (answer D). After having developed independent postural reactions on a stable surface, that is, the floor, the child can further refine sitting skills by learning to maintain posture when placed on an unstable surface (answer A). At first, the child should be left in control of the movement on this surface, and she should have both feet on the floor for maximal stability. Later, these skills can be refined by placing the child on more challenging surfaces, such as on a "hippity-hop" (answer C) or on a scooter pulled by another person (answer B). See Reference: Case-Smith (ed). Nichols, DS: The development of postural control.

101. (D) arm trough. An arm trough would provide a stable surface that would keep the individual's arm in a safe and appropriate position. In addition, an arm trough approximates the humeral head into the glenoid fossa at a natural angle. If the individual has edema in his hand, a foam wedge may be placed in the trough to elevate the hand. A lap tray (answer A) would provide support, but is more restrictive than an arm trough, which should be attempted first. The fact that the individual's arm was seen dangling by the side of the wheelchair indicates that the wheelchair armrest alone (answer B) is inadequate. Answer C, an arm sling, would provide support for his arm, but would immobilize it in adduction and internal rotation. Current literature supports the use of slings only when necessary, such as during ambulation when a flaccid upper extremity may sublux or cause loss of balance. See Reference: Pedretti and Early (eds). Gillen, G: Cerebrovascular accident.

102. (C) further decline. The prognosis for individuals with a progressive form of MS is gradually declining neurological function. Therefore, it is likely that the individual receiving a wheelchair will eventually decline further in functional performance. Improved wheelchair mobility and gains in strength (answers A and D) are not characteristic of progressive degenerative diseases. When ordering a wheelchair for a pediatric or adolescent client, it is important to anticipate growth of the individual (answer B). See Reference: Trombly and Radomski. Copperman, LF, Forwell, SJ, and Hugos, L: Neurodegenerative diseases.

103. (C) Provide project samples for individuals to duplicate. Individuals functioning at Cognitive Level 4 are able to copy demonstrated directions presented one step at a time. Providing a sample to copy (answer C) provides the visual cueing and situation-specific training that is needed at this cognitive level. Individuals functioning at Cognitive Level 3 are capable of using their hands for simple, repetitive tasks (answer A), but are unlikely to produce a consistent end product. Those functioning at Cognitive Level 5 can generally perform a task involving several familiar steps and one new one (answer B). Individuals functioning at Cognitive Level 6 can anticipate errors and plan ways to avoid them. These individuals would be capable of following written directions (answer D). See Reference: Bruce and Borg. Cognitive disability frame of reference-acknowledging limitations.

104. (D) Make sure the child's pelvis is secured in seat. The pelvis is one of the key points of control when positioning a child. Positioning the pelvis securely (answer D) against the back of the seat with a seat belt or an abductor wedge (or both) in the correct angle serves to break up the extensor pattern and facilitates the positioning of the other body parts (answers A, B, and C) so that the child can participate in family games. See Reference: Case-Smith (ed). Shepherd, J: Self-care and adaptations for independent living.

105. (C) Demonstrate how using a shower chair improves safety. Educating the client is the first response the OT practitioner should make. By describing and demonstrating the shower chair and how it makes showering safer, the therapist is conveying the concept that occupational performance is based on the interaction of performance contexts (physical environment) and performance components (the confidence to execute tasks safely). The therapist would then inquire about the client's desire to purchase a shower chair (answer B). Getting into a bathtub is even more dangerous than getting into the shower (answer A) so this is not a viable option. Answer D, explaining that the therapy will increase the client's confidence level, is a subjective belief of the therapist that may not be embraced by the client due to his very valid fear of falling. See Reference:

Piersol and Ehrlich (eds). Seibert, C: The clinic called home.

106. (C) Acknowledge that he uses rituals to cope with anxiety. Individuals with obsessive-compulsive disorder (OCD) perform unnecessary and meaningless actions repeatedly. The OT practitioner should "never criticize the patient's behavior. Instead, recognize that no matter how ridiculous the ritual may appear, it is one the patient uses to cope with anxiety" (p. 240). Telling him the behavior is unnecessary (answer A) will not help him to modify his behavior. Individuals with phobias should be encouraged to talk about their fears (answer B). Individual treatment (answer D) is indicated when an individual cannot tolerate a group environment. See Reference: Early. Responding to symptoms and behaviors.

107. (B) Obtain a raised toilet seat. The individual will most likely continue to require a raised toilet seat for several months in order to avoid flexing the hip past the designated range. A handheld shower (answer D) is not always necessary; however, a shower chair with adjustable legs and grab bars could be helpful. High contrast tape (answer C) may help to make ascending and descending stairs safer for individuals with limitations in vision. Moving items from low cabinets to higher locations may help this individual comply more readily with the necessary hip precautions, but moving objects from high to lower cabinets (answer A) would not. See Reference: Pedretti and Early (eds). Coleman, S: Hip fractures and lower extremity joint replacement.

108. (B) Place a seat belt at a 45-degree angle at the hips. A seat belt correctly placed at a 45-degree angle to the child's hips would inhibit extensor tone. Answer A is incorrect because trunk support from lateral trunk supports is for sideward movement only. Although a wedge-shaped seat insertion (answer C) increases hip flexion more than 90 degrees and inhibits extensor tone, it is not the best choice because it could have the undesirable side effect of tightening hamstrings over time. Answer D is incorrect because, although it may contribute to holding a child in a chair, it does not affect the angle of the hip joint, which is necessary for decreasing extensor tone when sitting. See Reference: Case-Smith (ed). Shepherd, J: Self-care and adaptations for independent living.

109. (D) position the person in an upright posture, making sure head is flexed slightly and in midline. Making sure that the resident is correctly positioned is the first step in addressing eating problems. Improper posture can result in difficulties with swallowing. Depending on the particular problems of the individual, providing adaptive devices (answer A)

may or may not be helpful, but nonetheless would not be the first step given without assessment of need. Observing for swallowing after each bite (answer B) and instructing caregivers as to proper setup (answer C) also would be important steps, but these would occur later in the intervention process. See Reference: Pedretti and Early (eds). Jenks, KN: Dysphagia.

110. (C) Relapse prevention. Relapse prevention (answer A) has become an important part of discharge planning with this population. This approach helps to make people "... aware of potential relapse situations" (p. 523), internal and external relapse triggers and how to use specific coping strategies to avoid relapse into substance abuse. Developing ADL and IADL routines, learning how to use leisure time, and developing social participation skills (answers A, B, and D) are all areas that would be addressed throughout hospitalization, and possibly after discharge as well. See Reference: Creek (ed). Chacksfield, J and Lancaster, J: Substance misuse.

111. (C) Use a tub transfer bench and leg lifter. The use of a tub transfer bench would allow the client to back up to the tub bench, sit, and manually lift the knee over the side of the tub, either by using her own hands or a leg lifter. Answer A, postponing bathing, is not considered a standard course of treatment. Answer B, use of a hand rail, would assist with transfers, but would not address the limitation of knee motion. Answer D, use of a low kitchen stool in the tub, even one with rubber tips, would not be considered a safe or stable selection for transfer training. See Reference: Pedretti and Early (eds). Coleman, S: Hip fractures and lower extremity joint replacement.

112. (D) Role playing a tea party with "Barbie" dolls. Answer D, role playing with dolls, is the most appropriate choice because the OT is encouraging the child to partake in pretend play. "Playfulness, like play, encompasses intrinsic motivation, internal control, and freedom to suspend reality" (p. 296). Role playing is focused primarily on the activity at hand, rather than the end product, such as in answer A (playing a game of "Go Fish") and answer B (playing a game of checkers). Answer C, jumping rope, might frustrate the child secondary to her difficulty with motor tasks. The end goal of an occupational therapy treatment would be to increase the child's play skills in the hopes that the child will begin to interact more comfortably within the home, school and peer environment. See Reference: Solomon (ed). Clifford-O'Brien, J: Play.

113. (B) Provide a large area of personal space, where the person is protected from physical contact with others. Patients who exhibit sexual behaviors may be more likely to think about, and act on, their sexual impulses when they experience close physical contact with others. Answer A would be an appropriate intervention environment for individuals with delusional thinking. The environment described in answer C would be best for people experiencing hallucinations. An environment where all distractions are reduced as much as possible (answer D) is most relevant for individuals exhibiting manic behaviors. See Reference: Early. Responding to symptoms and behaviors.

114. (B) A shower chair and terry bath robe. According to Huntley, "bathing is a particularly strenuous activity because the hot, humid air makes breathing difficult...using a chair in the shower and using a thick terry robe after showering instead of toweling off help to reduce energy expenditure" (p. 1087). Answers A and C would most likely be used by individuals with limited reach and limited grip strength respectively, while use of proper body mechanics (answer D) is important for individuals with back injuries. See Reference: Trombly and Radomski. Huntley, N: Cardiac and pulmonary diseases.

115. (A) Perform pursed-lip breathing when doing activities. Pursed-lip breathing is a technique that narrows the passage of air during expiration. This technique helps individuals with COPD keep the airway open and improves breathing efficiency. The overall effect is improved endurance and tolerance for activities. Taking hot showers and avoiding air conditioning during warm weather (answers C and D) are incorrect in that both activities are contraindicated for individuals with COPD. Using a long-handled bath sponge (answer B) may be helpful, but is not the most likely tip to be on a home program for an individual with COPD. See Reference: Pedretti and Early (eds). Matthews, MM: Cardiac and pulmonary diseases.

116. (C) Simple and highly structured activities. Projective media, isolation, and discussing delusions are all contraindicated for people with schizophrenia. Projective activities (answer A) are most useful for encouraging expression of feelings. It may be appropriate to separate individuals (answer B) who are violent or unable to tolerate the presence of others nearby, but this would not be part of the regular group routine. Discussing delusions (answer D) is undesirable because it is likely to reinforce them. See Reference: Creek (ed). Gardner, M: Cognitive approaches.

117. (D) Use a dust mitt to keep fingers fully extended. Using dust mitts prevents prolonged finger flexion and allows the fingers to remain straight while dusting. Pushing the vacuum (answer A) for-

ward by straightening the elbow completely, then pulling it back close to the body utilizes long strokes and promotes good elbow and shoulder range of motion. When ironing (answer B), trying to get the elbow into full extension helps to maintain elbow range of motion. Keeping lightweight objects (answer C) on high shelves encourages reaching, which helps maintain shoulder range of motion. See Reference: Pedretti and Early (eds). Buckner, WS: Arthritis.

118. (C) Encourage the child to wear a necklace with chewable objects attached. "Excessive biting of inedible objects is a problem often encountered in children with developmental disabilities...a chewy can be extremely helpful for children who bite excessively...the chewy can be worn as a necklace, attached to a belt, or even put in a pocket" (p. 227). Answers A, B, and D will most likely be ineffective when working with a young child with a developmental disability. Implementing answers A and B (verbal feedback and time-out periods) is unlikely to extinguish the behavior, while answer D (waiting until the child eventually gets bitten back) would be considered an ineffective and inappropriate solution to the problem. See Reference: Solomon (ed). Jones, LMW and Machover, PZ: Occupational performance areas: Daily living and work and productive activities.

119. (C) Give him a tour of the OT department and a schedule of activities. Becoming familiar with an environment in advance and knowing what to expect can help reduce anxiety. Reducing distractions and keeping lights low (answer A) may be useful environmental adaptations for individuals with mania or hyperactivity. Providing a stimulating environment and real life activities (answer B) is recommended for individuals experiencing delusions. OT practitioners should leave doors open and avoid being alone (answer D) with individuals who are hostile or violent. See Reference: Early. Responding to symptoms and behaviors.

120. (A) Transfer on and off a commode seat while using a walker. The patient will most likely utilize a walker to transfer on and off a commode seat. In this case, the assistive device (the walker) will permit the patient to adhere to the mandated "touchdown" precautions (10% to 15% of body weight on operated limb), while providing balance, decreasing pain, and encouraging safe transfers. Answer B, bed mobility, should not be performed by rolling and pushing with both heels, because this will most likely increase the patient's pelvic pain. In this case, the patient may benefit from the use of a trapeze attached to the bed to increase the use of both upper extremities, while performing bed mobility. Answer C, eating independently in bed, may be contraindicated. The patient would most likely be encouraged to get out of bed to prevent immobility and risk of pneumonia. Answer D, distal lower extremity dressing, is actually facilitated with devices such as a long handled shoehorn, sock aid, dressing stick, elastic shoelaces and reacher, which help prevent pain and increase independence. See Reference: Trombly and Radomski. Bear-Lehman, J: Orthopaedic conditions.

121. (C) On a tiltboard or bolster. Answer C is correct because "testing equilibrium and protective reactions has typically taken the form of placing the child on a tiltboard or other unstable surface (e.g., ball or bolster). The child's responses to displacement are observed in lateral, anterior, posterior, and diagonal directions" (p. 276). Answers A, B, and D would not permit the therapist to accurately assess equilibrium and protective reactions because of the compromising position in which the child is being placed. See Reference: Case-Smith (ed). Nichols, DS: Development of postural control.

122. (B) Discuss precautions necessary for sex when an indwelling catheter is present. Individuals with an indwelling catheter may safely participate in sexual intercourse when certain precautions are observed. If the catheter becomes kinked or closed off, pressure on the bladder must be avoided and the length of time urine flow is restricted should remain under 30 minutes. It also is advisable to avoid drinking fluids for 2 hours before intercourse and to void the bladder before sexual activity. Sexuality is a part of human performance that OT practitioners should be knowledgeable about and comfortable in discussing. When uncomfortable discussing the topic, the therapist may refer the patient to another team member, which may include the physician (answer A). It is not necessary to remove an indwelling catheter for participation in sexual activity and it is not within the scope of OT practice to teach an individual how to remove one (answer C). See Reference: Pedretti and Early (eds). Burton, GU: Sexuality with physical dysfunction.

123. (B) relaxation exercises while incorporating breaks into the day if using the keyboard frequently. Progressive relaxation exercises (answer B) are the most relevant to the client's shoulder tension. This technique involves "systematic tensing and relaxing of muscle groups to verbal cues" (p. 641). Answer A is for individuals who are unable to distinguish between assertive and aggressive behaviors, and therefore, do not respond assertively when necessary. Answer C is useful for individuals whose irrational beliefs and thought processes lead

to maladaptive behaviors. Answer D applies to individuals who have difficulty selecting effective solutions or identifying the source of their problems. See Reference: Crepeau, Cohn, and Schell (eds). Giles, GM: Stress management.

124. (A) Holding the hammer. Holding the hammer (answer A) is the only activity listed that requires gripping with the entire hand. Holding the stamping tools and needle (answers B and D) requires pinch patterns. Squeezing the sponge (answer C) offers less resistance than holding the hammer, and therefore, would be less effective for strengthening. See Reference: Breines. Folkcraft.

125. (C) An electric toothbrush. According to Case-Smith, "for the child who independently brushes, an electric toothbrush enables more thorough cleaning. This is a good solution for children with limited dexterity, although for children with weakness, an electric toothbrush may be too heavy to manage" (p. 516). Answer A, using a soft bristle brush, would most likely assist a child with tongue thrust, while answer B, attaching a Velcro strap to the toothbrush, would assist a child who has decreased grip strength in the hand. Answer D, encouraging the child to use a soft sponge-tipped toothette, is typically indicated in the child with oral hypersensitivity or defensiveness. See Reference: Case-Smith (ed). Shepherd, J: Self-care and adaptations for independent living.

126. (D) A buttonhook attached to a cuff that fits around the palm. Individuals with C6 quadriplegia may have a tenodesis grasp or no grasp available to them. Therefore, a buttonhook attached to a cuff or possibly, a buttonhook with a built-up handle, are the only appropriate choices. A buttonhook with a knob handle (answer B) or on a 5-inch dowel (answer C) is appropriate for an individual with a functional grasp, but limited dexterity. A buttonhook with an extra long, flexible handle benefits an individual with limited range of motion. See Reference: Trombly and Radomski. Atkins, M: Spimal cord injury.

127. (C) Install an alarm on the client's door. Installing an alarm on the client's door (answer C) would be the preferred intervention to address the issue of wandering. According to Toglia, "adaptation involves changing, altering, or structuring the activity demands or context to prevent disruptive behaviors or accidents" (p. 607). Keeping hallways clear of obstructions (answer B) results in a safer environment for wanderers, but does not prevent wandering. Modifying the environment is preferable to increasing demands on nursing staff (answer D), whereas answer A (applying restraints) would be the last choice for intervention because it interferes with a client's functional independence. See Reference: Crepeau, Cohn, and Schell (eds). Toglia, JP: Cognitive-perceptual retraining and rehabilitation.

128. (B) A dedicated device with 911 auto-dial backup. A dedicated device with 911 auto-dial backup (answer B) is necessary for a person with a high level spinal cord injury; "these systems can activate intercoms, unlock doors, and dial the phone. Individuals should be aware of their vulnerability in power outages and either install uninterruptible power supplies or have a 911 auto-dial back up system" (p. 410). A simple EADL (answer A) does allow independence in operating appliances, lights, and so on through the use of switches or voice control, but would not be a necessity for safety. A remote control power door opener that would allow a caretaker to enter would be useless if the individual is unable to call for assistance. An electric page turner (answer D) is useless without the ability to call for someone to position or replace reading material. See Reference: Trombly and Radomski. Angelo, J and Buning, ME: High-technology adaptations to compensate for disability.

129. (C) Foam tubing around the utensils. Foam tubing would be the best choice (answer C) because it increases the diameter of the utensils, thus permitting an easier grip. Answer A, swivel utensils, are most appropriate for children who experience incoordination or tremors, while answer B, pediatric universal holders, are commonly introduced when a child has no grip at all. In this case, the cuff can be directly attached to the child's hand while the utensils, are inserted into the sleeve of the cuff. Answer D, weighted utensils would not assist the child with decreased grip, but may assist a child with motor incoordination. See Reference: Solomon (ed). Jones, LMW and Machover, PZ: Occupational performance areas: Daily living and work and productive activities.

130. (B) determine if there are any motivational or cultural issues interfering with splint-wear compliance. Prior to fabricating another splint, the OT practitioner must determine if the individual is likely to comply with a new splinting program. Some individuals refuse to wear splints due to cultural norms, while others are simply embarrassed to wear a splint in public. Some people demonstrate a low motivational level in regard to regaining function, while others may overdo their splinting program in the hopes that it will facilitate healing. In the given case, it would not be indicated to fabricate a new splint, answer A, unless the individual agrees to adhere to wearing schedule. Answer C, requesting that the individual find the splint or you will threaten to call his physician, would not be the first step to take in the process. Contacting the physician regarding the individual's non-compliance, as well as providing documentation of performance is indicated, but not something to be used to threaten the individual. Answer D, discharging the individual, would not be appropriate until the therapist discusses the case with the physician and individual. See Reference: Pedretti and Early (eds). Belkin, J: Hand splinting: Principles, practice, and decision making.

131. (A) suggest the individual complete the activity in a seated position. Answer A best represents the process of activity adaptation. The OT practitioner effectively modified (adapted) the activity to address the individual's needs. "Adaptation is a change that facilitates performacne" (p. 481). Answer B, recommending the individual work on ironing prior to folding, is an example of upgrading an activity. However, in this case, the client is in need of downgrading, not upgrading. Answer C is an example of activity analysis. Activity analysis consists of breaking an activity apart in to smaller components, while examining each step of the task. Answer D is representative of clinical reasoning, the problem-solving process that a practitioner implements to reflect upon treatment. See reference: Early: Analyzing, adapting, and grading activities.

132. (A) decreasing the amount of energy expended while working with the computer through an alternative keyboard. According to Cook and Hussey, "the interface between the human and the device can be designed to minimize the amount of fatigue by requiring low energy expenditure. We also can design the device so it is flexible and reduces the amount of effort as the person tires" (p. 85). Answer B addresses other relevant factors in computer use, but none that would directly effect fatigue, while answers C and D do not coincide with the student's independent use of the computer. See Reference: Cook and Hussey. The disabled human user of assistive technology.

133. (C) Trim lines of the splint should extend proximal to the MCP crease. Trim lines of a splint that extend proximal to the MCP crease allow for adequate MCP digit extension and flexion. Answers A, B, and D fall distal to the MCP crease, thus restricting full extension and flexion of the digits at the metacarpal heads. See Reference: Pedretti and Early (eds). Bekin, J and Yasuda, L: Orthotics.

134. (A) rote repetition of the task sub-steps with gradually fading cues. Functional skill training focuses on mastery of a specific task. It requires the client to repeatedly practice the sub-steps of a task with the number of cues given for each step gradually decreasing or fading. Answer B, fine-motor activities, is incorrect because the functional training approach does not emphasize underlying performance components. Answer C, caregiver training, and answer D, use of instructional cards, represent adaptation and compensation approaches, rather than actual skill training. See Reference: Crepeau, Cohn, and Schell (eds). Toglia, JP: Cognitive-perceptual retraining and rehabilitation.

135. (A) 3 years. According to Solomon, "mobility devices can be introduced successfully at any age... therefore children should be introduced to mobility at as young of an age as possible...the younger the better" (p. 340). Since this child has no cognitive issues, answer A would be correct. Answers B, C, and D are incorrect because the power wheelchair can first be considered at a much earlier age since no cognitive delay is present. See Reference: Solomon (ed). Clayton, K. and Mathena, CT: Assistive technology.

136. (C) A phone with extra large buttons. "Phone companies offer adapted phone systems for children and adults who have various limitations... some phones have extra large buttons for those with incoordination or visual impairments" (p. 267). A phone with extra large buttons would most likely be the best solution for the child with mild visual impairments who desires to use the phone without assistance. Answers A, B, and C would assist individuals who are unable to hold the phone independently due to incoordination, weakness, or loss of function in the hand or upper extremity. See Reference: Solomon (ed). Jones, LMW and Machover, PZ: Occupational performance areas: Daily living and work and productive activities.

137. (C) train the client in the operation of the assistive technology system and in strategies for its use. Training activities in the use of the assistive devices are the next critical step after setup of the system, and are essential because the complex nature of assistive technologies can require many hours of practice to master. Evaluating how well the whole system works (answer A) usually occurs after training is completed during the follow-up phase. Evaluating the match between the client and the technology (answer B) is done earlier in the process to ensure maximum success and because expensive technological devices may only be ordered once. Funding sources (answer D) also are determined before ordering equipment. See Reference: Pedretti and Early (eds). Anson, D: Assistive technology.

138. (A) baking brownies. A correctly sequenced progression of difficulty in meal preparation is access a prepared meal; prepare a cold meal; prepare a hot beverage, soup, or prepared dish; prepare a hot one dish meal; and prepare a hot multi-dish meal. Making a fresh fruit salad (answer D) is a less challenging activity, because no cooking is involved. Although both involve heating an item, preparing toast (answer C) is simpler than heating soup because opening a plastic bag is a less complex task than opening a can. Baking brownies (answer A) is slightly more complex, because of the progression from stove top to oven, and the addition of several ingredients that need to be mixed. Therefore, this would be the appropriate upgrade. Making an apple pie (answer B) requires a higher level of task performance and complexity than brownies, and would be an appropriate task after the individual demonstrates competence in the less complex task of baking brownies. See Reference: Solomon (ed). Occupational performance areas: Daily living and work and productive activities.

139. (C) Lateral trunk supports. Lateral trunk supports (answer C) would help maintain correct alignment of the pelvis and trunk in the wheelchair. Answer A, a reclining wheelchair, would shift the child's weight posteriorly, but would not prevent lateral shifting of the trunk. An arm trough (answer B) would probably contribute to lateral shifting although bilateral arm troughs or a lapboard could help maintain a more centered trunk position. Lateral pelvic supports (answer D) would stabilize the pelvis and prevent it from shifting sideways, but would be too low to prevent the trunk from moving laterally. See Reference: Pedretti and Early (eds). Adler, C and Tipton-Burton, M: Wheelchair assessment and transfers.

140. (D) Recommend that the girl wear an emergency alert system pendant around her neck. An emergency alert system would be the most likely solution for the OT to recommend to the family. "Emergency alert systems, worn as pendants or stabilized on wheelchairs, are available for purchase with a service that places emergency calls when the system is activated" (p. 518). This intervention would be most effective because it can be placed on the client's body and does not require a great deal of dexterity to manipulate. This also would be especially appropriate if the teenager's parents were not home when the fire occurred. Answer A, positioning a wireless cell phone near the girl, may be an effective solution, but would not be of much assistance if her dexterity is limited, in that she may not be able to push the buttons effectively. Answer B, establishing a quick exit routine in the event of a fire, is something that the OT and the client's family should address, but in the event that no family members are home with the client when a fire occurs is potentially hazardous. While answer C, educating the client regarding fire prevention within the home, is something that should be reviewed by the OT, it does not address the immediate needs of responding to an actual fire via an emergency call system. See Reference: Case-Smith (ed). Shepherd, J: Self-care and adaptations for independent living.

141. (B) have the resident dress in bed with garments that are stretchy and one size larger than usual, and then preview each step of the process with the resident. The resident who is resuming the dressing activity has low endurance as well as cognitive deficits so they would most likely benefit from an adapted, structured approach. Dressing in bed will require less energy initially, and the larger, stretchy garments will make dressing easier. Reviewing each step before it occurs will provide cognitive cues. Answer A, having the client only select clothing, does not provide enough participation to be therapeutic. Answers C and D are too demanding and do not provide the structure necessary to ensure safety and successful performance. See Reference: Hellen. Daily living care activities.

142. (B) good hand strength, range of motion, and perceptual awareness. According to Shepherd (2001), "children performing catheterizations or bowel programs may have difficulty in any of the following areas: maintaining a stable yet practical position, hand dexterity, perceptual awareness, strength, range of motion, and stability and accuracy when emptying collection devices" (p. 509), answer B. Answer A is typically indicated in a child with mental retardation, while answers C and D (bidets and reducer rings) are toileting adaptations commonly utilized to assist with cleansing and positioning on the toilet. See Reference: Case-Smith (ed). Shepherd, J: Self-care adaptations for independent living.

143. (D) deeply inhale and slowly exhale. Deep breathing can be learned quickly and may be effective in reducing tension in the shoulders, trunk, and abdomen. Progressive relaxation exercises, another method of stress reduction, involve a series of isometric exercises of systematically contracting and relaxing selected muscle groups (answer A). Meditation, which may take many months to learn, involves focusing on a word or phrase to reduce stress (answer B). Aerobic activity (answer C), which can reduce pain and relieve stress, involves repetitive contraction of the large muscles of the arms and legs. See Reference: Crepeau, Cohn, and Schell (eds). Giles, GM: Stress management.

144. (D) Give the individual a rest break. Fatigue may cause additional structural damage in the acute stage of MS, and therefore should be avoided. Rest breaks need to be scheduled to avoid fatigue. Strengthening activities (answer C) do not need to be discontinued, but should be designed to benefit the patient without causing undue fatigue. See Reference: Dutton. Biomechanical postulates regarding intervention.

145. (A) elevate the arm on pillows so it rests higher than the heart. Elevation, contrast baths, retrograde massage, pressure wraps, and active range of motion are effective methods for managing edema. When massaging an edematous extremity, stroking should be performed from the distal area to the proximal, not the reverse (answer B). Because active and PROM can both be beneficial to managing edema, instructing the patient to avoid range of motion activities (answers C and D) would be incorrect. See Reference: Pedretti and Early (eds). Kasch, MC and Nickerson, E: Hand and upper extremity injuries.

146. (B) Resting pan splint. A resting pan splint is the most appropriate splint to fabricate for the maintenance of a functional hand position. Answer A, a bivalve cast is typically utilized when circumferential pressure of a body part is required to maintain a desired position. Areas that commonly benefit from bivalve casts are digits, wrists, and knees. Answer C, dynamic extension splint, is not considered to be a static splint, but a splint with moving parts (dynamic). This splint incorporates outriggers to maintain a position of function. Answer D, a wrist cock-up splint, does not impact the position of the entire hand due to the splints distal aspect terminating at the MCP crease. See Reference: Pedretti and Early (eds). Belkin, J, and English, CB: Orthotics.

147. (C) Work hardening. Work hardening programs (answer C) are designed to include and/or simulate job related tasks that gradually progress the individual to obtain the skills that meet the actual demands of a job. Continuing to perform a home exercise program and discontinuing OT services (answers A and D) would probably not enable the individual to return to the work force after a 3 month absence. Home health OT (answer B) is only appropriate for individuals who are unable to leave their homes to attend outpatient occupational therapy. See Reference: Pedretti and Early (eds). Burt, CM: Work evaluation and work hardening.

148. (B) Teach the child to sit in a chair with a back support, lift the affected leg onto a stool, and use socks with a wide opening. "For a child with hemiplegia or limited balance, sitting with back support may be the best starting position for putting on and removing socks. The child lifts the affected leg onto a box or step to bring the foot closer to the unaffected hand...a wide sock opening can prevent frustration during the most difficult part of putting on socks" (p. 235). Answer A, encourage the child to wear tight fitting socks, would make it more difficult for the child to put on and take off his or her socks. Answer C, encouraging the child to request assistance from his mother and answer D, placing the unaffected foot on a small stool, would not assist in dressing skills independence for this child. See Reference: Solomon (ed). Jones, LMW and Machover, PZ: Occupational performance areas: Daily living and work and productive activities.

149. (A) Give the individual a specific task such as filling up the water containers. Assigning a specific and concrete task allows the individual to focus on the task at hand, while sending the message that the individual is a valued member of the group. Giving the individual control over other group members (answer B) feeds into the individual's issues. Pairing the individual with another group member (answer D) will give the other person little opportunity for involvement. Limiting participation to observation (answer C) will only increase the individual's frustration and lead to feelings of isolation. See Reference: Early. Group concepts and techniques.

150. (D) Just before discharge. Because the prognosis for patients with Guillain-Barré syndrome is usually good, equipment should be ordered just before discharge to accurately determine the individual's needs. Equipment ordered during the first week of therapy, or as soon as approved (answers B and C), may not be necessary at the time the individual is discharged. Although collaborating with the patient and family on decisions about ordering equipment is essential, acceptance of the disability (answer A) may not necessarily correspond with the appropriate time for ordering equipment. See Reference: Pedretti and Early (eds). Lehman, RM and McCormack, GL: Neurogenic and myopathic dysfunction.

151. (A) increased wrist extension, such as carrying dishes on a tray at shoulder height. Intratunnel pressure is lowest with the wrist in the neutral position. Wrist extension (answer A) and wrist flexion both increase pressure and may increase symptoms. Ulnar deviation (answer C) and radial deviation (answer D) are unlikely to impact the median nerve as it passes through the carpal tunnel. See Reference: Mackin, Callahan, Skirven, Schneider, and Osterman (eds). Evans, RB: Therapist's management of carpal tunnel syndrome.

152. (D) Obtain a narrower wheelchair because this one is now too wide. The recommended wheelchair seat width is 2 inches wider than the widest point across the hips and thighs of the seated individual. If the seat is 2.5 inches wider than the individual, it is too wide, not too narrow (answer A). In addition, the width of the wheelchair should be kept as narrow as possible. The narrower the wheelchair, the easier it is to maneuver. Because a narrower wheelchair would be better, padding the sides (answer C) is a less desirable option. The need to lose or gain weight (answer B) should be discussed first with an individual's physician. See Reference: Pedretti and Early (eds). Creel, TA, Adler, C, Tipton-Burton, M, and Lillie, SM: Mobility.

153. (D) perform skin conditioning techniques. Skin conditioning techniques such as massage and lubrication with a water-based cream or lotion are essential in preventing damage to newly healed skin for individuals who take more than 2 weeks to heal. Wound debridement (answer A) begins in the acute phase of treatment, and does not necessarily need to be performed prior to ADL training. Compression garments (answer B) are worn constantly and should not be removed for anything other than bathing and skin care. Compression garments "are beneficial for desensitization, general skin conditioning, edema control, and early scar compression. Upper extremity strengthening (answer C) may be part of the treatment plan, but does not need to be performed prior to ADL activities. See Reference: Pedretti and Early (eds). Reeves, SU: Burns and burn rehabilitation.

154. (D) practitioner who encourages group members to share similar situations and reactions with one another. Answer D is an approach designed to develop cohesiveness and universality among members. Seeing others as similar has been identified by individuals as a curative factor. Answers A and C are approaches designed to impart information. Answer B is an example of catharsis, which may not be helpful to all members and requires the practitioner to understand precautions for the use of catharsis. See Reference: Posthuma. The small group in counseling and therapy.

155. (B) understand basic concepts related to money. According to Newman, "individuals who have moderate mental retardation are usually able to attain skills of a second-grade student, which include the following: writing names in cursive, reading simple texts...understanding basic concepts of money" (answer B) (p. 133). Answers A, C, and D are most representative of a child with mild mental retardation who is functioning at the fourth or fifth grade level. See Reference: Solomon (ed). Newman, D: Mental retardation.

**156. (D) "The client asks for more beverages during meals and appears surprised when the

OT practitioner indicates beverages in closed containers are on the meal tray." The subjective portion of the SOAP note should contain information gained through a chart review or communication with the patient, his or her family, or staff. This information is not measurable, and therefore is considered subjective (answer D). Answer A would be in the program plan. Answers B and C would be in the objective portion of the notes because they are either measurable or based on specific observations. See Reference: Borcherding. Writing the "S" - Subjective.

157. (A) Postural hypotension. A frequent side effect of neuroleptic drugs is a decrease in blood pressure in response to sudden movements, specifically up and down, resulting in faintness or loss of consciousness. The parachute activity involves significant up and down body movements, and therefore, warrants the therapist's full attention with this patient population. Answers B, C, and D also are potential side effects of antipsychotic medications, but would usually not be problematic with parachute activities. See Reference: Stein and Cutler. Medications related to psychosocial issues.

158. (D) identify alternative methods for meeting sexual needs that do not cause pain. Because the individual's pain cannot be seen or felt by the sexual partner, communication is particularly important. The couple can discuss alternative positions and methods for achieving sexual fulfillment that are acceptable to them and do not cause pain, such as alternate positions, masturbation, and fantasy. Good communication will ensure the needs of both partners are met and will prevent misunderstandings. Therefore, answer C is inappropriate. A pain-free position is important for successful sexual expression, but there is insufficient information to determine whether answer A, a side lying position, is a pain-free position for this individual. Timing sex for periods of high energy (answer B) is an appropriate strategy for individuals with low endurance. However, timing sex for periods of lessened pain, such as after taking pain medication, may be a useful strategy for individuals with severe pain. See Reference: Pedretti and Early (eds). Burton, GU: Sexuality and physical dysfunction.

159. (D) Finishing a prefabricated wood birdhouse from a kit. A person experiencing a manic episode is likely to exhibit high energy levels, short attention span, poor frustration tolerance, difficulty delaying gratification, and making decisions. Finishing a prefabricated wood birdhouse would be the most appropriate activity because it is a short-term, concrete, predictable activity with a few steps which provides high likelihood of success. It also can be carried with the person if he or she needs to get up and move around during the activity. Answer A, a needlepoint project, would require too high a degree of attention to detail for guaranteed success. Answer B, making a clay object, uses an unpredictable material and requires creative decisions, both of which are qualities that should be avoided. Answer C, watercolor painting, would not be a good choice because it is an unfocused activity involving artistic skill performance that could lead to frustration. See Reference: Cara and MacRae (eds). Cara, E: Mood disorders.

160. (A) flex the child's hips. Flexing the hips breaks up the extensor pattern, and combined with knee flexion, reduces tone in the lower extremities, thus facilitating dressing. Flexing more distal joints first (answers B, C, and D), is ineffective in reducing tone and may lead to excessive stress on the joints involved. See Reference: Case-Smith (ed). Shepherd, J: Self-care and adaptations for independent living.

161. (D) An electronic augmentative communication device. An augmentative communication keyboard is a high-technology aid that can compensate for expressive deficits and assist a student with communication, answer D. Answer A is incorrect because an environmental control unit is a device that allows a person with severe disabilities to operate appliances or devices. It may be used to turn on a tape recorder for note taking, but it would not be used as the primary method for conversation and graphics in the classroom. Answers B and C are incorrect because both the Wanchik's writer and a head pointer are low-technology aids for communication, rather than high-technology devices. See Reference: Trombly and Radomski. Angelo, J. and Buning, ME: High-technology adaptations to compensate for disability.

162. (B) offer even-tempered acceptance, reflecting back what is heard without agreeing that the situation is hopeless. Answer B is a good example of an empathetic response that validates the individuals' feelings. This is the best approach to use with individuals with depression. In contrast, a cheerful approach (answer A) can be perceived as denying the importance of the person's feelings. Silence (answer C) also may be perceived as unaccepting. Answer D is incorrect because the OT practitioner needs to provide the structure because initiating and maintaining discussions is often difficult for depressed individuals. See Reference: Cara and MacRae (eds). Cara, E: Mood disorders.

163. (B) detachable armrests. Detachable armrests (answer B) need to be removed to allow the individual to move sideways out of the wheelchair. Footrests (answer A) may be swung away, but do not need to be detached to perform a transfer. Anti-tip bars (answer C) prevent a wheelchair from tipping over backwards (such as when performing a "wheelie" or when going up or down a step), but not when transferring. Brake handle extensions (answer D) allow the brakes to be locked more easily, but would be in the way of a board transfer. See Reference: Pedretti and Early (eds). Adler, C and Tipton-Burton, M: Wheelchair assessment and transfers.

164. (A) whether the areas of concern to the OT interfere with the child's education. Related services are defined as services needed to help a student benefit from education. If the student's disability no longer interferes with education, OT as a related service can be discontinued. Functional skills (answer B) and independence in ADL (answer C) may be ongoing goals in therapy as provided in a rehab setting or hospital, but would not be provided as a related service in schools. Accessibility of the learning environment (answer D) is an important concern, but it would be covered by consultation with the school or teacher, not through direct service provision. See Reference: Case-Smith (ed). Case-Smith, J, Rogers, J, and Johnson, JH: School-based occupational therapy.

165. (B) 1 foot of ramp for every inch of rise in height. According to the ADA Accessibility Guidelines for Buildings and Facilities, the maximum slope for a ramp should be 1:12. A foot of ramp for every inch of rise in height would be the maximum amount of incline to allow for independent and safe navigation by an individual using a wheelchair. Answers A, C, and D would all make extremely short and steep ramps, which would be either unsuitable or unsafe for an individual independently entering or exiting a home. See Reference: Trombly and Radomski. Pierce, S: Restoring competence in mobility.

166. (D) suggest a more realistic activity. Manic individuals are often unaware of their problem areas, and therefore tend to make grandiose or inappropriate choices. This lack of awareness may make it difficult for the individual to recognize or accept anyone telling him that his attention span is too limited (answer B). Whereas a depressed individual may need support for his choices (answer A), a manic individual may need to be redirected. However, it is not the type of tool that is problematic (answer C), but the qualities of building a clubhouse related to cost, space, time, complexity, and possibly skill. See Reference: Early. Responding to symptoms and behaviors.

167. (B) Pants with an elastic waistband. According to Solomon, "pants or skirts with elastic waistbands are the easiest to put on and remove. Waistbands may need to be fairly loose for children

with severe weakness, abnormal movement patterns, or incoordination" (p. 232). Answers A, B, and C typically make dressing and undressing easier, but due to this particular child's incoordination and weakness, elastic waistbands would be the most effective method to introduce in order to promote independence with this particular dressing skill. See Reference: Solomon (ed). Jones, LMW and Machover, PZ: Occupational performance areas: Daily living and work and productive activities.

168. (D) Block out all areas of a page except important words. Answer D is correct because this compensatory technique is a way of dealing with visual figure-ground or visual discrimination problems. The child needs to learn how to rule out extraneous stimuli and focus on the important area of a task, such as reading. Answer A is not correct because this is a technique used to orient a child with left-right visual tracking problems. Answer B is not correct because it is a technique used to deal with visual attention problems. Answer C is not correct because it is a technique used to help children deal with visual memory problems. See Reference: Kramer and Hinojosa (eds). Todd, VR: Visual information analysis: Frame of reference for visual perception.

169. (B) Adaptive equipment/ADL needs in the classroom. The most essential information for parents and teachers to receive from the OT is how to provide adaptations for the child in the classroom, along with information on the client's ADL status and how JRA symptoms may affect the child's ability to participate in school activities. Information on the OT evaluation (answers A and C) and progress in OT (answer D) are of lesser importance, and may be unimportant in terms of the child's current functional problems. See Reference: Case-Smith (ed). Rogers, SL, Gordon, CY, Schanzenbacher, KE, and Case-Smith, J: Common diagnoses in pediatric occupational therapy practice.

170. (A) ease the patient onto the floor. Proper body mechanics must be used when transferring patients, and OT practitioners should not attempt a transfer that seems unmanageable because of the discrepancy between the patient's size and her own or because of the patient's level of dependency. Attempting to continue or reverse the transfer of an obese patient who has already begun to slip (answers B and C) is likely to result in injury to the OT and perhaps to the patient as well. Once the patient has started to slip, the OT should immediately begin easing him to the floor. Although calling for assistance is an appropriate action, the higher priority action is to begin easing the patient to the floor to prevent injury to the individuals involved. See Reference: Trombly and Radomski. Pierce, S: Restoring competence in mobility.

171. (B) Tell the client that you don't mind appropriately discussing sexuality-related questions as long as his parents are comfortable with the idea. "While working with adolescents on personal self-care tasks such as bathing or personal hygiene, sexuality questions may arise. Children and adolescents of all disabilities are sexual beings. Their parents may be receptive to discussing their child's sexuality, or they may feel unprepared to address these issues. When the child is less than 18 years of age, parental permission to discuss sexuality issues is necessary" (p. 518). Answer A, referring the client to a psychologist, would be an appropriate response if the parent's agreed to the idea, and if the treating clinician did not feel comfortable or knowledgeable regarding the topic of sexuality. Answer C, attempting to change the subject, may encourage the child to feel inadequate, frustrated or more confused regarding his sexuality. It is important to remember that "children of all disabilities are sexual beings" (p. 518). Answer D, answering the client's questions, would only be appropriate after seeking the permission of the child's parents to discuss the topic of sexuality. See Reference: Case-Smith (ed). Shepherd, J: Self-care and adaptations for independent living.

172. (D) Encourage group members to share similar experiences and reactions with each other. Answer D is a strategy designed to develop cohesiveness among members and facilitate learning new skills from others by hearing their experiences and offering feedback in a trusting environment. Many people have reported that recognizing one's similarities with other people is a very valuable experience. Answers A and C are designed to impart information. Answer B is an example of catharsis, which may not be helpful to all members. Moreover, the OT practitioner must be aware of, and understand, the precautions necessary for the use of catharsis. See Reference: Cara and MacRae (eds). Cara, E: Groups.

173. (B) Tip the wheelchair backward and guide it down the ramp forward. This is the recommended technique for going down a steep ramp. The individual sitting in the wheelchair also can help to control the wheels if capable of doing so, by grasping the hand rims. It would be difficult for the person guiding a wheelchair backward down a ramp (answer A) to see where he or she is going. Only extremely strong individuals can propel themselves independently down a steep ramp (answer C). Using two peo-

ple to move a wheelchair down a steep ramp could be awkward and dangerous (answer D). See Reference: Pedretti and Early (eds). Adler, C and Tipton-Burton, M: Wheelchair assessment and transfers.

174. (D) Having him place his feet through loops of therapeutic band. Preparatory methods, "Prepare the client for occupational performance. Used in preparation for purposeful and occupation based activities" (p. 628). Answer D is an example of an activity that simulates the activity of putting pants on and so provides practice in the necessary motor patterns needed to attempt the occupation of donning pants. Answers A and B are examples of purposeful activity. Removing socks (answer C) is an activity that practices the opposite skill, removing feet from something. See Reference: AOTA: Practice Framework. Table I. Types of occupational therapy interventions.

175. (A) Modifying the environment to protect the infant from overstimulation and inappropriate stimuli. Answers B and D represent traditional OT rehabilitation with an emphasis on specific diagnoses, developmental delay, immature sleep-wake state acquisition, limited ROM, and splint fabrication. This approach will continue to be of importance within the NICU. However, the developmental support care approach has expanded the traditional rehabilitation model to include and focus upon a protective and preventative component, which best defines occupational therapy in the NICU in the year 2000. Therefore, answer A best describes a protective and preventative approach to intervention in the NICU. Answer C, educating parents and staff, is a crucial aspect of both the traditional rehabilitation model and the Developmental Support Care approach to implementing services in the NICU. However, it is not the best descriptor of an occupational therapist's scope of practice. See Reference: Case-Smith (ed). Hunter, JG: Neonatal Intensive Care Unit.

176. (B) providing staff education, recommendations, and support for restraint alternatives. Providing education on the effects of restraints, and recommendations, and program support for alternatives to the use of restraints, such as activities, distraction techniques, and environmental adaptations would be the most appropriate functions for the OT practitioner to provide. Answers A, C, and D would be elements of a facility's restraint reduction efforts, but would not be likely to be performed by the OT practitioner. See Reference: Hellen. Physical wellness: Mobility and exercise.

177. (C) recommend activities to develop fine coordination that teachers can incorporate into

classroom programming. The role of the consultant is to provide services that will help to solve problems by, "identifying and analyzing issues, developing strategies to address problems, identifying resources..." (p. 938). Recommending classroom activities that will develop the performance skill area of fine motor coordination would be an appropriate consultant recommendation of strategies to address the problem and the best population-based intervention because it involves addressing the occupational performance needs of many students. Answers A, B, and D focus OT efforts on individual or direct intervention approaches. See Reference: Crepeau, Cohn, and Schell (eds). Jaffe, EG and Epstein, CF: A consultative approach to occupational therapy practice.

178. (C) Programs emphasizing engagement in social and productive activities. Engagement in social and productive activities, answer C, have been shown in research to "lower the risk of all causes of mortality as much as fitness activities do" (p. 41), and are more appropriate for the capabilities of this population than physical fitness programs (answer A). Answer B, educational programs for safety and answer D, assistive technology training, may both be useful to segments of the multiply-handicapped the population in addressing specific issues, but will not have the overall impact on wellness that the focus on social and productive activities will have. See Reference: Crepeau, Cohn, and Schell (eds). Wilcock, AA: Occupational therapy practice Section II: Population interventions focused on health for all.

179. (C) Work simulation to increase strength and endurance for necessary work-related skills. Work simulation is considered to be a primary goal of work hardening, in addition to increasing productivity and feasibility through work-simulated activities. Answers A and B, ADL retraining and progressive resistive exercises, are not typical goals associated with the description of a work hardening program. Answer D, vocational retraining, is incorrect. It is vital that a work hardening program be viewed as an adjunct to vocational retraining, not as a vocational training program in and of itself. OT practitioners typically measure and assess a client's overall physical ability to perform the requirements of a particular job. See Reference: Pedretti and Early (eds). Burt, CM: Work evaluation and work hardening.

180. (A) negotiate a contract. Many OT practitioners have moved into consultation roles. Once the practitioner has gained entry into the system, the next step in the consultation process should include negotiation of a contract. This immediately establishes the general terms of agreement and a focus of the activities that are to be completed by the therapist. Establishing trust (answer B), assessing the problem (answer c), and developing goals (answer D) should follow after the contract has been negotiated. See Reference: McCormack, Jaffe and Goodman-Lavey (Eds). Epstein, CF and Jaffe, EG: Consultation: Collaborative interventions for change.

181. (A) Reminiscence groups. In a reminiscence group, the focus is on providing social opportunities for sharing life stories and feelings, expressing pride in past life experiences, and gaining support for past life difficulties, all of which would enhance self-esteem and help the residents achieve acceptance of past and present life. Answers B, C, and D would address some of the goals stated, but not as comprehensively as a reminiscence group. See Reference: Hellen. Appendix 9-10: Activity therapy care conference report form information: Therapeutic value.

182. (B) develop a plan with staff to change the social environment to one that will enhance motivation and activity levels. Answer A, "provide occupational therapy treatment to increase occupational performance in the areas identified," would represent direct service; answer C, "design a range of living skills groups so that every resident will be included," would represent a program development approach, and answer D, "help the residents to achieve personal goals, make decisions or change behaviors," would be more typical of a counseling role. All of these are levels of occupational therapy intervention, but answer B, "develop a plan with staff to change the social environment to one that will enhance motivation and activity levels," is correct because it best reflects the scope of the consultant with populations in community-based practice, which is to provide, "problem solving in [the] area of concern" (p. 350). See Reference: Scaffa, ME (ed). Scaffa, ME, Russel, V and Brownson, CA: Future directions in community-based practice.

183. (A) Activities that promote mother-child communication and foster attachment. When working with the mother of infants, it is most important to develop the bond between mother and baby. Many of the mothers in this type of program engage in high-risk behaviors, including unprotected sex and substance abuse. They often have poor leisure skills, limited or no knowledge of child development, and do not know how to play appropriately with their children. Low frustration tolerance and limited awareness can result in inappropriate responses to problems with their children. Modeling and discussing appropriate disciplinary techniques (answer B) is an effective way of developing this skill for parents of toddlers and young children. Answers C and

D also include important concepts for these teenage mothers and their children, who are at risk for cognitive, psychosocial and emotional deficits; however, in infancy, the mother-child bond is paramount. See Reference: Cottrell (ed). Zeitz, MA: The mothers' project: A clinical case management system.

184. (C) tai chi. Tai chi would be the best activity because it incorporates slow stretching and provides graduated challenge to coordinated movements which can help improve balance. Answer A, safe transfer training, is useful to teach safety precautions but would not have as much impact on motor skills. Answer B, walking, is a good general exercise, but would not provide stretching movement or challenge balance. Answer D, gardening, would not be particularly useful because it can be performed while in a stationary position. See Reference: Bonder and Wagner (eds). Tideiksaar, R: Falls.

185. (C) no longer makes substantial progress regardless of several adjustments made to intervention techniques. According to Case-Smith, "it may be appropriate to discontinue occupational therapy when the student...is no longer making significant progress on established objectives despite changes in intervention strategies or service-delivery models" (p. 773), answer C. Answers A and B would most likely indicate to the OT practitioner that changes/adjustments are necessary in order to assist the student in attaining identified objectives. Whereas answer D, transitioning from elementary to middle school, would not be a reason to terminate OT services if the student continues to demonstrate a need for OT services within the classroom setting. See Reference: Case-Smith (ed). Case-Smith, J, Rogers, J, and Johnson, JH: School-based occupational therapy.

186. (A) Controlled stimulation with meaningful sensory cues. An environment that provides controlled stimulation with visual, tactile, and auditory cues that are meaningful to the resident, is preferable because it will best facilitate correct perception of the environment. Difficulty in perceiving or misunderstanding environmental cues can lead to behavioral problems or agitation. Environments that are too stimulating (answer B) or too unstimulating (answer C) can increase confusion. Answer D is incorrect because while dementia units should have a homelike atmosphere, and residents should have familiar objects near them to maintain links with memories, the more important consideration in overall environmental design is to incorporate the special environmental adaptations that will enhance function. See Reference: Bonder and Wagner (eds). Corcoran, MA: Dementia.

187. (D) Obtain the same results as another OT practitioner who has demonstrated service competency. To establish service competency, it is necessary to obtain the same results as a competent OT practitioner when performing a treatment technique or evaluative procedure. Demonstrating service competency often requires more than one trial in order to refine techniques to obtain the same results. Answers A, B, and C are methods for developing service competency, but do not provide the opportunity for the OT practitioners to compare and contrast their techniques and measurements in order to obtain the same results. See Reference: Crepeau, Cohn, and Schell (eds). Sands, M: The occupational therapist and occupational therapy assistant partnership.

188. (A) completing the chart reviews. An identified role of the COTA is to complete data collection records such as a record review, general observation checklist, or behavior checklist. Answers B and C suggest that the COTA is independently collecting non-standardized data and interpreting the data. These roles are not appropriate for an assistant. A COTA can contribute to the development of a treatment plan, but it is not within the COTA scope of practice to develop treatment plans independently. See Reference: AOTA: Guidelines for Supervision, roles, and responsibilities during the delivery of occupational therapy services.

189. (C) assist the student in developing a general comfort level with client needs. According to AOTA, "the goal of level I fieldwork is to introduce students to the fieldwork experience, and develop a basic comfort level with and understanding of client needs." While Answers A, B, and D are all significant objectives that are developing with the OT student, they are most representati\ve of the expectations of a level II fieldwork experience. See Reference: AOTA: Standards for an accredited educational program for the occupational therapist. AOTA (1999c). Standards for an accredited educational program for the occupational therapist. AJOT 53, 575-582.

190. (A) referral. A referral is a request for OT services. OT services may be requested verbally or in writing, depending on the policies of the facility. Referrals from a physician typically include some or all of the following information: date of request, patient or client name, diagnosis and precautions, desired goals, duration and frequency of treatment, and physician signature. Screening (answer B) is the process of observing and collecting information about the individual to determine the need for OT services. Goals (answer C) should be included in OT documentation and should be objective and measurable. Treatment planning (answer D) is the process of analyzing and determining what the individual's problems are and deciding how to solve them. See Reference: AOTA: Standards of practice for occupational therapy.

191. (B) Based on his refusal, do not treat the individual and document the interaction in the chart. As stated in principle 3 of the Code of Ethics, "Occupational therapy personnel shall respect the individual's right to refuse professional services or involvement in research or educational activities." Answers A and C are incorrect because the therapist proceeded to treat the patient against his wishes. Answer D is incorrect because it does not meet with principle 5 of the Code of Ethics, "Occupational therapy practitioners shall record and report in an accurate and timely manner all information related to professional activities" (p.). See Reference: AOTA: Occupational Therapy Code of Ethics.

192. (C) Obtain a physician's plan of care identifying services to be provided. Within the home care setting, the therapist must have a physician's order, which identifies the services that are to be provided. After the OT's assessment, identification of deficits as well as short- and long-term goals (answers A and B) can be established. The individual's history of the current illness (answer D) is contained within the initial assessment. See Reference: Piersol and Ehrlich (eds). Zahoransky, M: The system and its players.

193. (A) When the COTA consistently obtains the same results as the OTR. The term "service competency" indicates an interrater reliability between two OT professionals. Service competency is determined by skill level, not by years of experience (answer D). Passing the NBCOT examination (answer B) establishes entry-level competence, not service competence in a particular area. OT practitioners have a professional responsibility to maintain competence, and continuing education (answer C) is one method for maintaining competence and promoting lifelong learning. See Reference: Crepeau, Cohn, and Schell (eds). Cohn, ES: Interdisciplinary communication and supervision of personnel.

194. (D) health promotion. Health promotion is the advancement of healthy lifestyles, which may include education, behavioral change, and cultural support. Answer A, occupational behavior, is the developmental continuum of play to work. Answer B, intervention, is actually the provision of treatment. Answer C, self-efficacy, would be promoting the positive effects of OT services. See Reference: Crepeau, Cohn, and Schell (eds). Jaffe, EG: and Epstein, CF: A consultative approach to occupational therapy practice.

195. (B) a formal, public disapproval of a practitioner's conduct. A censure differs from a reprimand in that it is more serious and is public. A reprimand is a formal written expression of disapproval against a practitioner's conduct and is retained in the NBCOT's files (answer A). This information also is communicated privately with the individual. Probation is when a practitioner is given a period of time to retain the counseling or education (answer C). Revocation is permanent loss of NBCOT certification (answer D). See Reference: Crepeau, Cohn, and Schell (eds). Hansen, RA: Ethics in occupational therapy.

196. (C) CARF. The Commission on Accreditation of Rehabilitation Facilities (CARF) is the regulatory agency for the provision of rehabilitation services. AOTA (answer A) was formed in March of 1917 as the National Society for the Promotion of Occupational Therapy. JCAHO (answer B) is the Joint Commission on Accreditation of Hospital Organizations. The JCAHO reviews the medical care provided by hospital organizations. The NBCOT (answer D) is the agency that develops and administers the examination for registration as an OT; therefore, answers A, B, and D are incorrect. See Reference: Crepeau, Cohn, and Schell (eds). Evanofski, M: Occupational therapy reimbursement, regulation, and the evolving scope of practice.

197. (C) Creating effective communication via weekly staff meetings, voice mail, and faxes. According to Zahoranksy, within the home care environment, "the key to any effective team effort is communication...commonly used modes of communication are pagers, voice mail, faxes, phone calls and written communication forms" (answer C) (p. 35). Countersignature alone for documentation (answer B) does not necessarily constitute adequate supervision. Individual states may have additional specific guidelines. A handout (answer D) may provide useful information to the client and caregivers about OT services, but is not a critical component in establishing a collaborative relationship. Determining reimbursement criteria (answer A) would be something that should transpire as a result of effective communication/collaboration between the OT and COTA. See Reference: Piersol and Ehrlich (eds). Zahoransky, M: The system and its players.

198. (B) A presentation to physicians. Answer B, a presentation to physicians, is correct because this is an example of internal marketing. Other internal marketing strategies are site-based open houses, progress notes, service reports, and in-services for nursing staff. Answers A, C, and D are all examples of external marketing strategies. See Reference: Jacobs and Logigian (eds). Jacobs, K: Marketing occupational therapy services.

199. (B) The COTA updates the OTR on the progress a patient has made in the past week, and both provide information to update the goals. A collaborative relationship between an OTR and a COTA supports sharing of information and the use of each professional's skills. In this type of relationship, communication is two-way, and both individuals work as a team to the benefit of the patient. Answers A and D demonstrate one-way communication in which the OTR tells the COTA what to do. In answer C, the OTR takes information from the progress note, but does not get input or recommendations from the COTA for the patient's discharge summary. See Reference: AOTA: Guidelines for Supervision, roles, and responsibilities during the delivery of occupational therapy services.

200. (C) Program evaluation. "Program evaluation is an outcome-monitoring system that reflects the results of services on consumers by defining and reviewing the outcomes of care" (p. 902). Final evaluations of clients involved in the program and client satisfaction surveys (answers A and B) may both be components of the program evaluation. Utilization review (answer D) evaluates the care that is provided to ensure that services were appropriate and not overutilized or underutilized. Utilization review also analyzes the services to ensure that the interventions were provided in an economical manner. See Reference: Crepeau, Cohn, and Schell (eds). Perinchief, JM: Documentation and management of occupational therapy services.

Simulation Examination 3

Directions: Circle the correct answer to the following questions. When you have completed this examination, check your answers against the answer key that follows. As you will see, an explanation is given for each answer along with a reference for further study. The book author is listed as well as the chapter author. See the bibliography for complete references. Study the areas in which your comprehension was low then test yourself again by taking Simulation Examination 4.

■ EVALUATION

1. An individual who has recently had a stroke seems to have difficulty with selecting utensils while he eats and the OT practitioner would like to perform a screening for agnosia. Which of the following screening techniques would be MOST appropriate for this purpose?
- A. Ask the person to demonstrate to you how they would use a knife and fork.
- B. Ask the person to pick out a spoon and fork from a drawer containing many utensils.
- C. Ask the person to tell you the steps involved in using the utensils.
- D. Ask the person to identify several common objects by sight only.

2. During an interview following a total hip replacement, it is CRITICAL that the OT practitioner determine the individual's:
- A. marital status.
- B. cognitive status.
- C. leisure interests.
- D. work responsibilities.

3. In the subjective section of a daily progress note in a mental health facility, an OT practitioner documents an individual's initial refusal to participate in OT activities. Which of the following subjective statements would MOST likely cause the therapist to consider depression as a factor in the evaluation process?
- A. "I had an argument with another group member and I'm too angry."
- B. "I do not want to participate because I do not know how to do the activity."
- C. "I'm just too tired."
- D. "I'm waiting for my visitors to come."

4. Evaluations MOST appropriate for an individual beginning a community re-entry program following a TBI would include:
- A. bed mobility and transfers.
- B. dressing, feeding, and grooming skills.
- C. cognition, sensation, and motor skills.
- D. use of an ATM machine and public transportation.

5. A home-care OT is assessing a child who has a pervasive developmental disorder. Which of the following would be the MOST effective way for the OT to engage in skilled observation?
- A. Request that the child and his parents partake in a questionnaire and/or interview.
- B. Attempt to determine and compare the child's developmental milestones with those determined by predetermined performance standards.
- C. Refer to the child's medical records, portfolio, and school performance records.
- D. Watch the child engage in dressing, eating, and bathing activities.

6. An OT practitioner is working with a motivated and alert adult who recently had a cerebrovascular accident (CVA). Despite many ADL training sessions, the individual still seems unaware of his limitations, is unsafe and unable to learn compensation techniques for neglect, leading the therapist to assess that the individual is MOST likely exhibiting:
- A. a visual field cut.
- B. apraxia.
- C. aphasia.
- D. anosognosia.

7. An OT practitioner is evaluating a group of individuals with Parkinson's disease in an aquatic therapy program. Which of the following would be MOST important for successfully walking across the pool?
- A. Strength, fine motor coordination, and kinesthesia
- B. Auditory processing, postural control, and gross motor coordination
- C. Vestibular processing, postural control, and muscle tone
- D. Normal range of motion, praxis, and crossing the midline

8. An OTR is evaluating a child with cerebral palsy. Which of the following would the OT MOST likely organize in order to assess parallel play skills?

   A. Encourage two or more children to play next to each other while sharing finger paint supplies.

   B. Initiate a game of "Go Fish" where the child who wins the most of five games is declared the winner.

   C. Instruct the child to work in a distraction free environment while completing a paint-by-number picture.

   D. Encourage several of the children to partake in an air hockey match in the school gym.

9. While evaluating an individual with left hemiparesis, the OT practitioner notes limited AROM throughout the LUE. When analyzing the reason for this, the therapist should consider which combination of factors?

   A. Muscle tone, edema, sensation, and diadochokinesis

   B. Edema, proprioception, and muscle tone

   C. Edema, contracture, muscle tone, and pain

   D. Contracture, stereognosis, and sensation

10. An OT practitioner observes an individual having difficulty trying to find a white sock on a bed with white sheets. This behavior MOST likely indicates a deficit in the area of:

   A. figure-ground discrimination.

   B. unilateral neglect.

   C. position in space.

   D. cognitive mapping.

11. Which of the following instructions should the OT practitioner follow when administering standardized tests to young children?

   A. Test in a stimulating environment.

   B. Follow test manual directions.

   C. Always administer tests in a single session.

   D. Carry on a conversation with the child.

12. An individual diagnosed with major depressive disorder is late for the inital OT evaluation; arriving with hair uncombed, clothing disheveled, and smelling badly. Which of the following methods is MOST appropriate for assessing this individual's self-care skills?

   A. Have the individual demonstrate dressing, hygiene, and grooming skills to the OT practitioner.

   B. Interview the individual using open-ended questions that encourage the client to describe how she is doing with things like personal hygiene, bathing, dressing, and grooming.

   C. Briefly interview the individual using closed-ended questions, targeting the individual's premorbid and current self-care performance levels.

   D. Based on observation of the individual's appearance, the OT practitioner can determine that the individual demonstrates significant self-care deficits.

13. An OT practitioner is participating in the evaluation of an older adult in the early stage of Alzheimer's disease. Evaluation of which deficit area is MOST essential because of its association with early stage Alzheimer's disease?

   A. Disorientation to time and place

   B. Incontinence

   C. Memory impairment

   D. The inability to dress and undress

14. An OT performing a motor skills evaluation observes that a child is awkward at many gross motor tasks. Though able to skip rope forward, the child is unable to skip rope backward, even after several attempts. This information would lead the therapist to be particularly observant for additional signs of:

   A. delayed reflex integration.

   B. inadequate bilateral integration.

   C. developmental dyspraxia.

   D. general incoordination.

15. When performing a pre-prosthetic evaluation of a patient who is s/p long above elbow amputation, the OT practitioner should measure the circumference of the stump at the:

   A. distal radio-ulnar joint.

   B. proximal radio-ulnar joint.

   C. distal humerus.

   D. proximal humerus.

16. Which type of assessment would an OT practitioner be MOST likely to begin with for the developmentally disabled client preparing for transition from school to the workforce?

A. Vocational assessment
B. Environmental assessment
C. Prevocational assessment
D. Assistive technology assessment

17. A preteen with a diagnosis of spastic cerebral palsy (CP) desires to use a computer. Prior to evaluating computer needs, the OT should FIRST assess:

A. physical, cognitive, and sensorimotor abilities.
B. the family's ability to finance a computer terminal.
C. computer learning programs.
D. appropriate keyboard and screen options.

18. An OT is assessing hand function in an individual with arthritis. While making a peanut butter sandwich, the individual is unable to remove the lid from a peanut butter jar, but is able to stand at the counter, spread peanut butter on the bread with a knife, and replace the lid. These observations would MOST likely reflect a deficit in which of the following?

A. Range of motion
B. Coordination
C. Endurance
D. Strength

19. An OT practitioner needs to assess whether an individual who had a traumatic brain injury can transfer learning from one activity to another. The MOST appropriate way to assess this patient's learning ability would be to:

A. describe situations that might be unsafe and ask the individual how he would respond.
B. give the individual a simple jigsaw puzzle to solve.
C. have the individual perform a simple cooking task, then use a different food at the next session.
D. give the individual simple calculations to perform.

20. An occupational therapist is evaluating sitting balance with a child who has cerebral palsy. Which of the following positions would the OT MOST likely implement to facilitate muscle co-contraction?

A. Place the child on their stomach with shoulders abducted and legs extended and time how long the child can maintain this position.
B. Position the child on their back with arms crossed across the chest and time how long the child can maintain this position.
C. Seat the child in an unsupported chair and ask the child to grab the OT's thumbs, gently rock the child to see how long they can maintain the seated position.
D. Have the OT sit opposite of the child and request the child to supinate and extend both forearms, then guide the child to place the wrists into a stretched position.

21. When evaluating an individual for phantom limb pain, the OT practitioner would expect the individual to report:

A. feelings of numbness and tingling at the stump site.
B. a perception that the amputated limb is actually intact and painful.
C. feelings of sharp pain at the stump site.
D. a perception that the amputated limb is actually intact, but not terribly uncomfortable.

22. While assessing a child diagnosed with CP, the OT practitioner observes that the child's movements appear writhing, purposeless, and uncontrollable. These movements would BEST be described as:

A. athetoid.
B. hypertonic.
C. spastic.
D. hypotonic.

23. An OTR provided information about adaptations that will assist in resuming sexual activity to a patient with a spinal cord injury. Afterward, the patient confides to the OT that there are serious personal issues affecting his sexual relationship with his wife. What is the BEST action for the OT to take?

A. Encourage the patient to explain further about the problems he is having with his wife.
B. Explain that this is normal, and that divorce rates are actually higher after serious injuries.
C. Direct the patient to speak with his physiatrist about his concerns.
D. Encourage the patient to speak with the rehabilitation psychologist to discuss his concerns.

24. What should an acute care OT practitioner do FIRST to obtain accurate information about a patient's family situation and about their occupational, cultural, and educational backgrounds?

    A. Read the medical history record.

    B. Interview the patient's family.

    C. Interview the patient.

    D. Read the social worker's report.

25. A child with a pervasive developmental disorder engages in restrictive-repetitive acts during an OT evaluation. Which of the following would the OT MOST likely document regarding the child's behavior?

    A. "The child rocks and bangs his head against the wall throughout the evaluation."

    B. "The child frequently cries, although there does not seem to an obvious reason that creates the tearfulness."

    C. "The child does not verbally respond to the questions initiated by the OT."

    D. "The child does not make eye contact with the OT throughout the evaluation."

26. An OT is evaluating problem-solving and sequencing skills of a woman with a long-standing history of mental illness as she makes brownies from a mix. The OT observes the individual put the whole egg, shell and all, into the bowl. Which of the following actions should the therapist take FIRST?

    A. Evaluate the individual's cognitive function.

    B. Determine that the individual is interested in meal preparation as a goal, then develop short- and long-term goals and a treatment plan.

    C. Schedule the individual for meal preparation group sessions to improve skill level.

    D. Determine the individual's home environment and her need for meal preparation skills.

27. An individual who uses a wheelchair is being discharged from a rehabilitation facility to home. In determining accessibility of the interior home environment, the area the OT practitioner should be MOST concerned with is:

    A. location of telephones and appliances.

    B. arrangement of furniture in bedrooms.

    C. steps, width of doorways, and threshold heights.

    D. presence of clutter in the environment.

28. Using the Model of Human Occupation as a frame of reference, evaluation of an individual should focus PRIMARILY on which of the following?

    A. Identification of problem behaviors that need to be extinguished

    B. Clarification of thoughts, feelings, and experiences that influence behavior

    C. Cognitive function, including assets and limitations

    D. The effect of personal, behavior, values, routines, performance capacity and the environment on role performance

29. An OT observes a child climb into a high-chair and jump up and down on a toy trampoline. However, when presented with a new rocking horse, the child is unable to determine how to mount the horse. This MOST likely indicates a problem in the area of:

    A. fine motor skills.

    B. gross motor skills.

    C. reflex integration.

    D. motor planning.

30. When evaluating self-care performance with an individual with functional limitations in shoulder abduction and external rotation, which of the following is MOST essential for the OT practitioner to assess?

    A. Buttoning a shirt

    B. Combing the hair

    C. Tucking in a shirt in the back

    D. Tying a shoe

31. During a coloring activity, an OT practitioner observes a preschooler stabilizing a crayon between the thumb and first two fingers. The practitioner MOST accurately documents this grasp as:

    A. pincer grasp.

    B. radial-digital grasp.

    C. palmar grasp.

    D. lateral pinch.

32. While measuring the active range of motion of a patient's metacarpophalangeal (MCP) joints, it is MOST important for the OT practitioner to provide stabilization:

    A. proximal to the MCP joints.

    B. distal to the MCP joints.

    C. at the wrist.

    D. on top of the MCP joints.

33. The BEST method for the OT practitioner to evaluate the presence of unilateral neglect is by using which of the following evaluations?

A. Six-block assembly
B. Line bisection
C. Proverb interpretation
D. Identification of the square in four overlapping figures

34. An infant has begun to sit and is leaning forward onto his arms. The OT practitioner notes that the infant is able to coactivate muscle groups around the shoulder and arm in order to bear weight on arms in sitting. This demonstrates that the infant has MOST likely developed which type of reactions?

A. Protective
B. Equilibrium
C. Rotational righting
D. Support

35. The OT practitioner is assessing an individual who demonstrates normal range of motion when flexing the elbow, but hyperextends by 15 degrees when the elbow is extended. The practitioner will MOST LIKELY record the measurement as:

A. −15 to 0 to 140 degrees.
B. 0 to 140 degrees.
C. 15 to 140 degrees.
D. −15 to 120 degrees.

36. An individual with a TBI is able to pick up a toothbrush and apply toothpaste independently, but takes 15 minutes to brush his teeth. This behavior most likely indicates difficulty in which of the following areas?

A. Sequencing
B. Following directions
C. Problem solving
D. Termination of activity

37. When assessing the sense of proprioception at an individual's joint, movement within the range would BEST be performed:

A. until pain is elicited.
B. until the stretch reflex is elicited.
C. at the end ranges of the joint.
D. at the midrange of the joint.

38. A child avoids playground equipment that requires her feet to be off the ground. This behavior MOST likely indicates:

A. tactile defensiveness.
B. developmental dyspraxia.
C. gravitational insecurity.
D. intolerance for motion.

39. When evaluating light touch of the primary somatic system, the OT practitioner will MOST likely use:

A. light perception and visual field tasks.
B. alternating pressure of both ends of a safety pin on the client's skin.
C. warm and cold water tubes placed on the client's skin.
D. a cotton swab to apply light touch to a small area of the client's skin.

40. A withdrawn preschooler diagnosed with developmental delay reaches out for a toothbrush and starts to brush her hair with it. The OT practitioner interprets the PRIMARY significance of this behavior as:

A. demonstrating attention-getting behavior.
B. a sign of cognitive limitation.
C. indicating initiative and beginning task-directed behavior.
D. demonstrating misinterpretation of cues because of a visual deficit.

41. An individual who works as a nurse reports difficulty squeezing the bulb of the sphygmomanometer when taking blood pressures and difficulty opening pill bottles. Which of the following instruments would be MOST appropriate for assessing this individual?

A. Goniometer
B. Aesthesiometer
C. Volumeter
D. Dynamometer

42. An OT practitioner is performing a non-standardized assessment on a preschool child who has an autism spectrum disorder. The OT is MOST likely to rely upon:

A. results from a one-to-one interview with the child.
B. observation of the child in a social, gross motor, and self-feeding task.
C. performance on the Miller Assessment for Preschoolers.
D. observation of the child's performance skills while outside on the playground.

43. When a new patient is referred for psychiatric services, the OT practitioner reviews the chart, completes performance measures, and performs an interview. The practitioner relies on the interview part of the assessment to address the individual's:

A. diagnosis.
B. current medications.
C. ability to concentrate and solve problems.
D. view of the problem and overall goals.

44. Which of the following is BEST to use when assessing three-jaw chuck strength?

    A. An aesthesiometer
    B. A pinch meter
    C. A dynamometer
    D. A volumeter

45. Which of the following BEST represents a normally developing 1–1.5-year-old child's functional mobility?

    A. The child uses a narrow base of support, low arm guard position, and takes big steps.
    B. The child uses a wide base of support and can navigate uneven ground.
    C. The child uses a narrow base of support and low arm guard position.
    D. The child uses a wide base of support and can walk well for very short distances.

46. Upon initial evaluation of an individual who sustained lacerations to the flexor tendons of the right index, middle, and ring fingers, the OT practitioner should FIRST be concerned with the individual's:

    A. attitude toward the use of adaptive equipment.
    B. skin integrity, pain, ROM, and sensory loss.
    C. ability to engage in fine motor coordination tasks with his right hand.
    D. ability to perform resistive tasks with his right hand.

47. During evaluation, the OT practitioner responds to an individual who recently lost her spouse in a car accident by paraphrasing. The OT is MOST likely implementing this technique to:

    A. refocus or redirect the individual's comments.
    B. show acceptance and understanding regarding the individual's situation.
    C. persuade the individual to make a choice.
    D. encourage the individual to provide additional information.

48. A 4-year-old child with spina bifida has a lesion at the lumbar level resulting in a flaccid bladder. The parents are requesting a bladder training program. The MOST appropriate response would be to:

    A. explain to the parents that toilet training is not a feasible option.
    B. recommend waiting until the child is 5 years old.
    C. begin a toilet training program.
    D. assess the child's ability to remove lower extremity garments.

49. While evaluating an individual's ADL status on the first day of treatment following open heart surgery, it is MOST important for the OT practitioner to:

    A. keep the MET level below 3.0.
    B. observe for shortness of breath.
    C. listen for complaints of chest pain.
    D. monitor heart rate, blood pressure, and symptoms.

■ INTERVENTION PLANNING

50. The office doorway of an individual using a wheelchair has a clear opening of 28 inches. According to ADA guidelines, which of the following recommendations would be the MOST appropriate to facilitate clear passage of the wheelchair through the doorway?

    A. The doorway width needs to be expanded to have a minimum clearance of 32 inches when the door is open.
    B. The client needs to obtain a wheelchair narrower than 28 inches.
    C. The doorway width needs to be expanded to have a minimum clear opening of 45 inches.
    D. The doorway width is satisfactory and needs no modification.

51. A child's long-term goal is to increase fine motor skills. The assessment has revealed a deficit in tactile discrimination, specifically stereognosis. The MOST relevant short-term goal would be that the:

    A. child will correctly identify five out of five fingers touched when given tactile stimulus.
    B. child will correctly identify five out of five shapes drawn on the dorsum of her hand.
    C. child will correctly identify five out of five matching textures.
    D. child will correctly identify, by feel only, five out of five common objects.

52. An individual with a history of chronic obstructive pulmonary disorder has limited endurance. The long-term goal for this individual is to prepare three meals a week. The MOST relevant short-term goal for the OT practitioner to focus on is:

    A. the use of energy conservation.
    B. work-hardening activities.
    C. graded activities to increase strength.
    D. safety in the kitchen.

53. An OT is working with a child whose poor visual attention is affecting his ability to perform school work. An adaptation of the sensory environment that would MOST improve attention during a visual task is to have the child:

A. work with lively background music to increase competing sensory input.

B. work against a patterned background to increase competing visual input.

C. use headphones during work to reduce competing sensory input.

D. use dim lighting to reduce the visual input.

54. When treating individuals in the acute phase of cardiac rehabilitation, it is important for the OT practitioner to FIRST select activities that:

A. can be accomplished without causing fatigue.

B. decrease the effects of prolonged inactivity.

C. promote strength, ROM, and endurance.

D. can be carried out independently after discharge.

55. A child with Asperger's syndrome presents with gross motor skill deficits. The OT can BEST intervene by providing activities that facilitate:

A. vestibular reactions.

B. fine motor skills.

C. oral motor activities.

D. pincer skills.

56. An individual with a C6 spinal cord injury has been referred to OT 2 days post-injury. Immobilized with a halo brace, the individual demonstrates fair plus wrist extension and poor minus finger flexion. Which of the following interventions should be implemented FIRST?

A. Volar resting pan splints to prevent flexion contractures

B. Wrist support with universal cuff to promote independence

C. Wrist splints to promote development of tenodesis

D. Instruction in bed mobility techniques to prevent decubiti

57. In a psychiatric treatment facility, an individual with a low level of arousal has been referred to occupational therapy. Which type of activity would be BEST for helping the individual to reach a more appropriate level of arousal?

A. Slowly rocking in a rocking chair

B. Listening to melodious and soft sounds

C. Looking at pastel colors

D. Rubbing different textures on the skin

58. An individual is dependent with self-care and transfers with the assistance of two people. Since the individual's goal is to return home with an ADL status requiring the assistance of one person, the MOST appropriate long-term goal would be for the individual to:

A. complete upper-extremity sponge bathing with setup of equipment and verbal cues.

B. perform lower-extremity dressing with the maximal assistance of one person.

C. complete upper-extremity self-care using appropriate adaptive equipment with supervision by a family member.

D. complete a modified sit-pivot transfer to the commode with moderate assistance of two people.

59. An OTR is concerned about a child's inability to control flexion and extension of the arm when reaching for toys. The child flexes or extends the arm too much, making placement of the hand very difficult. A goal for this child would be to improve the:

A. ability to isolate movement.

B. ability to grade movement.

C. ability to control how fast movement occurs.

D. bilateral integration of arm movements.

60. The goal for a patient who has had a CVA is to be able to put on a shirt independently. The MOST effective way for the OT practitioner to structure dressing training for maximum learning retention and generalization of this skill is:

A. teaching and practicing each segment of the dressing procedure during consecutive treatment sessions.

B. practicing the whole task of putting on a shirt in a setting similar to the real environment.

C. providing dressing simulation activities (button boards, etc.).

D. allowing the client to view a videotape on how to put on a shirt and providing written directions for completing steps for dressing.

61. An individual with depression is collaborating with his OT practitioner to help the practitioner identify goals for treatment, but is able to describe only vague and general goal areas. It is MOST important for the OT practitioner to guide the goal development process so that the finished treatment goals include:

    A. objective and measurable statements of what will be accomplished with time frames.

    B. description of the client's reasons for the goals.

    C. specific measurements of the individual's skill and performance.

    D. identification of the intervention approach to be used.

62. The mother of a physically disabled 3-year-old has a goal that her child will be walking independently around the house. This is an unrealistic goal for the child, but one that would be helpful to the mother who is finding her child difficult to lift. The BEST way to assist in the development of family-centered intervention for this child would be to:

    A. support and work on the parent's goal as is.

    B. suggest an alternative, realistic OT goal of improving sitting balance for playing.

    C. propose a modified goal that still meets the parent's needs.

    D. empower the child to set her own goals.

63. Which of the following are the MOST appropriate interventions for the OT to plan in treating a person following a total knee replacement?

    A. Providing range of motion and strengthening activities for the upper extremities

    B. Providing range of motion and strengthening activities for the lower extremities

    C. ADL training in use of adaptive techniques for LE dressing and transfers

    D. Providing an evaluation of homemaking activities

64. An OT practitioner is developing a stress reduction and management program for an individual recently diagnosed with multiple sclerosis. One stressor that the individual has identified is that his teenage children are resistive to helping with chores that were previously his responsibility (e.g., mowing the lawn and taking out the trash). Which coping strategy could the OT recommend that would be MOST effective in dealing with this stressor?

    A. Using effective communication skills

    B. Applying time management techniques

    C. Deep breathing and muscle relaxation

    D. Laughter

65. The BEST position in which the OT can place a 15-month-old child to provide opportunity to further develop trunk rotation is in the:

    A. supine position.

    B. prone position.

    C. side-lying position.

    D. sitting position.

66. A toddler with feeding difficulties due to deficient oral-motor control and oral defensiveness now demonstrates the ability to eat dry cereals with milk. The OT practitioner can now progress the child to which of the following foods?

    A. Applesauce and mashed bananas

    B. Cut up meats and sandwiches

    C. Strained fruits and vegetables

    D. Scrambled eggs

67. An OT practitioner is simulating cylindrical grasping activities with an individual who desires to work on the skills necessary to be a carpenter. Which of the following activities would MOST likely address these needs?

    A. Positioning a nail on a piece of wood

    B. Hammering a nail into a piece of wood

    C. Carrying a pail of bolts

    D. Unscrewing a lunchbox thermos

68. Which of the following statements would BEST explain the purpose of a prevocational evaluation program to a new participant?

    A. "The program will help you to learn about your interests, talents, and skills for assembly jobs."

    B. "This program will help you to learn about the skills you have that are needed on MOST jobs and about your potential for work."

    C. "This program will help you identify the responsibility you have to your employer while you are in treatment and to inform your employer of these responsibilities."

    D. "This program will help you to develop skills for getting a job."

69. An OT is planning treatment activities to use for a child with postural instability. The activities selected would MOST likely address:

    A. weight shifting and equilibrium reactions.

    B. discomfort with motion activities.

    C. anxiety when his or her feet are off the ground.

    D. gravitational insecurity.

70. When planning treatment for a patient who has recently experienced a traumatic amputation of his right upper extremity at the short below-elbow level, which of the following areas of patient education would the OT practitioner address FIRST?

   A. Training to put on and take off the prosthesis
   B. Training in residual limb wrapping
   C. Activities to teach grasp and prehension functions
   D. Training to resume vocational activities

71. Following hospitalization for an acute schizophrenic episode, a college student in a day program is uncomfortable in social settings, has difficulty sustaining conversations, is unable to make eye contact, and responds to others with bizarre comments. Which of the following would be the MOST effective treatment approach?

   A. Vestibular stimulation and gross-motor exercises
   B. Modification of the social environment
   C. Pleasurable activities that do not require conscious attention to movement
   D. Social skills training

72. An OT practitioner is working with a group of 3-year-old children in a preschool setting. The OT has decided to initiate a group that facilitates symbolic play. Which of the following would be the MOST appropriate activity to introduce first?

   A. Scissors and cutting activities with construction paper
   B. Jump rope games
   C. Make-believe group with stuffed animals and imaginary friends
   D. Building towers with blocks that resemble pictures in books

73. An OT practitioner is making a home visit to an elderly individual who lives alone and has severe hand weakness resulting from arthritis. When planning to address safety in the home, the MOST important area to consider is the individual's ability to:

   A. work locks and latches on doors and windows.
   B. use built-up utensils while eating.
   C. use energy conservation techniques.
   D. manipulate fasteners on clothing.

74. An individual demonstrates a left visual field cut as a result of a TBI, and demonstrates difficulty crossing the midline during many self-care activities. Which of the following activities would MOST effectively promote this individual's ability to cross the midline?

   A. Making a coil pot out of clay
   B. Making a macramé planter
   C. Stringing a bead necklace
   D. Weaving on a frame loom

75. The OT practitioner is working on feeding skills with an individual with amyotrophic lateral sclerosis who is in the late stages of the disease process. Which of the following is the MOST appropriate intervention for this individual?

   A. Provide a rocker knife, plate guard, and nonskid mat.
   B. Implement a pureed diet and allow adequate time for eating.
   C. Emphasize upper extremity strengthening.
   D. Minimize the use of adaptive equipment.

76. An OT practitioner is working with an individual who complains of hypersensitive fingers following a crush injury to the hand. Which of the following methods would be MOST appropriate for achieving desensitization?

   A. Textured material, rubbing, tapping, and prolonged contact
   B. Massage, facilitory electrical stimulation, and a progressive desensitization program
   C. Pressure, percussion, vibration, icing, and edema massage
   D. Visual compensation and functional use of the extremity

77. An individual with a cognitive disability in a sheltered workshop setting demonstrates the ability to copy demonstrated directions when presented one step at a time, and to visualize an end-product, but is unable to recognize errors, and may not be able to correct them when they are pointed out. According to Allen's Cognitive Disability Theory, the MOST appropriate placement for this individual is in a group involved with:

   A. sorting plastic utensils into separate containers.
   B. assembling packets that include a knife, fork, spoon, and napkin based on a sample.
   C. selecting matching shoelaces from a mixed pile and lacing them onto a display card.
   D. gluing labels onto cans and placing them in an appropriate container according to color.

78. **When teaching children with moderate mental retardation to feed, groom, and dress themselves, the OT is MOST likely to use which technique?**
    A. Chaining
    B. Practice and repetition
    C. Demonstration
    D. Role modeling

79. **After a radial nerve injury, an individual initially had trace muscle strength in elbow extension. One week later, strength is noted to have increased to poor minus. The individual is ready for which activity?**
    A. Passively self-ranging the injured arm
    B. Extending the elbow in mid range 30 to 40 degrees with the forearm resting on the table
    C. Pushing a cup filled with pennies with the back of the hand, with arm resting on the table
    D. Lifting a book placed on the back of the hand up off the table

80. **A sales executive is participating in a time-management program. Which of the following would be the expected outcome for the individual?**
    A. To control anxiety when arriving late for a meeting.
    B. To take responsibility when late with reports.
    C. To cope with feelings of inadequacy when missing a deadline.
    D. To arrive at work on time consistently.

81. **An individual with Alzheimer's disease has limitations in shoulder range of motion. The OT goal for this individual is to improve active shoulder motion in order to resume self-care activities. Which strategy would be MOST effective in actively engaging the individual?**
    A. Telling the individual to perform repetitions of active UE range-of-motion exercises independently
    B. Training the individual to use long-handled adaptive devices to compensate for decreased shoulder motion
    C. Incorporating simple, familiar activities such as hanging up clothing or catching a ball
    D. Performing PROM exercises on the individual

82. **A child has low muscle tone resulting in problems in the following printing and hand-writing subskill areas: (1) postural stability, (2) shoulder stability, and (3) grasp of the pencil. If the OTR uses a proximal-to-distal approach to skill development, which of the following treatment sequences is BEST?**
    A. Improve posture, then improve shoulder stability, then improve grasp.
    B. Improve shoulder stability, then improve posture, then improve grasp.
    C. Improve grasp, then improve posture, then improve shoulder stability.
    D. Improve shoulder stability, then improve grasp, then improve posture.

83. **An individual diagnosed with Guillain-Barré syndrome exhibits good upper extremity strength. The activity that would be MOST appropriate for further strengthening and endurance building would be:**
    A. peeling potatoes.
    B. bedmaking.
    C. polishing furniture.
    D. washing windows.

84. **An OT practitioner is working with three individuals in a cooking group who demonstrate difficulty attending to tasks, frequently ask to leave the room, and do not interact with each other. Based on the developmental group frame of reference, which of the following is the MOST appropriate goal for this group?**
    A. Each member will experiment with trying one different group role.
    B. Each member will share materials and tools with at least one other group member.
    C. Each member will express two positive feelings about himself within the group session.
    D. Each member will share space while working on a task without disrupting the work of others for 15 minutes.

85. **A child with a learning disability has significant problems with visual memory. An OT practitioner may use which of the following to better enhance visual memory?**
    A. Provide memory tasks that are of low interest to the child.
    B. Decrease visual attention before doing memory tasks.
    C. Combine task with additional sensory input (tactile, proprioceptive, and auditory).
    D. Repeat the visual memory task once.

86. A long-term goal for an individual with back pain is to be able to return to work as an illustrator, which requires long periods of sitting. Which of the following is the BEST example of a short-term goal for this individual?

A. Client will draw sitting at a work table.

B. Client will draw for 1 hour, taking stretch breaks every 20 minutes.

C. Instruct client in stretching techniques to be performed every 20 minutes.

D. Instruct client in the use of proper body mechanics that apply to prolonged sitting.

87. An OT practitioner is starting an inpatient group for individuals with schizophrenia whose psychosis has been controlled through medication, but who continue to display negative symptoms, including difficulty sustaining attention, limited ability to express feelings and ideas, depressed affect, low interest and energy levels. Which type of activities would the OT be MOST likely to plan for the members of the group at this beginning stage?

A. Skill building activities with concrete goals, such as time management training

B. Self-management activities, such as relaxation training

C. Expressive/projective activities such as journal writing

D. Verbal activities such as discussing movies or current events

88. Results of an OT evaluation show that a young child has many tactile defensive behaviors. The MOST appropriate beginning activity for intervention to normalize sensory processing would require that:

A. the therapist has the child play "sandwich" between heavy mats.

B. the therapist applies a feather brush lightly to the child's arms and legs.

C. the child is blindfolded and must guess where he or she is touched on the body.

D. the therapist has the child play the "Duck, duck, goose" circle game.

89. An OT practitioner is working with an individual in a work program setting. What is the FIRST step to achieving the program objective of preventing reinjury?

A. Performing a prework screening

B. Learning proper body mechanics

C. Participating in work hardening

D. Engaging in vocational counseling

90. An individual is receiving OT to promote independence in meal preparation and cleanup activities. Which method of structured activity practice would BEST promote retention of learning and transfer of skills?

A. Practice preparing a variety of foods using different cooking methods and recipes.

B. Practice cooking one meal from beginning to end in the same kitchen setting several times.

C. Practice making a sandwich until that is mastered, then practice preparing another part of a meal until the person has mastered that skill, and so on.

D. Practice performing each step of the food preparation process, such as cutting vegetables.

91. An OT is introducing sensory integration activities to a child with autism; however, the child does not appear to be enjoying a gentle swinging activity. How should the OT intervene NEXT?

A. Abandon the swinging intervention and introduce another activity.

B. Attempt to push the child higher and slightly harder.

C. Ask the child what activity they would prefer to do next.

D. Evaluate the child's level of adaptive responses.

■ IMPLEMENTING INTERVENTION

92. An individual with ALS swims three times a week to maximize strength and endurance. Initially able to swim for only 10 minutes, the individual is now able to swim 20 minutes without becoming fatigued. The NEXT step is to:

A. continue the program of swimming 20 minutes, three times a week.

B. decrease swimming frequency to two times a week.

C. increase swimming time to 25 minutes or to tolerance.

D. provide adaptive equipment that will enable the individual to swim using less energy.

93. An OT practitioner is advising the parents of a 5-year-old child with athetoid cerebral palsy about the type of construction toy they should buy the child to facilitate play. The BEST type of construction toy to recommend for this child is a set with:

A. large, easily interlocking pieces.
B. blocks that are small and have a firm surface.
C. lightweight and soft-textured building blocks.
D. colorful blocks in a variety of shapes.

94. An individual covered by Medicare who has been receiving OT and PT in the home is now able to transfer in and out of the car with supervision of a caregiver and visit friends 30 minutes away. OT services are still required to improve mobility, upper extremity function, and home management skills. Which of the following actions should the OT practitioner take FIRST?

A. Provide a home program and discharge the individual.
B. Explain to the individual and caregiver that one must be "homebound" in order to be eligible for home care services.
C. Refer the individual for outpatient therapy and provide a comprehensive discharge summary to the outpatient setting.
D. Inform the PT of the individual's status.

95. An individual with strong dependency needs is able to lace a leather wallet only with consistent verbal cueing. Which is the BEST way to grade this activity in order to decrease dependency?

A. Provide written instructions on lacing techniques and ask the individual to continue on her own.
B. Ask the individual to try some lacing with distant supervision and praise her for what she has been able to do.
C. Ask the individual to take the lacing to her room and continue without the OT's assistance.
D. Tell the individual to complete a small amount of lacing while the OT assists another patient in the same room.

96. An OT practitioner is working on keyboarding activities with an individual with asymmetrical muscle tone who keeps falling to the side while sitting in a wheelchair. Which adaptation would MOST effectively stabilize the upper body in a midline position?

A. Change to a reclining wheelchair.
B. Use an arm trough.
C. Provide lateral trunk support.
D. Provide lateral pelvic support.

97. An OT practitioner is working with a school-age child to improve her power grasp technique. Which of the following activities would the OT MOST likely request the child perform in order to elicit this grasp?

A. Pegboard activities
B. Brushing her own hair
C. Carrying a light-weight briefcase
D. Throwing a ball

98. An OT practitioner working with an individual to develop meal preparation skills observes that the individual demonstrates minimal to moderate difficulty figuring out, sequencing, and organizing the steps needed to prepare a macaroni and cheese dish. Which cooking activity is MOST appropriate to use for the next OT session?

A. Making baked chicken and mashed potatoes
B. Making a peanut butter and jelly sandwich
C. Preparing a frozen dinner
D. Making instant pudding

99. An OT practitioner is implementing a self-feeding session with an individual with a C5 spinal cord injury. Which piece of feeding equipment would be MOST appropriate for the OT to introduce?

A. A wrist-driven flexor hinge splint
B. A mobile arm support
C. An electric self-feeder
D. Built-up utensils

100. The MOST effective method of compensation for both unilateral neglect and absence of sensation in an upper extremity with good motor control is to:

A. avoid the use of sharp tools or scissors and to avoid extreme water temperatures.
B. provide a warning tone, such as noisy bracelets on the wrist, or as a reminder to visually scan toward the affected side.
C. use an electric shaver.
D. wear elbow pads on the affected side.

101. An individual with depression finishes making a poorly constructed Christmas tree ornament, and tells the OT practitioner he wants to throw it away because it is "such a sorry looking thing." What is the BEST way for the therapist to respond?

A. Suggest that he give it to a family member.
B. Tell him it is beautiful and ask to keep it.
C. Ask if it is OK to hang it on the tree on the unit.
D. Accept his decision.

102. The BEST way for an individual with hemiparesis and mild perceptual deficits to button a shirt is to:
  A. button all the buttons before putting the shirt on.
  B. get the shirt all the way on, then line up the buttons and holes, and begin buttoning from the top.
  C. get the shirt all the way on, then line up the buttons and holes, and begin buttoning from the bottom.
  D. use a buttonhook with a built-up handle.

103. An OT practitioner consults with the parents of a child with attention deficit disorder regarding modifications to the child's bedroom. To BEST help the child with self-organization skills, the therapist should recommend:
  A. providing open storage space for clothing and school supplies for easy access.
  B. painting walls and furniture in bright colors to help visual focus.
  C. adding cabinets with labeled compartments to store items out of sight.
  D. placing the bed on the floor for ease of transfer out of bed.

104. In preparing a patient with a unilateral below-knee amputation for discharge from a rehabilitation facility, the MOST important adaptive equipment for the OT practitioner to recommend is:
  A. lightweight cooking utensils.
  B. a tub bench and toilet rails.
  C. long-handled dressing devices.
  D. a reacher.

105. A child with CP tends to flex forward while riding her adapted tricycle, even though her lower extremities are correctly positioned. Which of the following adaptations should the OT recommend to BEST enable the child to maintain an upright position while riding?
  A. Raising the seat height
  B. Raising the handlebars
  C. Lowering the seat height
  D. Lowering the handlebars

106. An individual requires supervision for ambulation, but consistently leaves her cane in her room. When asked where her cane is, she replies, "Oh, that cane, it's just so ugly." Which of the following actions is MOST appropriate to take?
  A. Discuss issues related to self-concept with the individual.
  B. Evaluate the individual's short-term memory.
  C. Evaluate the individual's long-term memory.
  D. Devise strategies to address time management.

107. During the course of treatment, a young individual diagnosed with depression tells the OT practitioner that he leads a very isolated lifestyle and often feels alone and afraid. The BEST therapeutic response would be to:
  A. reassure the client that they can be friends.
  B. tell the client, "I know how you feel."
  C. encourage the client to socialize more often.
  D. use active-listening techniques.

108. An OT is positioning a child with low muscle tone and postural instability into a prone stander to develop head righting. The child rapidly shows fatigue and associated reactions. How can the OT BEST adjust the stander to decrease these reactions while continuing to address the goal of head righting?
  A. Place the child in prone on the floor.
  B. Position the stander at 45 degrees from the floor.
  C. Position the stander at 75 to 80 degrees from the floor.
  D. Position the child upright in a prone or supine stander.

109. An OT practitioner is instructing an individual in how to perform stand-to-sit transfers after a total hip replacement. Prior to sitting down from a standing position, the therapist should instruct the individual to:
  A. extend the operated leg forward, reach back for the armrests, then slowly sit.
  B. extend the nonoperated leg forward, reach back for the armrests, and slowly sit.
  C. extend the operated leg forward, hold the walker securely, and slowly sit.
  D. extend the nonoperated leg forward, reach back for the armrest with one hand while holding the walker securely with the other, and slowly sit.

110. An OT practitioner in a psychosocial setting is documenting a client's responses to an activity. Which of the following should the therapist write in the chart in order to relay the objective portion of the note?

A. The client did not want to finish her stenciling activity.
B. The client was hostile to another client in the activity group.
C. The client independently selected one of six craft designs presented.
D. The client demonstrated an appropriate level of frustration tolerance during most of the activity.

111. A child currently uses compensatory arm and hand movements while seated because of the inability to sit independently. Which aspect of therapeutic positioning should the OT stress?

A. Stabilizing the trunk
B. Placing weight on the arms
C. Stabilizing the pelvis, hips, and legs
D. Stabilizing the head and neck

112. An individual with advanced lung cancer is about to be discharged from an acute care setting to home. She is depressed, and although she remains ambulatory and independent in basic ADLs, she tires very quickly and no longer participates in most of her life roles. Which of the following is the BEST action for the OT practitioner to take?

A. Provide her with a home program.
B. Recommend home health OT.
C. Recommend discontinuation of OT services.
D. Recommend hospice OT.

113. A school-age child with fine motor skill difficulties is ready for discharge from outpatient OT services. The MOST important information to include in the discharge summary concerns the:

A. child's interests and hobbies.
B. child's writing, dressing, and self-feeding skills.
C. child's academic achievement.
D. availability of the child's parents for follow-up services.

114. An individual who is several days s/p myocardial infarction experiences nausea during a bathing evaluation. Which of the following is the FIRST action the OT practitioner should take?

A. Stop the activity.
B. Document the symptoms.
C. Instruct the individual to sit and then continue the activity.
D. Ask the individual if he feels he can continue the activity.

115. What type of interactive play would an OT MOST likely recommend to a mother of a 5-year-old child?

A. Coloring on paper
B. A simple board game of checkers
C. Looking at picture books
D. Participation in an organized sport such as softball

116. A person with a long history of Parkinson's disease is experiencing considerable fatigue during the day. The BEST way to enable the individual to maintain his level of function is to teach him how to:

A. "work through" the fatigue.
B. perform desired activities in a simplified manner to conserve energy.
C. utilize pursed-lips breathing.
D. eliminate activities or reduce activity level as much as possible.

117. The OT practitioner is planning a simple meal preparation activity that will result in success for a patient with cognitive deficits. The SIMPLEST activity would be preparing:

A. a can of soup.
B. a casserole.
C. brownies from a box mix.
D. a meal with two side dishes and an entree.

118. An OT is working on hand function with a school-age child diagnosed with juvenile rheumatoid arthritis. To prevent hand fatigue, the OT recommends the use of a:

A. Reacher
B. Jar opener
C. Pencil gripper
D. Plate guard

119. An individual with joint changes that limit finger flexion would be MOST comfortable using utensils with:

A. regular handles.
B. weighted handles.
C. a universal cuff attachment.
D. built-up handles.

120. During the interview with the parents of a 3-year-old child with mild CP, the OT practitioner learns that the child is regularly fed by his grandmother and does not have any independent feeding skills. The FIRST issue the OT practitioner needs to explore further is:

A. the degree of abnormal muscle tone in the UEs.
B. the possibility of developmental delay.
C. the cultural context and family interaction patterns.
D. the need for adapted equipment.

121. An individual with C4 quadriplegia is able to independently use a mouth stick to strike keys on a computer keyboard for 3 minutes. To upgrade this activity, the OT practitioner should:

A. provide a heavier mouth stick.
B. have the individual work at the keyboard for 5 minutes.
C. progress the individual to a typing device that inserts into a wrist support.
D. teach the individual how to correctly instruct a caregiver in use of the keyboard.

122. A COTA and OTR are planning for the discharge of a child from an early intervention program. What advice to the parents will MOST likely result in effective carryover of a therapeutic home program?

A. Set aside a certain time daily to focus on therapeutic activities.
B. Incorporate therapeutic activities into family routines.
C. Provide therapeutic activities on an as-needed basis.
D. Do therapeutic activities daily, but vary the time of day.

123. An OT practitioner is working with an individual who is at risk for aspiration during swallowing. The BEST position for the individual to maintain during feeding activities is:

A. slight neck extension.
B. reclined in bed.
C. head erect, chin slightly tucked.
D. full neck flexion.

124. An OT practitioner is leading a cognitive skills group with adolescents diagnosed with schizophrenia. Which of the following is the BEST method to use to facilitate problem-solving?

A. Begin with activities that have obvious solutions and a high probability of success, and then gradually increase the level of complexity.
B. Begin with activities that require gross motor responses, and then gradually progress to fine motor responses.
C. Select activities that require interaction with others, and then provide opportunities to discuss and analyze how the group went.
D. Gradually increase the time used in the activity by 15-minute increments.

125. The OT practitioner is educating the parents of a small child with sensory defensiveness regarding hair grooming. The parents report that each time they shampoo their child's hair she becomes anxious, restless, and agitated. The OT would MOST likely recommend that the parents:

A. wash the child's hair with water only and avoid shampoo.
B. have the child's hair washed thoroughly each time she gets a haircut.
C. use a calm and soothing voice while informing the child about each step of the hair wash prior to doing it.
D. use cool water when shampooing the child's hair.

126. An individual confides to the OT practitioner that he is concerned that lower extremity flaccidity may cause problems during sexual activity. The BEST strategy to recommend is to:

A. use a side-lying position.
B. use pillows to prop up body parts into the desired position.
C. incorporate slow rocking into movements.
D. avoid movements that elicit a quick stretch.

127. Members of an OT group at a mental health day program who have physical disabilities in addition to mental illness began expressing anger about the lack of accessibility in the building where the day program is housed. Which of the following offers the action that will MOST empower the group members?

A. Employ an OT practitioner to assess the facility for ADA compliance.

B. Incorporate advocacy skill training into the group format.

C. Bring a lawsuit against the facility for violating the ADA.

D. Involve the clients in a stress management group.

128. A child has poor sitting balance, which interferes with seated tabletop activities. Which intervention should the OT suggest to the child's teacher for the promotion of ongoing postural adjustments in sitting?

A. Use a sturdy chair with lateral trunk supports while the child is doing homework.

B. Use a corner floor seat with built in desk surface while the child is self-feeding.

C. Provide a bolster for back support while the child is coloring.

D. Provide a therapy ball to sit on while the child is playing a game of checkers.

129. A child is able to bring her hand close to her mouth for feeding, but cannot orient the utensil directly into her mouth. The MOST helpful adapted utensil for this child would be a:

A. spoon with an elongated handle.

B. "spork."

C. spoon with a built-up handle.

D. curved spoon and fork.

130. An individual with an L4 spinal cord injury wishes to become independent in driving an automobile. The MOST appropriate piece of adaptive equipment for this individual is:

A. a palmar cuff for the steering wheel.

B. a spinner knob on the steering wheel.

C. pedal extensions for acceleration and braking.

D. hand controls for acceleration and braking.

131. An individual who uses an augmentative communications system wishes to increase his conversational communication skills. Which of the following BEST represents this form of communication?

A. Paper and pencil or written forms of communication

B. Calculator skill development

C. Telephone conversations

D. Keyboard skill development

132. An individual with rheumatoid arthritis complains of joint pain and inflammation. The individual reports continuing with the home program despite the pain, and demonstrates a series of briskly executed active range of motion movements. The OT should instruct the individual to:

A. continue performing the program as demonstrated.

B. perform gentle active range of motion with weights as tolerated.

C. eliminate all range of motion exercises for a week.

D. perform only gentle active range of motion.

133. A child with athetoid CP is working in OT to develop self-feeding skills. When the child attempts to pick up food, it slides off the plate. Which adaptation should the OT provide to solve this problem?

A. A swivel spoon

B. A nonslip mat

C. A mobile arm support

D. A scoop dish

134. After fabricating an antispasticity splint, the MOST important thing for the OT practitioner to determine is that:

A. the fingers are flexed.

B. the thumb is in an opposable position.

C. the patient is wearing the splint at all times.

D. any pressure marks or redness from the splint disappears within 20 minutes.

135. An occupational therapy practitioner is using a motivational interview approach with a client who has a history of substance abuse. When the client seems reluctant to discuss how his drinking habits interfered with his daily activities in the past, the MOST appropriate and therapeutic response for the therapist to make would be to:

A. confront the client about the impact drinking had on his life.

B. help the client to interpret why he finds drinking necessary.

C. avoid opposing the client or arguing for change.

D. discuss how daily activities could be improved if the client stops drinking.

136. A high-functioning child with a behavior disorder has an innately difficult temperament. Which of the following treatment approaches is MOST appropriate for the OT practitioner to initiate?

A. Emphasize limit-setting with the child during activities.

B. Help the child develop cognitive strategies for anxiety-producing activities.

C. Help care providers develop an unpredictable routine in order to develop problem-solving strategies with the child.

D. Provide a play environment in which the parent and child can act out conflicts.

137. An OT practitioner is providing instruction to caregivers in a long-term care facility about how to assist a resident whose severe attention span deficits impair the ability to participate in self-feeding. The therapist is MOST likely to recommend which method?

A. Demonstration of feeding process for the resident

B. Providing verbal feedback to the resident about how he or she is progressing

C. Hand-over-hand assistance

D. Chaining

138. While participating in the first session of a relapse prevention group, an individual reports that he often misses a dose of his medication because he forgets when to take it. Which of the following actions should the OT practitioner take FIRST?

A. Ask group members to discuss how they feel about taking their medications.

B. Suggest using a diary to record each dose of medication.

C. Instruct him in the use of a timer to assist in medication management.

D. Make sure he knows what his medication schedule is.

139. An infant born 15 weeks prematurely has a history of multiple medical issues, including retinopathy of prematurity, mechanical ventilation for 5 weeks, and poor feeding skills. The infant is now chronologically a 58-week-old (43 weeks old corrected) medically stable and engaging infant, with a G-tube and oxygen supplement of 2 liters by nasal cannula. The MOST appropriate intervention to provide at this time would be:

A. positioning and handling.

B. PROM of all extremities.

C. multisensory input.

D. music therapy.

140. An individual uses a mouthstick when working with a computer. Which of the following devices will prevent the mouthstick from accidentally striking other keys?

A. A moisture guard

B. A key guard

C. An auto-repeat defeat

D. One-finger-access software

141. Following a heart attack, an inpatient tells the OT practitioner that there is really nothing wrong with him and his nurse reports that the individual is not complying with cardiac precautions. Which of the following is the MOST important action for the OT to take?

A. Monitor the individual's response to activities to prevent him from performing at activity levels that are too high and unsafe.

B. Instruct the individual in energy conservation techniques to minimize energy expenditure.

C. Emphasize the consequences of not observing cardiac precautions, and provide concrete proof of the myocardial infarction to the individual.

D. Refer the individual for psychological services.

142. An OT practitioner observes that a child moves from a completely prone position to a prone-on-elbow position. In reporting the child's progress, the OT documents that the child is gaining control in the midline position through the development of:

A. primitive reflexes.

B. prehensile reactions.

C. righting reactions.

D. equilibrium reactions.

143. When working on cooking skills, an individual with a history of traumatic brain injury exhibits moderate upper extremity incoordination. Which of the following recommendations would be MOST beneficial for this individual?

A. Use built-up utensil handles.

B. Use heavy utensils, pots, and pans.

C. Use a high stool to work at counter height.

D. Place the most commonly used items on shelves just above and below the counter.

144. A splint for an individual with carpal tunnel syndrome should position the wrist in:

A. 2 degrees of flexion.

B. 10 degrees of flexion.

C. 5 to 10 degrees of extension.

D. 10 to 15 degrees of extension.

145. An OT practitioner is instructing a family how to observe for sensory overload when carrying out a sensory integration home program. The MOST important autonomic responses to watch for are:

A. crying and the child's refusal to participate.
B. self-stimulation and screaming.
C. head banging and hand flapping.
D. flushing and perspiration.

146. An OT practitioner is teaching an individual who recently sustained an above-elbow amputation how to tie shoelaces with one hand. Which of the following methods would the OT practitioner MOST likely implement to facilitate success with shoe tying?

A. Problem-solving method
B. Retraining method
C. Altered task method
D. Compensation method

147. An individual with severe cognitive limitations frequently chokes while drinking liquids. Which of the following is the MOST appropriate course of action?

A. Use a straw for drinking liquids.
B. Use a "sippy cup" for drinking liquids.
C. Monitor fluid intake.
D. Add a thickening agent to liquids.

148. A 17-year-old individual who wears a hip brace is being measured for a wheelchair. The correct seat dimension for the OT to recommend would be:

A. 2 inches wider than the widest point across the child's hips with the brace on.
B. 2 inches wider than the widest point across the child's hips.
C. 2 inches more than the distance from the back of the bent knee to the buttocks.
D. the same as the distance from the back of the bent knee to the buttocks.

149. An artist recently diagnosed with MS is interested in pursuing a leisure activity that will promote physical fitness. Because the individual's symptoms are limited to mild upper extremity numbness and slight weakness in the dominant hand at this point, the BEST activity to recommend is:

A. volleyball.
B. painting with the dominant hand.
C. swimming in a cool water pool.
D. jogging on a track or treadmill.

150. An OT practitioner working on laundry skills with an adult with cognitive disabilities has determined that the individual is unable to recognize or judge when clothing is dirty. What is the NEXT step that should be taken to maximize the individual's independence in doing laundry?

A. Instruct the individual to wear clothes for 2 days and to then launder those items.
B. Assess the individual's ability to recognize dirty clothing.
C. Recommend that the individual take clothes for dry cleaning rather than wash them at home.
D. Recommend to the staff that they do the individual's laundry from now on.

151. An individual with hand weakness has difficulty holding a fork. Using a biomechanical frame of reference, the OT practitioner should:

A. elicit functional grasp using reflex inhibiting postures.
B. stimulate the hand flexors using quick stretch to promote a functional grasp.
C. have the individual repeatedly squeeze with the hand against increasing amounts of resistance.
D. build up utensil handles.

152. Task-specific training is being used to train an individual with severe cognitive limitations to put on a tee shirt. This training will be MOST effective if it takes place:

A. in the individual's home.
B. in the OT department.
C. at least twice a week.
D. when the client is feeling cooperative.

153. An OT practitioner is preparing an individual with burns to perform a home program of positioning and splinting. The MOST appropriate recommendation to prevent deformity would be to:

A. discontinue the positioning and splinting program upon returning home.
B. continue the same positioning and splinting program that was indicated before discharge.
C. continue with the positioning and splinting program only during the day.
D. continuing with the positioning and splinting program only at night.

154. A student has been working on learning to activate a switch for a communications device. Although the switch is mounted on the wheelchair tray, the student continues to have difficulty operating it because of excessive muscle tone. Despite practicing for extended periods of time, the student is not making any progress. The OT practitioner decides to:

A. position the switch to facilitate easy access and reposition as needed.

B. passively stretch the student's upper extremity to increase range of motion.

C. use a brightly colored switch to increase visibility.

D. use systematic behavioral reinforcement through shaping.

155. During a kitchen activity, an individual with decreased shoulder ROM demonstrates difficulty retrieving items from the higher shelves. Which of the following recommendations will BEST facilitate home management for this individual?

A. Store the most frequently used items on shelves just above or below the counter.

B. Use the largest joint available to move or lift items from high shelves.

C. Perform shoulder range-of-motion exercises 10 times each, twice a day.

D. Continue reaching for items on high shelves because it will help improve range of motion.

156. An OT practitioner is instructing a patient with left hemiplegia and unilateral neglect to put on a tee shirt. The MOST effective dressing sequence to teach the patient is to:

A. (1) place left hand into sleeve and pull up sleeve past elbow; (2) place right hand into sleeve and pull up sleeve; (3) pull shirt up over head; (4) pull shirt down over trunk.

B. (1) position shirt on lap; (2) place left hand into sleeve and pull up sleeve past elbow; (3) place right hand into sleeve and pull up sleeve; (4) pull shirt up over head.

C. (1) position shirt on lap; (2) place right hand into sleeve and pull up sleeve past elbow; (3) place left hand into sleeve and pull up sleeve; (4) pull shirt up over head.

D. (1) pull shirt up over head; (2) place left arm into sleeve; (3) place right arm into sleeve; (4) pull down shirt over trunk.

157. A 6-year-old has been receiving OT for dressing skill development and is now independent. At discharge, the BEST advice for the OT to give the child's parents in order to maintain the child's independence in dressing at home is:

A. give assistance when the child asks for it to provide a successful experience.

B. give praise for completed dressing; do not help the child get dressed.

C. give him oversize clothing with Velcro closures and large snaps.

D. give him verbal prompts when needed and help with closures only.

158. Which of the following is the BEST example of "objective" information as written by an OT practitioner for the objective section of a discharge summary?

A. Patient reports he can work at the computer much longer and more comfortably than he could initially.

B. Patient's ability to work at the computer has increased from 10 minutes to 3 hours with stretch breaks every 30 minutes.

C. Patient has improved significantly in his ability to work at the computer.

D. Patient reports he is now able to work at the computer for 3 hours, where initially he was only able to tolerate 10 minutes.

159. An individual with cognitive deficits exhibits little transfer of skills from one activity to the next. Which intervention would be BEST to assist this individual in performing the steps of doing laundry?

A. Performing memory drills of the steps involved in doing a laundry activity

B. Placing serial pictures of a laundry activity in sequence

C. Making a checklist of steps in the process, then consulting the list while doing laundry in the actual setting

D. Reading a story about a person doing laundry with the individual, then discussing the story

160. A mother of three young children complains of severe low back pain. The BEST way for her to get her toddler up from the floor to the changing table for a diaper change is to:

A. carry the child as close to her body as possible.

B. lift the child from the floor using a wide base of support, one foot slightly in front of the other.

C. lift the child from the floor by bending the knees, not the back.

D. have the child climb up onto her lap.

161. What is the appropriate level of assistance for an OT practitioner to provide within a parallel group to address the psychosocial needs of the group members?

A. Encourage experimentation among group members.

B. Observe from the sidelines and not act as an authority figure.

C. Participate as an active member.

D. Assist clients in the selection of simple, short-term tasks.

162. A child is on a pureed diet because of an inability to chew food. The MOST effective method to facilitate the child's ability to chew would be to:

A. encourage the child to remove food from the spoon with his teeth.

B. stimulate the management of texture by using vegetable or beef soup.

C. increase the management of texture by slowly increasing texture of food with a baby food grinder.

D. stimulate biting and chewing by placing a raisin between the child's teeth.

163. When transferring an individual from one seat to another, OT practitioners can BEST protect themselves from injury by:

A. stepping back from the individual.

B. keeping the back in a flexed position.

C. keeping the knees bent.

D. maintaining a narrow base of support.

164. According to the independent living movement (ILM), which nonresidential facility would the OT MOST likely recommend to an elderly individual with a disability who has no resultant functional limitations?

A. A cradle-to-grave home

B. A transitional living center

C. An adult day program

D. A center for independent living.

165. An OT practitioner is considering possible topics for a discharge planning group for individuals on an inpatient psychiatric unit. Which of the following topics would be MOST important to cover because it is significantly related to the possibility of rehospitalization?

A. Management of household and finances

B. Living skills needed for keeping aftercare appointments

C. Coping strategies for continuing medication compliance

D. Education about alcohol and substance abuse

166. An OT practitioner working in a school system is part of a multidisciplinary team that contributes to an individualized education program. An individualized education program is MOST APPROPRIATELY completed for:

A. occupational therapists as part of the continuing education plan.

B. adults who have sustained a head injury.

C. all children with disabilities before they receive special education services.

D. families before discharge of a significant other from OT services.

167. The goal for an elderly individual with lower extremity weakness is to be independent with bathing, but this requires the tub to be more accessible to the individual, who uses a walker. Which environmental adaptation would the OT practitioner MOST likely recommend to achieve this?

A. Tear out the tub and install a walk-in shower.

B. Install shower doors for privacy and support getting in and out of tub.

C. Provide a transfer tub bench and install grab bars.

D. Place nonskid decals in the tub and mats on the floor to prevent slipping on the wet floor.

168. An OT practitioner is running a community re-entry group in which individuals discuss their personal feelings and concerns about returning to the community. Which of the following would be the BEST method to facilitate this process in a nonthreatening manner?

A. Individuals write fears and concerns on index cards and then the therapist collects and reads the cards to the group for discussion.

B. Individuals write fears and concerns on index cards and then take turns reading their cards to the group.

C. Individuals each take a turn verbalizing their fears and concerns to the group.

D. The psychologist speaks to the group about discharge fears in general.

169. A young child with hypertonicity is unable to bring his hands to midline to reach for a toy while in the supine and sitting positions. The BEST position to use in order to reduce the effects of abnormal patterns and facilitate midline grasp is:

A. the standing position.

B. the prone position.

C. the side-lying position.

D. the quadruped position.

170. Which adapted technique would the OT practitioner MOST likely select in order to teach an 8-year-old girl with hemiparesis who wishes to dress independently?

- A. Encourage the child to do most of her dressing while lying in her bed.
- B. Teach the child to dress her hemiparetic extremities first.
- C. Educate the child's mother regarding how to assist with dressing skills.
- D. Teach the child to dress her non-hemiparetic extremities first.

171. A high-school-age patient is being discharged from a burn center to his home environment after an 8-month inpatient stay for severe burns. In educating the parents about common psychological reactions, the OT would MOST likely address:

- A. the possibility of decreased range of motion and sensation.
- B. the potential for noncompliance, apathy, and depression.
- C. the likelihood of violent behavior and sexual acting out.
- D. the potential for delirium and fatigue.

172. An individual who uses a wheelchair and has limited financial support is moving into a new apartment and wants to select a floor surface for easy maneuverability. Which of the following surfaces is the MOST appropriate for this situation?

- A. Vinyl floor
- B. Short pile carpeting
- C. Deep pile carpeting
- D. Several area rugs

173. A young child exhibits tactile defensiveness with all dressing tasks. The MOST effective handling technique would be to:

- A. tickle the child prior to dressing and undressing.
- B. play loud music when undressing the child.
- C. lightly stroke the child's arms and legs during dressing tasks.
- D. hold the child firmly when dressing him.

174. An OT practitioner who needs to transfer an obese man is not confident she can manage the transfer alone. The BEST action for the practitioner to take is to:

- A. use proper body mechanics.
- B. ask someone from PT to do the transfer.
- C. ask another person for assistance.
- D. refrain from transferring the patient.

■ OCCUPATIONAL THERAPY FOR POPULATIONS

175. A multidisciplinary team is conducting a needs assessment to develop a fall prevention program for the frail hospital population. The MOST likely section of the needs assessment for the OT practitioner to perform would be:

- A. analysis of statistical data on the number of falls occurring each year.
- B. environmental hazard analysis and fall risk during performance of ADL.
- C. evaluation of gait and mobility device use of those at high risk for falls.
- D. assessment of medication impact on fall incidence.

176. An OT who is employed by a senior center has been asked to develop groups to address the motor needs of people with Parkinson's disease. Which of the following activities would be MOST appropriate to include?

- A. A game of rhythmic exercises performed to music
- B. Creating time capsules for their grandchildren
- C. Wheelchair races performed in pairs
- D. Taking turns reading out loud from the newspaper

177. A school-based OT works with children who require assistance with upper and lower extremity strengthening to facilitate safe mobility on the playground and in the cafeteria. The need to strengthen arms and legs is MOST likely identified by the OT during the assessment of:

- A. motor performance
- B. sensory processing
- C. visual perception
- D. cognition

178. Which of the following reflects a primary goal area appropriate for wellness programs with the elderly population?

- A. improving strength following strokes.
- B. increasing overall physical activity levels and fitness.
- C. improving social interactions for depressed elders.
- D. increasing independent performance of ADL and mobility.

179. An OT practitioner has developed a work conditioning program for men and women who were previously homeless and exhibit generally decreased endurance. The FIRST part of the work conditioning program would be to have the individuals perform:

A. adapted work activities.
B. nonspecific job-simulated work tasks.
C. job-specific work tasks.
D. range of motion and strengthening exercises.

180. An OT practitioner is employed by a school district to provide consultation to vocational instructors in a high school program for students with moderate developmental disabilities. Which of the following activities would be MOST appropriate for the OT to provide?

A. Developing an in-house prevocational work program
B. Bringing in outside speakers from different job settings
C. Teaching the vocational instructor different assessment tools and scoring procedures
D. Meeting the vocational instructor weekly to discuss adaptations to work tasks

181. An OT practitioner has been hired to develop social skills training programs for persons with long-term mental illness in a community mental health facility and needs to select a behavior to assess as an outcome measure. Which would BEST indicate that the program was successful in achieving goals for this population?

A. Improved ability to balance rest, work, play, and leisure
B. Improved verbal and nonverbal communication skills
C. Improved ability to identify areas for vocational exploration
D. Improved ability to perform daily self-care and home management activities

182. An OT practitioner consulting to a drop-in shelter for homeless women is developing a leisure activity group protocol. One of the goals of this group is to foster a sense of competence and mastery over the environment. Which of the following types of activity BEST addresses this goal?

A. Small group collage activities
B. Leather lacing change purses from kits
C. Outings to see movies
D. Presenting resident talent shows

183. The goals of an occupational therapy health promotion program for a well elderly population include enhancing life satisfaction and preventing loss of physical and social function. What is the MOST important type of activity to include in this program?

A. Activities that promote home and community safety
B. Socialization activities
C. Balance and ambulation activities
D. Activities to promote the skills of caregivers

184. An OT practitioner working for an assisted living corporation needs to design programs to engage residents with dementia who wander and pace the halls throughout the day. The BEST type of activity program to plan for these residents would be:

A. reminiscing about previous jobs.
B. walking as part of a walking club.
C. singing oldies in a group.
D. a craft activity requiring concentration.

185. An OT practitioner providing accessibility consultation services to a local library finds a reference room with a doorway that has a threshold height of 2 inches, making wheelchair access difficult. Which of the following recommendations would be MOST appropriate?

A. Keep the threshold as is, and place a sign near the door alerting people to the threshold.
B. Provide a throw rug that covers the threshold.
C. Remove the threshold altogether.
D. Ramp the threshold.

186. The director of an assisted living facility has asked an OT to help them develop a falls prevention program. The OT should FIRST:

A. evaluate residents of the facility who have fallen in the last 6 to 12 months.
B. interview facility administration and staff to determine goals for the program.
C. determine how frequently falls occur, how many individuals are affected, and how the problem is currently being addressed.
D. provide the director with a menu of recommendations that will address the problem of falls in the facility and determine a starting point.

■ SERVICE MANAGEMENT AND PROFESSIONAL PRACTICE

187. An OT practitioner has recommendations concerning adaptations for a child's artificial limb. This would require that the therapist consult the:

A. physiatrist.

B. orthotist.

C. prosthetist.

D. physical therapist.

188. While preparing for a presentation at a professional conference, an OT realizes he does not have the name of the author of an article containing critical information he planned on photocopying and distributing. Which of the following is the MOST appropriate action for the OT to take?

A. Distribute the handout and apologize for not having the author's name.

B. Show the handout with an overhead projector and apologize for not having the author's name.

C. Use the handout only as a resource while developing the presentation.

D. Use the article without mentioning the author.

189. An OT practitioner is asked, "What is the primary emphasis of occupational therapy services?" by another health professional. The MOST accurate response for the OT to give is that the emphasis is on:

A. skill acquisition.

B. compensation for deficits.

C. environmental adaptation.

D. reinforcement and enhancement of performance.

190. A clinical manager of OT supervises an employee who has demonstrated specialized skills in treatment and serves as an expert for her peers. This practitioner has completed research, leadership training, and assisted in continuing education activities. The manager of the department is MOST likely to supervise this individual at what level?

A. Close supervision

B. Intermediate supervision

C. Advanced supervision

D. Educator supervision

191. An OT manager is providing an in-service to the OT staff pertaining to medical conditions and payment. Which of the following BEST represents the process of the federal government recommending a standardized payment for health-care services?

A. DRGs

B. PPS

C. PAMs

D. cost shifting

192. An OT practitioner is working with an individual who tests positive for HIV. The individual accidentally cuts his finger with a knife while helping with a meal preparation activity. Which of the following are the MOST appropriate precautions to follow?

A. Suicide precautions

B. Universal precautions

C. Escape from unit precautions

D. Medical precautions

193. An OT practitioner evaluating a child notices a bruise on the child's shoulder that looks like an adult's hand and fingerprints. Which of the following actions is MOST critical for the OT practitioner to take?

A. Discuss this with the family member who picks up the child.

B. Observe for additional injuries.

C. Make a report to appropriate authorities.

D. Avoid becoming involved in personal family matters.

194. An OTR arrives for a home health visit, but the individual is not feeling well so they reschedule for the following day. The practitioner's charges for the week are due that afternoon. Anticipating a follow-up visit with the individual the next day (1/15/05) and reluctant to wait another 2 weeks to submit for payment, the practitioner bills for treatment using the 1/14/05 date. The OT practitioner's action is:

A. acceptable because treatment has been scheduled for the next day.

B. acceptable if the agency she works for allows it.

C. unacceptable because it violates the Code of Ethics.

D. unacceptable because if the individual is still ill and unable to participate in therapy on 1/15/01, a delay of more than 1 day is unacceptable for billing purposes.

195. When working within a school system to assist the mainstreaming of a child with spina bifida into a regular classroom, the OT consults with the classroom teacher. The nature of this "consultation" relationship is BEST characterized by the following statement:

A. the OT teaches the teacher.

B. the OT provides therapy to the child.

C. the OT directs the teacher.

D. the OT problem-solves with the teacher.

196. Which of the following BEST represents the disciplinary action that designates a time frame in which an OT practitioner is required to attain counseling or additional education in order to remain certified?

A. A reprimand

B. A censure

C. Probation

D. Revocation

197. An OT practitioner is writing a job description for an aide position in the OT department. According to AOTA guidelines, which of the following is BEYOND the scope of practice of an aide?

A. Cue an individual with schizophrenia to maintain attention to task during a weekly cooking group led by an OT.

B. Practice use of a sock aid and shoe horn in the OT department with a patient who has had a hip replacement and is able to perform the task safely, but takes an excessive amount of time.

C. Help place food on the spoon for a patient practicing the use of a universal cuff in the patient's room at lunchtime, while the OT supervisor runs a lunch group in the dining room.

D. Help a child maintain correct positioning during paper and pencil activities next to the OTR who is working with another client.

198. An OT learns that a nursing home resident fell during the night and may have sustained a new fracture. The individual still wishes to engage in therapy. What is the BEST course of action for the OT to take?

A. Provide treatment as originally planned, based on the wishes of the individual.

B. Withhold treatment, but gather information on the course of events for documentation and consultation with the treatment team.

C. Provide treatment by observing performance in self-feeding, an area not listed as an OT treatment goal, but an ADL activity that the individual continues to perform despite the possible fracture.

D. Withhold treatment and leave all information gathering and treatment decisions to the OT director, despite the fact that the OT director may not be in the facility until the following week.

199. During OT treatment, a child has a seizure. The MOST important action for the OT practitioner to take during the seizure is to:

A. check breathing and administer mouth-to-mouth resuscitation if necessary.

B. attempt to restrain the child's movements to prevent injury.

C. ease the child to a lying position, remove or pad nearby objects, and loosen clothing.

D. take no action except observation of the child.

200. One of the core values of the American Occupational Therapy Association's Code of Ethics is related to OT practitioners and their ability to respect the well-being of their clients. This aptitude is commonly referred to as:

A. prudence.

B. beneficence.

C. justice.

D. fidelity.

Answers for Simulation Examination 3

1. (D) Ask the person to identify several common objects by sight only. Asking the person to identify various objects by sight, answer D, would identify if the person has difficulty with recognition of objects through visual input alone, called agnosia. Answer A, asking for a demonstration of using utensils, would be a screening technique to reflect if the person has a deficit in planning purposeful movement, called apraxia. Picking out utensils from a drawer of similar items in various positions could provide information about the person's visual perception in the areas of form constancy or figure ground discrimination. Answer C, asking for the steps of the process, would provide some information on the person's cognitive ability to sequence steps of a task rather than a perceptual function. See Reference: Pedretti and Early (eds). Wheatley, CJ: Evaluation and treatment of perceptual and perceptual motor deficits.

2. (B) cognitive status. The individual's ability to learn how to safely perform ADLs and IADLs is directly related to cognitive status (answer B). Poor memory, poor judgment, or impulsive behavior can interfere with safe occupational performance after discharge. While it also is important to know what type of support the individual will have upon returning home, which can include marital status (answer A), this information could be obtained from the medical chart or other sources. Leisure interests and work responsibilities (answers C and D) are important areas to identify, but are secondary to cognitive status because of its relationship to safety. See Reference: Trombly and Radomski. Bear-Lehman, J: Orthopaedic conditions.

3. (C) "I'm just too tired." One of the main symptoms of major depressive disorder is decreased energy; therefore, the response of "I'm too tired" indicates fatigue. Answer A reflects a level of feeling that is higher than the usual subdued feelings associated with depression. Answer B reflects the individual's perceptions of his or her ability or competence. Answer D is a response reflecting interests or values that conflict with the proposed activity. See Reference: Cara and MacRae (eds). Cara, E: Mood disorders.

4. (D) use of an ATM machine and public transportation. Money management, shopping, and community mobility skills are the areas most likely to be addressed in a community reintegration program. Bed mobility and transfers (answer A), self-care skills (answer B), and cognition, sensation, and motor skills (answer C) are all areas that would have been addressed initially during the inpatient phase of rehabilitation. See Reference: Pedretti and Early (eds). Gutman, SA: Traumatic brain injury.

5. (D) Watch the child engage in dressing, eating, and bathing activities. Watching the child engage in dressing, eating, and bathing tasks within the home would be the only choice that reflects the components of skilled observation. According to Clark, Miller-Kuhaneck, and Watling, one must "observe variables (contextual, activity, client factors) that support or hamper participation" (p. 112). Answer A, performing a questionnaire, is most representative of interviewing, not observing, while answer B, obtaining performance information, is considered to be a measurement assessment method. And lastly, answer C, referring to medical/performance data, reflects those items most closely linked to record review, not skilled observation. See Reference: Miller-Kuhaneck. Clark, G, Miller-Kuhaneck, S, and Watling, R: Evaluation of a child with an autism spectrum disorder.

6. (D) anosognosia. Anosognosia is a form of neglect in which an individual denies any deficits. Compensation techniques cannot be taught to someone who has no awareness of his or her deficits. A person with a visual field cut (answer A) has a loss of a specific area of vision related to an area of the visual system that has been damaged. When there is an awareness of the loss, compensatory techniques can be taught. A person who has apraxia (answer B) is unable to perform a purposeful movement on command, but is able to understand a loss of ability and can perform activities spontaneously or follow some cues. Aphasia (answer C) is an impairment of receptive or expressive communication verbally, but a person with this is able to comprehend gestures or pictures and use them as a compensatory technique. See Reference: Trombly and Radomski. Quintana, LA: Assessing abilities and capacities: vision, visual perception, and praxis.

7. (C) Vestibular processing, postural control, and muscle tone. Vestibular processing and postural control are required for maintaining balance. Muscle tone that is too high or too low will limit an individual's ability to move the lower extremities for ambulation. Therefore, vestibular, postural and adequate muscle tone (answer C) are important for successfully walking across the pool. Fine motor coordination (answer A) is not required to walk across the pool. In addition, although walking in water requires some strength, it can still be successfully performed with significantly decreased strength, because the body weighs much less when submerged. Answer B includes postural control and gross motor coordination, which are both important for walking in the pool, but it also includes auditory processing, which is not necessarily indicated for this particular aquatic activity. Answer D includes range of motion and praxis, both of which are required to some degree for walking in the pool, but it also includes crossing the midline, which is not required. See Reference: Pedretti and Early (eds). Creel, TA, Adler, C, Tipton-Burton, M, and Lillie, SM: Mobility.

8. (A) Encourage two or more children to play next to each other while sharing finger paint supplies. Encouraging the child to play next to another child while finger painting is most representative of a parallel play situation. According to Mulligan, "parallel play occurs when children play comfortably next to each other, possibly sharing materials and conversing, but their play agendas and activities are separate" (p. 100). Answers B and D are most representative of social play. "Social play involves play activities that are shared and requires children to interact directly with one another during play. Social play involves cooperation, mutually agreed upon roles or rules, social interchange, and (often) competition" (p. 100). And lastly, answer C is viewed as a form of solitary play, where the child is simply playing in isolation of other children. See Reference: Mulligan. Mulligan, S: Typical Child Development.

9. (C) Edema, contracture, muscle tone, and pain. Edema limits range of motion because of the increase of fluid in the extremity. A contracture can result when joint motion is limited by a prolonged spasticity or change in the tissues, causing resistance to passive stretch. Muscle tone also may be a limiting factor in one's ability to complete range of motion. If an individual is unable to move a part through full range against gravity, the therapist may put the individual in a gravity-eliminated position to attempt the same movement. Finally, pain may be a limiting factor. This may particularly be seen in individuals with arthritis or changes in joint structure. Pain generally occurs in the end ranges of motion. Other options listed (proprioception, stereognosis, sensation, and diadochokinesis) may affect the quality of active movement or coordination, but do not limit or PROM. See Reference: Trombly and Radomski. Trombly, CA and Podolski, CR: Assessing abilities and capacities: Range of motion, strength, and endurance.

10. (A) figure-ground discrimination. Figure-ground discrimination is the ability to distinguish an object from the background. A person with impaired figure-ground discrimination would have difficulty finding the sock despite its position on the bed (answer A). Other deficits that may be demonstrated by the person would be an inability to see the sock on one side of the bed (unilateral neglect), to find it in relation to the bed (position in space), and to know how to get back to the bed to look for the sock (cognitive mapping). See Reference: Trombly and Radomski. Quintana, LA: Assessing abilities and capacities; vision, visual perception, and praxis.

11. (B) Follow test manual directions. When administering a standardized test, directions from the test manual should be followed closely to ensure reliability of test results. The test environment should be free of visual or auditory distractions or the child may have difficulty concentrating; therefore, answer A, "test in a stimulating environment" is incorrect. Answer C is incorrect because there are times when "...a child's fatigue, behavior, or time constraints" make it impossible to give the complete test in one session, and "most tests provide guidelines about how the test can be administered in two sessions" (p. 239). Answer D is wrong because, although the overall success of an evaluation can depend on the

OT practitioner's ability to establish a rapport with the child and the family, too much conversation with the child may be distracting and prevent optimal performance. See Reference: Case-Smith (ed). Richardson, PK: Use of standardized tests in pediatric practice.

12. (C) Briefly interview the individual using closed-ended questions, targeting the individual's premorbid and current self-care performance levels. Severely depressed individuals often exhibit low self-esteem, lack of interest in personal appearance and hygiene, difficulty concentrating, and low energy, in addition to many other possible symptoms. A brief assessment would be indicated for an individual with a short attention span, and closed-ended questions (answer C) are usually easier to answer and require less energy to answer than open-ended questions (answer B). Having to demonstrate self-care tasks (answer A) would likely be frustrating for this individual, and a poor performance level could reinforce feelings of low self-esteem. Basing an initial assessment on observation (answer D) could prove a valid method; however, many factors other than limited ability could account for this individual's appearance. For example, this appearance may be typical of this individual's premorbid appearance, or the individual may not have had time to prepare herself prior to the scheduled evaluation. See Reference: Early. Responding to symptoms and behaviors.

13. (C) Memory impairment. Cognitive abilities such as memory (answer C) are most often the first to be affected in individuals with Alzheimer's disease. Disorientation to time and place (answer A), personality changes, and loss of independence in ADL (answer D) appear in the middle stage of the disease. Incontinence (answer B), the inability to recognize family members, and the inability to walk are evident in the late stage of Alzheimer's disease. See Reference: Cara and MacRae (eds). Mental health of the older adult.

14. (C) developmental dyspraxia. The motor problem described as it occurs during the evaluation is characteristic of developmental dyspraxia. Children with dyspraxia often learn tasks such as jumping rope with great difficulty, effort, and considerable practice. However, when the task is altered, such as in this case by asking the child to skip backward, the child is unable to adapt the task for a long while. Answer A is incorrect because the child with delayed reflex integration would have difficulty with all aspects of the task. Answer B is incorrect because a problem of bilateral integration would affect both aspects of this task, jumping rope forward and backward. Answer D also is incorrect because general incoordination would probably affect performance of both forward and backward rope jumping. See Reference: Case-Smith (ed). Parham, LD, and Maillous, Z: Sensory integration.

15. (C) distal humerus. An individual who has undergone a long above elbow amputation has lost the limb at the level of the distal humerus. This results in loss of hand and wrist function, all pronation and supination, and elbow flexion and extension. See Reference: Pedretti and Early (eds). Keenan, DD and Morris, PA: Amputations and prosthetics.

16. (C) Prevocational assessment. Prevocational assessment, answer C, is particularly effective if conducted before entrance to the workforce and focuses on examining a client's vocational readiness in terms of "...the skills involved with getting and keeping a job, social- and community-living competencies, personal care, and leisure activities" (p. 302)." Prevocational assessment also helps to identify work preferences and would be the most appropriate area of work-related assessment with which to begin before the actual work begins. Answer A, vocational assessment, is incorrect because this assessment focuses on work performance within a specific work situation. Answer B, environmental assessment, and answer D, assistive technology assessment, are both essential parts of the overall job analysis process that helps match workers with appropriate jobs, but would occur later in the transition phase. See Reference: Ross and Bachner (eds). Wysocki, DJ and Neulicht, AT: Work is occupation: what can I do as an occupational therapy practitioner?

17. (A) physical, cognitive, and sensorimotor abilities. According to Buning and Schmeler (2003), "before assessing computer needs, the primary therapist should complete, a holistic evaluation of the client's physical, cognitive, psychological, and sensorimotor abilities" (p. 673). While answers B, C, and D do address other relevant factors regarding computer use, they would most likely be initiated after assessing client ability. See Reference: Crepeau, Cohn, and Schell (eds). Buning, ME and Schmeler, MR: Contextual Modification and Assistive Technology.

18. (D) Strength. Exerting enough pressure to twist off a jar lid requires strength. The client demonstrates adequate range of motion (answer A) when he grasps the knife. He demonstrates adequate coordination (answer B) by spreading peanut butter on the bread and accurately positioning the lid onto the jar opening, and he demonstrates adequate endurance (answer C) by standing during the entire activity of making a peanut butter sandwich. See Reference: Pedretti and Early (eds). Pedretti, LW: Muscle strength.

19. (C) have the individual perform a simple cooking task, then use a different food at the next session. Giving the individual a functional task, then changing it, and observing how he responds, will tell the therapist how well the individual can transfer learning to new situations. If the individual cannot perform the activity when it is changed slightly, it suggests there may be difficulty transferring learning. If the patient can perform the activity with many changes and in a different setting, it suggests that he has more aptitude for transfer of learning to new situations. Answers A, B, and D could be ways of assessing different aspects of cognition (judgment, perceptual problem-solving, and ability to calculate figures), but as described, would not provide evidence of transfer of learning. See Reference: Crepeau, Cohn, and Schell (eds). Giuffrida, CG and Neistadt, ME: Overview of learning theory.

20. (C) Seat the child in an unsupported chair and ask the child to grab the OT's thumbs, gently rock the child to see how long they can maintain the seated position. Because the child is being evaluated for sitting balance, the most appropriate position to assess for muscle co-contraction would be answer C. According to Mulligan, "co-contraction is the ability of opposing muscle groups to contract at the same time, providing stability around a joint...push and pull in an arc-type motion, up and toward the child, and down and away from the child. Do not let the child lock elbows; if the child has good co-contraction, he should be able to stay relatively still" (p. 222). Answer A is the ability to maintain the prone extension position, while answer B is an example of supine flexion. And lastly, answer D is a position used to determine hyper-extensibility and subsequent low tone of the arms. See Reference: Mulligan. Mulligan, S: Interviews and Observations.

21. (B) a perception that the amputated limb is actually intact and painful. Phantom limb pain is present when the amputated limb is perceived to be present with accompanying pain (answer B). Answers A and D, feelings of numbness and tingling or an intact limb, are associated with the sensation of a phantom limb, but not phantom limb pain. Answer C, feelings of sharp pain at the stump site may be due to a neuroma, which can be related to nerve tissue issues. See Reference: Pedretti and Early (eds). Keenan, DD and Morris, PA: Amputations and prosthetics.

22. (A) athetoid. Athetoid cerebral palsy is characterized by widely fluctuating tone (answer A). When tone rapidly shifts from hypertonic to hypotonic, movements appear writhing and uncontrolled. Hypertonic muscle tone or spasticity (answers B and C) results in impaired ability to control movement or force of movement. Hypotonia or low tone (answer D) results in flaccid muscles and floppy movements. See Reference: Solomon (ed). Wandel, JA: Cerebral palsy.

23. (D) Encourage the patient to speak with the rehabilitation psychologist to discuss his concerns. OT practitioners often need to address functional issues related to sexuality when working with individuals who have been seriously injured or disabled, and should be well versed and comfortable with the topic. Rather than moving into an area requiring skills beyond the scope of the OT (answer A), the OT should refer the individual to the psychologist, whose role is to provide more extensive sexual or marital counseling, which appears to be what is required in this situation. The physiatrist (answer C), a physician specializing in rehabilitation, is responsible for attending to the medical needs of the individual and coordinating the rehabilitation process. Discussing the increased chances of divorce (answer B), while true, would not be helpful to this individual at this vulnerable time. See Reference: Crepeau, Cohn, and Schell (eds). Cohn, ES: Interdisciplinary communication and supervision of personnel.

24. (D) Read the social worker's report. The social worker's report typically includes details about the patient's family situation, occupational, educational, and cultural background, and expected environment. Referring to this document eliminates the need to duplicate this information. Reviewing the medical history would be valuable (answer A) prior to an initial evaluation, but the social worker's report would most likely provide information related to social/cultural issues. Interviews with the patient and family by OT practitioners (answers B and C) are designed to obtain information concerning role and task performance, and performance levels in work, self-care, and leisure. See Reference: Early. Data gathering and evaluation.

25. (A) "The child rocks and bangs his head against the wall throughout the evaluation." Answer A is most representative of restrictive-repetitive acts such as rocking, hand flapping, biting, dumping, throwing, and self-talk. According to Audet, "the diagnostic criteria for disorders on the PDD spectrum include the presence of restrictive and repetitive acts" (p. 53). Answers B, C, and D

are most representative of behaviors related to socialization deficits frequently seen in cases of PDD. According to Audet, "children with PDD often have difficulty with the range and quality of social acts" demonstrated by the child crying, laughing inappropriately, and not responding to others' initiations for no apparent reason (p. 49). See Reference: Miller-Kuhaneck. Audet, L: The pervasive developmental disorders: A holistic view.

26. (D) Determine the individual's home environment and her need for meal preparation skills. It is important to include the context in which an individual performs, or will need to perform, work, self-care, and leisure activities as part of the evaluation process, as well as the individual's needs, interests, strengths, and weaknesses. It is possible that this individual has always lived in environments where others cooked for her and that she may never need to cook for herself. If indeed meal preparation skills are important to this individual, it may then be necessary to evaluate her cognitive level (answer A) in order to develop appropriate short- and long-term goals (answer B). After evaluation is complete and goals are established, the individual can be scheduled for an intervention such as a meal preparation group (answer C). See Reference: Early. Data collection and evaluation.

27. (C) steps, width of doorways, and threshold heights. The first area of evaluation would be the steps, width of doorways, and presence and height of door thresholds (answer C) to determine whether the wheelchair user will be able to enter and exit interior spaces in the wheelchair or whether structural modifications are required. Answers A, B, and D reflect areas that also will need to be evaluated; however, they are not as critical to initial interior access. See Reference: Pedretti and Early (eds). Foti, D: Activities of daily living.

28. (D) The effect of personal, behavior, values, routines, performance capacity, and the environment on role performance. Evaluation, according to the Model of Human Occupation, would focus on the holistic understanding of how personal factors such as interests, values, personal causation (volitional subsystem), habits, roles and routines (habituation subsystem), and performance systems (brain, mind, body) affect one's choices in occupational behavior and role performance. Evaluation according to the Behavioral frame of reference identifies problem behaviors that need to be extinguished (answer A). The Object Relations frame of reference attempts to clarify thoughts, feelings, and experiences that influence behavior (answer B). An OT using the Cognitive Disability frame of reference should evaluate cognitive function, including assets and limitations (answer C). See Reference: Bruce and Borg. Model of human occupation-systems perspective of occupational performance.

29. (D) motor planning. Motor planning or praxis problems are often seen in young children when they are dealing with novel equipment. Motor planning (answer D) requires an adequate body concept and the ability to cognitively plan movements. Fine motor skills (answer A) are required for dexterity and manipulation and are not required for mounting a rocking horse. In order to climb into the high-chair and jump on a trampoline, the child must have integrated reflexes (answer C) and adequate gross motor skills (answer B). See Reference: Case-Smith (ed). Appendix 12-A.

30. (B) Combing the hair. An individual normally abducts and externally rotates the shoulder to comb his or her hair; therefore, the individual is more likely to have difficulty in this area than any of the others. Shoulder abduction is not required for buttoning a shirt (answer A) or tying a shoe (answer D). Tucking in a shirt in the back (answer C) requires shoulder abduction and internal rotation. Tying shoelaces (answer D) is less dependent on shoulder motion than on hip and spine flexibility. See Reference: Pedretti and Early (eds). Foti, D: Activities of daily living.

31. (B) radial-digital grasp. Children usually develop a radial-digital grasp (answer B) at the age 9 months; they use the grasp for precision control. A pincer grasp (answer A), or tip pinch, is characterized by opposition of the thumb and index fingertips to allow the child to make a circle with the fingers. The palmar grasp (answer C) is a power grasp, in which the individual flexes the fingers around an object while stabilizing it against the palm. In a lateral pinch (answer D), the individual places the pad of the thumb against the radial side of the index finger near the DIP joint. This pattern is used as a power grip on small objects. See Reference: Case-Smith (ed). Exner, CE: Development of hand skills.

32. (A) proximal to the MCP joints. Stabilization is applied proximal to the MCP joints to isolate the joint movement being measured and to eliminate any combined movements. Answers B, distal to the MCP joints, and C, at the wrist, would allow combined movements of the joints and would invalidate the individual joint measurements. Answer D, on top of the MCP joints, would block joint movement and make any individual joint measurements incorrect. See Reference: Crepeau, Cohn, and Schell (eds). Kohlmeyer, K: Sensory and neuromuscular function.

33. (B) Line bisection. Line bisection is used as a method of determining unilateral neglect. The block assembly (answer A) is used for evaluating constructional apraxia. Proverb interpretation (answer C) evaluates an individual's ability to think abstractly. The overlapping figures (answer D) test figure-ground discrimination. See Reference: Unsworth (ed). Corben, L and Unsworth, C: Evaluation and intervention with unilateral neglect.

34. (D) Support. Answer D is correct because the term "support reaction" refers to the ability to coactivate muscle groups of the appropriate extremity or about the midline in order to support the body weight or posture in a certain position. Answer A is incorrect because protective reactions follow the development of support reactions in the arms (which protect the child when falling) and require that the body is free from support. Answer B is not correct because equilibrium reactions are compensatory movements used to regain stability, not to maintain stability. Answer C is not correct because rotational righting reactions involve turning of the head or trunk in order to maintain body alignment. See Reference: Crepeau, Cohn, and Schell (eds). Kohlmeyer, K: Sensory and neuromuscular function.

35. (A) −15 to 0 to 140 degrees. Negative range of motion documentation may vary from one setting to another. However, this range may be written as a negative (minus) sign preceding the degree (−15 degrees) or as a positive number preceding the neutral position (15 degrees to 0 degrees to 140 degrees). Therefore, answers B, C, and D are incorrect. See Reference: Pedretti and Early (eds). Pedretti, LW: Joint range of motion.

36. (D) Termination of activity. This individual demonstrated difficulty ending the task of brushing his teeth. Trying to put toothpaste on the toothbrush before taking off the cap would be an example of a deficit in sequencing (answer A). Difficulty following directions (answer B) could be evident if the individual attempted to brush his hair or shave rather than brush his teeth. An example of impaired problem solving ability (answer C) would be if the individual tried to squeeze the tube of toothpaste too softly so that nothing came out, and then gave up on the task. See Reference: AOTA: Practice Framework. Table 2. Performance Skills—Process Skills.

37. (D) at the midrange of the joint. Proprioception (or position sense) is demonstrated when an OT practitioner passively positions the joint being tested and the individual is able to imitate the position with the opposite extremity. The joint should not be moved through range to an extent that would elicit a stretch or pain response (answers A and B), which would be at the end ranges of the joint. Movement should be at a rate of approximately 10 degrees per second to prevent the stretch reflex from being elicited. The endpoints of the range (answer C) are used as the starting positions from which proprioception testing is initiated, because it is in these positions that the stretch or pain response would occur. See Reference: Pedretti and Early (eds). Iyer, MB and Pedretti, LW: Evaluation of sensation and treatment of sensory dysfunction.

38. (C) gravitational insecurity. Gravitational insecurity is described as "excessive fear during ordinary movement activities" (p. 352). The child easily experiences a fear of falling and prefers to keep her feet firmly on the ground. Tactile defensiveness (answer A) is a term used to describe discomfort with various textures and with unexpected touch. Developmental dyspraxia (answer B) is a term used to describe a problem with motor planning. Intolerance for motion (answer D) refers to a very similar and often related problem of inhibition of vestibular impulses, but it is usually associated with sensory information received from the semicircular canals. Gravitational insecurity, on the other hand, is associated with the utricle and saccule. See Reference: Case-Smith (ed). Parham, LD and Mailloux, Z: Sensory integration.

39. (D) a cotton swab to apply light touch to a small area of the client's skin. The senses included in the somatosensory system are touch, movement, pain, and temperature. The auditory, olfactory, visual gustatory, and vestibular systems are special systems that directly give input into the brain. Answer D, the use of a cotton swab, is a test commonly used to determine a client's ability to feel light touch, whereas answer A is a component for the assessment of vision. Answer B is typically used to determine pain perception and answer C is a technique commonly used to distinguish the client's ability to perceive temperature. See Reference: Crepeau, Cohn, and Schell (eds). Kohlmeyer, K: Sensory and neuromuscular function.

40. (C) indicating initiative and beginning task-directed behavior. Because this child is very withdrawn, any spontaneous action should be seen as a very positive sign. It is important to encourage the child in independent exploratory behavior to develop task competence and to become less withdrawn. Her use of a toothbrush instead of a hairbrush may indicate cognitive limitations (answer B), possibly caused by a lack of exposure; it also could be caused by a visual deficit (answer D), but the primary signifi-

cance of the observation lies in answer C. Attention-getting behavior (answer A) is unlikely in such a withdrawn child. See Reference: Case-Smith (ed). Cronin, AS: Psychosocial and emotional domains.

41. (D) Dynamometer. This individual exhibits difficulty in the area of strength. A dynamometer measures grip strength through gross hand grasp. A volumeter (answer C) is a container used to measure edema in the hand by measuring the amount of water displaced when the hand is placed into the container. A goniometer (answer A) is a tool with two arms used to measure movement at a joint. One arm is held stationary while the other arm moves around an axis of 360 degrees. An aesthesiometer (answer B) measures two-point discrimination with a movable point attached to a ruler that has a stationary point at one end. See Reference: Trombly and Radomski. Trombly, CA and Podolski, CR: Assessing abilities and capacities: Range of motion, strength, and endurance.

42. (B) observation of the child in a social, gross motor, and self-feeding task. Observation of the child's social play, motor processes, and self-feeding skills (answer B) would be the most appropriate nonstandardized form of assessment of a preschool child. Answer A, relying upon a one-on-one interview, would not be the most valuable choice, because preschool children are not always a reliable source for obtaining detailed information. It would be more helpful to combine an interview of the child in conjunction with a parent/teacher interview. Whereas answer C, relying upon the results of a standardized test, such as the Miller Assessment of Preschoolers, would not be considered a nonstandardized assessment. And lastly, answer D, observation of the child on the playground, could be something the OT might consider, but a more comprehensive picture can be drawn from a combined observation of the child's social, motor, and feeding skills. See Reference: Mulligan. Mulligan, S: A guide to evaluation.

43. (D) view of the problem and overall goals. The interview is generally the component of the assessment process in which the OT practitioner asks about the individual's goals for treatment, and gains an understanding of the problems from the person's perspective. Diagnoses and medications (answers A and B) are most often found in a review of the chart. Abilities (answer C) are determined through performance measures. See Reference: Early. Data collection and evaluation.

44. (B) A pinch meter. A pinch meter is used to measure the strength of a three-jaw chuck grasp (also known as palmar pinch), in addition to key (lateral) pinch and tip pinch. These tests are performed with three trials that are averaged together and then compared with a standardized norm. Answer A, the aesthesiometer, measures two-point discrimination. Answer C, the dynamometer, measures grip strength. Answer D, the volumeter, measures edema in the hand. See Reference: Pedretti and Early (eds). Kasch, M and Nickerson, E.: Hand and upper extremity injuries.

45. (D) The child uses a wide base of support and can walk well for very short distances. Answer D is correct because according to Mulligan, the child, "walks well for very short distances; may use a wide base of support, and falls frequently, especially over uneven ground" (p. 132). Answers A, B, and C are not considered typical for a normally developing child. See Reference: Mulligan. Mulligan, S: Typical child development.

46. (B) skin integrity, pain, ROM, and sensory loss. Upon initial evaluation of a client with a tendon injury, the OT must document "typical signs and symptoms of hand injury...disruption of skin integrity, localized pain, decreased ROM, possible sensory loss, and decreased functional use" (p. 803). Documenting the client's attitude toward adaptive equipment (answer A) is imperative although not as important as answer B because the client most likely has not been educated regarding the various types of equipment available to date. Answers C and D are typically contraindicated after a tendon injury until the extent of the injury is identified by the client's physician and/or tendon repair initiated. See Reference: Crepeau, Cohn, and Schell (eds). Spenser, EA: Upper extremity musculoskeletal impairments.

47. (B) show acceptance and understanding regarding the individual's situation. Paraphrasing is used to clarify and relay acceptance of what an individual has communicated. The OT paraphrases by repeating in her or his own words what the client has said. Redirection (answer A) is used to promote healthier thoughts and behaviors. Forcing the individual to make a choice (answer C) may be accomplished by providing a question that includes two possible choices. An individual is encouraged to provide additional information (answer D) when the OT asks open ended questions. See Reference: Crepeau, Cohn, and Schell (eds). Henry, AD: Introduction to evaluation and interviewing Section II: The interview process in occupational therapy.

48. (A) explain to the parents that toilet training is not a feasible option. Answer A is correct because "when the lesion is in the lumbar region or below, the bladder is flaccid (lower motor neuron bladder)...the reflex arc is not intact, and the bladder

has lost all tone...Children with a flaccid bladder cannot be trained because the bladder has no tone to empty" (p. 508). As toilet training is not appropriate (answer C), these children are commonly provided with some type of catheterization after medical testing is performed. Although nighttime bowel and bladder control may not be accomplished until the normally developing child is 4 or 5 years of age, waiting another year (answer B) would not change anything for this child. Independence in lower extremity dressing (answer D) is an appropriate goal for this child, but it is not relevant to the issue at hand. See Reference: Case-Smith (ed). Shepherd, J: Self-care and adaptations for independent living.

49. (D) monitor heart rate, blood pressure, and symptoms. "It is important to assess the patient's heart rate, blood pressure, ECG, and symptoms to establish the patient's tolerance for exercise" (p. 1077) when working with individuals with cardiac conditions (answer D). Shortness of breath and chest pain (answers B and C) are symptoms associated with exercise intolerance, and are subsumed within answer D. Additional symptoms may include pain referred to the teeth, jaw or ear, excessive fatigue, lightheadedness and dizziness, and nausea or vomiting. MET values are units of measurement associated with how much oxygen is required to perform various activities. Light ADL activities such as eating, shaving, and standing up require approximately 1.5 to 2.0 METS. Initial ADL evaluation would usually be at this level. Dressing and undressing require about 3.0 to 4.0 METS. A MET level of 3.0 (answer A) may be too high for individuals on the first day of therapy following open heart surgery. See Reference: Trombly and Radomski. Huntley, N: Cardiac and pulmonary diseases.

50. (A) The doorway width needs to be expanded to have a minimum clearance of 32 inches when the door is open. According to ADA accessibility guidelines, a doorway needs to have a minimum clear opening of 32 inches with the door open 90 degrees, measured between the face of the door and the opposite stop. In an environmental evaluation process, according to ADA guidelines, the doorway rather than the individual's wheelchair (answer B) needs to be adapted. See Reference: Trombly and Radomski. Shamberg, S: Optimizing access to home, community, and work environments.

51. (D) child will correctly identify, by feel only, five out of five common objects. Identifying an object by touch (answer D) is termed "stereognosis" or "identification of solids." Stereognosis is a tactile discrimination skill needed for the development of fine hand manipulation. Answer A demonstrates localization of tactile stimuli, answer B demonstrates graphesthesia, and answer C is an example of the tactile discrimination of textures. See Reference: Case-Smith (ed). Exner, CE: Development of hand skills.

52. (A) the use of energy conservation. Energy conservation techniques reduce the amount of energy expenditure an individual requires to perform various activities. For a client with COPD and limited endurance, energy conservation techniques should be taught early so they can be implemented and reinforced while performing other activities, such as preparing meals. Work hardening (answer B) and graded activities to increase strength (answer C) would not address the need to perform meal preparation in the most energy efficient manner. Safety in the kitchen (answer D) would be more relevant to individuals with sensory or balance loss rather than limited endurance. See Reference: Pedretti and Early (eds). Matthews, MM: Cardiac and pulmonary diseases.

53. (C) use headphones during work to reduce competing sensory input. Reducing competing sensory input is helpful in increasing visual attention. Increasing competing input (answers A and B), or reducing the amount of visual input (answer D), may reduce the ability to attend to visual stimuli. See Reference: Case-Smith (ed). Schneck, CM: Visual perception.

54. (B) decrease the effects of prolonged inactivity. Some of the main objectives of inpatient cardiac rehabilitation include decreasing the effects of prolonged inactivity, such as thromboembolism, orthostatic hypotension, and muscle atrophy; safely providing a program of monitored activity performance to maximize function; reinforcing cardiac precautions; and providing instruction in energy conservation techniques. It is acceptable and expected to encounter fatigue in this population after activity (answer A); however, activities that produce cardiac symptoms should be avoided. Activities that promote endurance and strength are beneficial, but ROM (answer C) is not usually an area of concern. Most individuals do not need to relearn activities, other than applying energy conservation techniques; therefore, independent performance (answer D) is not a primary concern. See Reference: Pedretti and Early (eds). Matthews, MM: Cardiac and pulmonary diseases.

55. (A) vestibular reactions. According to Miller-Kuhaneck (2004), "children with a PDD can demon-strate significant gross motor skill deficits...children with a PDD often are highly active yet might have difficulty perceiving where their heads and bodies are in relation to the pull of gravity because of their inefficient sensory processing" (p. 60). Answer A is the correct answer because vestibular activities pro-vide "opportunities for movement through space" (p. 231). However, it is important to monitor a child's reaction since the activity can either calm or disorganize the child's vestibular/proprioceptive sys-tems. Answers B and D are considered to be fine, not gross motor interventions, while answer C is oral, not gross motor in nature. See Reference: Miller-Kuhaneck. Chapter 3: The pervasive develop-mental disorders: A holistic view.

56. (C) Wrist splints to promote development of tenodesis. Hand splinting to promote tenodesis is implemented in the acute phase of rehabilitation. A tenodesis grasp is developed by allowing the finger flexors to shorten. The patient is then able to achieve a functional grasp by extending the wrist. This improves the ability of an individual with a C6 or C7 spinal cord injury to grasp and hold objects. A volar pan splint (answer A) would not allow finger flexors to shorten, and would interfere with the development of tenodesis. Interventions related to promoting independent performance (answer B) should begin as soon as possible, but issues related to positioning must be addressed first. An individual would not be instructed in bed mobility (answer D) until after the acute phase. See Reference: Pedretti and Early (eds). Adler, C: Spinal cord injury.

57. (D) Rubbing different textures on the skin. Based on the concept that stimuli which is novel or fast results in alerting responses (p. 309), then answer D, rubbing different textures on the skin, is correct because this activity would provide novel stimulation that would result in alerting responses and an increase in level of arousal. Answers A, B, and C all reflect types of activity stimuli which are routine, familiar or slow, and that would result in calming responses. See Reference: Bruce and Borg. Sensory motor model-physiological basis for improved function.

58. (C) complete upper-extremity self-care using appropriate adaptive equipment with supervision by a family member. A long-term goal is written in conjunction with the individual and family to specify the end result of a longer period of treatment. A short-term goal breaks the long-term goal into manageable steps to be accomplished by the individual within a certain time frame or number of treatment sessions. Performing upper-extremity bathing, lower-extremity dressing, or a commode transfer were all short increments toward the stated goal of the individual returning home with the assistance of one person. The goal that encompassed the long-range plan was to complete upper-extremity self-care with the supervision of a family member. See Reference: Trombly and Radomski. Radomski, MV: Planning, guiding, and documenting therapy.

59. (B) ability to grade movement. The grading of movement goal (answer B) best addresses the difficulty with control of the midrange of a movement pattern (common in children with athetosis). Answer A is incorrect, because this goal would be appropriate for a child who cannot break up a flexion or extension pattern during a movement. Answer C is not correct, because this goal is appropriate for a child who has difficulty with an arm or hand movement being too fast or too slow (graded movements are also too fast). Answer D is also incorrect, because this goal is appropriate for a child who has difficulty bringing both arms to midline and using them effectively together. See Reference: Case-Smith (ed). Exner, CE: Development of hand skills.

60. (B) practicing the whole task of putting on a shirt in a setting similar to the real environment. Retention of a skill will be enhanced if the task is practiced in its entirety during each performance trial, because whole task performance is easier to recall than separate steps. Generalization of skills is enhanced when an activity has been acquired in a setting that resembles the natural environment where the skill will be performed. Answer A, practice of each segment of the process, may be useful for improving performance of the activity segments practiced, but will not enhance retention and generalization of the skill. Providing simulation activities (answer C) may improve some performance components involved in the dressing process, but will not enhance learning of the whole task of putting on a shirt. Answer D, showing a videotape and providing written directions, is a useful instructional technique for client education from a cognitive perspective, but they do not provide the motor component necessary for learning a motor skill. See Reference: Gillen and Burkardt (eds). Sabari, JS: Activity-based intervention in stroke rehabilitation.

61. (A) objective and measurable statements of what will be accomplished with time frames. The purpose of a goal is to provide a specific measurable statement that addresses "..the desired targeted outcomes," (p. 617) and indicates what is to be ac-

complished. Clients and significant others play vital roles in working with the therapist to establish goals that are meaningful and realistic, but it is an essential aspect of the therapist's role to synthesize information provided by the client to help formulate finished goals which also are measurable and include time frames for achievement. Description of the client's reasons for the goals are a component of the evaluation information (answer B) and would not be included in goals. Specific measurements of the client's skill and performance (answer C) are parts of the assessment information that assist the therapist in establishing goals and treatment, but are not included in goals. Treatment approaches to be used (answer D) are included in the treatment plan, not the goal statements. See Reference: AOTA: Practice Framework. p. 617.

62. (C) propose a modified goal that still meets the parent's needs. "In family-centered intervention the occupational therapist addresses the needs of the entire family rather than only concentrating on specific deficits in the child" (p. 722). Proposing a modified goal of functional mobility with an adaptive mobility device, would best address both the parent's need for decreased carrying, and the child's need to improve functional mobility within the environment. Agreeing to work on an unrealistic and possibly unachievable goal (answer A), would not meet the child's needs for developmentally appropriate intervention. Answer B, offering an alternative goal, would not be responsive to the problems identified by the family. Answer D is incorrect because this child is too young to establish her own goals, though this might be encouraged at later stages of therapy. See Reference: Case-Smith (ed). Stephens, LC and Tauber, SK: Early intervention.

63. (C) ADL training in use of adaptive techniques for LE dressing and transfers. The primary role of the occupational therapist in working with the person with a total knee replacement is answer C, ADL training in use of adaptive techniques for LE dressing and transfers, as needed. Decreased knee movement may require the person to use adaptive equipment for tub transfer or special devices for lower extremity dressing (if the person cannot touch his toes), including practicing putting the knee immobilizer on and off. Answer A, improving strength of the upper extremities would not necessarily be an aspect of treatment. Answer B would be an area that the physical therapist would address. A homemaking evaluation, answer D, might be performed, but would not be a primary focus of intervention because the person would be expected to resume homemaking at the same level without difficulty once the period of recovery is over. See Reference: Pedretti and Early (eds). Coleman, S: Hip fractures and lower extremity joint replacement.

64. (A) Using effective communication skills. Clarifying expectations, honestly defining needs, and providing tactful and constructive feedback are communication skills that promote understanding. Successful communication with the client's children will most likely help them deal with their fears and concerns, increase their understanding of their father's condition, and elicit greater cooperation, which should help to decrease some stress for the father. Although time management techniques, deep breathing, progressive muscle relation, and laughter (answers B, C, and D) are all useful and valid stress reduction techniques, they do not address the issue at hand, which is communication between the father and his children. See Reference: Crepeau, Cohn, and Schell (eds). Giles, GM: Stress management.

65. (D) sitting position. Answer D is correct because an upright sitting position provides the child with the opportunity not only to further control head movement (stability has developed in horizontal positions), weight-bearing, and weight-shifting, but also to rotate the trunk as he or she reaches toward the opposite side of the body. Answers A and B are not correct because head and neck stability have most likely developed primarily in the prone and side-lying positions, before the child has attained a seated position. See Reference: Kramer and Hinojosa (eds). Schoen, SA and Anderson, J: Neurodevelopmental treatment frame of reference.

66. (B) Cut up meats and sandwiches. To increase oral tolerance and control of food, textures are gradually modified from smooth and consistent (answer C), to smooth and slightly varied (answers A and D), to increasingly resistive foods and a combination of contrasts, for example, hard and crunchy mixed with soft or liquid. After the child has mastered this level of control and tolerance, he or she can safely proceed to an even greater variety of textures, tastes, and temperatures, such as cut up meats and sandwiches, answer B. See Reference: Case-Smith (ed). Case-Smith, J, and Humphry, R: Feeding intervention.

67. (B) Hammering a nail into a piece of wood. Hammering a nail into a piece of wood requires the individual to stabilize the object against the palm and fingers, while the thumb is positioned to perform as an opposing force. Answer A is a form of prehension commonly referred to as tip prehension. Answer C, carrying a pail of bolts, requires a hook grasp. This requires the MCP joints to be placed in extension,

the PIP and DIP joints to be flexed, and may not include the use of the thumb. Answer D is considered a spherical grasp pattern that requires the fourth and fifth digits to assume a more flexed position for enhanced cupping of the palm. See Reference: Pedretti and Early (eds). Belkin, J and Yasada, L: Orthotics.

68. (B) "This program will help you to learn about the skills you have that are needed on MOST jobs and about your potential for work. Prevocational evaluation programs are designed to assess work skills that the client possesses, to identify their potential for work, and to help participants acquire skills by practicing skills that are important in the work environment. Vocational evaluation programs identify the actual interests and skills for specific types of work, such as assembly line work (answer A). Work role maintenance programs are for individuals who are employed, but whose involvement in treatment has temporarily interrupted their employment (answer C). Developing job search skills (answer D) is needed for clients who have job skills but who have difficulty finding employment. See Reference: Cara and MacRae (eds). Vocational programming.

69. (A) weight shifting and equilibrium reactions. According to Bundy, et al. (2002), "We discuss intervention to develop five aspects of postural control, including: tonic postural extension, tonic flexion, postural instability, weight shifting, righting and equilibrium reactions, and oculomotor control" (p. 281). Possible symptoms of an overreactive vestibular system are given in answers B, C, and D, which are problems of intolerance for motion, and gravitational insecurity. See Reference: Bundy, Lane, and Murray (eds). Koomar, J and Bundy: Creating direct intervention from theory.

70. (B) Training in residual limb wrapping. Residual limb wrapping would help prepare the residual limb to fit in the prosthesis by shrinking and shaping it. Training in how to put on and take off the prosthesis (answer A), and activities to improve grasp and prehension (answer C), come later in the intervention process when the prosthesis has been selected, prescribed, and fitted. Training to resume vocational activities (answer D) also would normally occur later in rehabilitation process after the patient has mastered the basics of prosthetic use. See Reference: Pedretti and Early (eds). Keenan, DD and Morris, PA: General considerations of upper and lower extremity amputations.

71. (D) Social skills training. Answer D, social skills training, is the correct answer because it can be used to develop the ability to relate appropriately and effectively with others (p. 60). The sensory integration treatment approach, which aims to improve the reception and processing of sensory information within the central nervous system, uses vestibular stimulation and gross-motor exercise (answer A). This approach involves the use of pleasurable activities that do not require conscious attention to movement (answer C), and is best suited to individuals with chronic schizophrenia who have proprioceptive deficits. Modification of the social environment (answer B) will not help in developing social skills and is most appropriate for individuals with cognitive disabilities. See Reference: Early. Some practice models for occupational therapy in mental health.

72. (C) Make-believe group with stuffed animals and imaginary friends. Encouraging a drama/make-believe group with 3-year-old children is the most suitable answer. Symbolic play is typically imaginative in nature, thus making any activity that involves pretending that dolls and stuffed animals are real appropriate. "The child also may imitate the actions of parents, teachers, and peers. At age 3 to 4 years, pretend play becomes more abstract, and objects, such as a block, can be used to represent something else" (p. 85). Answer A, scissors and cutting tasks, would most likely be used to facilitate fine motor and in-hand manipulation skills, while answer B, jumping rope, would involve gross motor skills typically seen in older children. Answer D, building towers to resemble an actual picture, is an activity that would be more representative of constructive play and/or manipulation skills. See Reference: Case-Smith (ed). Case-Smith, J: Development of childhood occupations.

73. (A) work locks and latches on doors and windows. The ability to manipulate the locks and latches is a safety concern because the individual may be unable to open them to let family members into the home or close them to keep intruders from entering. Built-up handles (answer B), energy conservation techniques (answer C), and adaptations to clothing fasteners (answer D) are not safety issues. See Reference: Trombly and Radomski. Yasuda, YL: Rheumatoid arthritis and osteoarthritis.

74. (D) Weaving on a frame loom. Use of and attention to the entire loom area is essential for weaving on a frame loom. The shuttle must slide across the entire width of the loom, which involves crossing the midline. It is possible to build a coil pot (answer A), to make macramé objects (answer B), and string beads for a necklace (answer C) without crossing the midline. See Reference: Breines. Folkcraft.

75. (B) Implement a pureed diet and allow adequate time for eating. As ALS progresses, speaking and swallowing become more difficult and a pureed diet becomes necessary. The individual runs the risk of aspiration or choking if meals are rushed. Adaptive equipment (answers A and D) are provided much earlier in the disease process. The independence achieved with adaptive equipment has a positive psychological effect on the individual who most likely sees his or her independence slipping away. Answer C, upper extremity strengthening, would be contraindicated in the late stages of the disease. See Reference: Pedretti and Early (eds). Schultz-Krohn, W, Foti, D, and Glogoski, C: Degenerative diseases of the central nervous system.

76. (A) Textured material, rubbing, tapping, and prolonged contact. Sensory desensitization helps the individual recalibrate altered sensory perceptions in order to decrease discomfort associated with touch. This type of intervention "...generally includes contact of the of hypersensitive skin with items that provide a variety of sensory experiences, such as textures ranging from soft to coarse" (p. 591), much like the graded tactile stimuli listed in answer A. Treatment is most successful when carried out and controlled by the individual. With a severe injury such as a burn, it also is necessary to train the individual in protective precautions. Answers B and C, techniques that provide an ungraded or nonspecific level of touch, would not be well tolerated by a person with hypersensitivity because much of the input is facilitatory and would be interpreted as painful. Visual compensation and functional use of the extremity (answer D) are techniques used with individuals who have impaired sensation. See Reference: Trombly and Radomski. Bentzel, K and Quintana, LA: Optimizing sensory abilities and capacities.

77. (B) assembling packets that include a knife, fork, spoon, and napkin based on a sample. Answer B is correct because this individual's abilities suggest that he is functioning at Allen's Cognitive Level 4. At this level of functioning, he is able to copy demonstrated directions presented one step at a time and may find it easier to copy a sample than to follow directions or diagrams, as would be the case for the activity of assembling packets that include a knife, fork, spoon, and napkin based on a sample. Answer A reflects functioning at Allen's Cognitive Level 3, where individuals are capable of using their hands for simple, repetitive tasks and sorting tasks, but are unlikely to produce a consistent end product. The shoelace task (answer C) is more appropriate for those functioning at Allen's Cognitive Level 5.

because these individuals can identify the relationships between objects and generally perform three-step tasks. Answer D, gluing labels onto cans and placing them in an appropriate container according to color, describes a task that can be performed by an individual who has the ability to anticipate errors and plan ways to avoid them; this is a also a generally more complex task and requires attention to detail, all of which requires that an individual be able to function at Allen's Cognitive Level 6. See Reference: Early. Some practice models for occupational therapy in mental health.

78. (A) Chaining. Chaining with a child who demonstrates a cognitive disability shows all sequences in the entire process of a task. Initially, the child performs only the beginning or end of a task. Thus, the child initially concentrates on only a small part of the task and gradually increases participation in all sequences in their correct order. Answers B, C, and D are other methods that can be used, but forward and backward chaining are instructional methods that have been particularly successful with individuals who are mentally retarded. See Reference: Early. Medical and psychological models of mental health and illness.

79. (B) Extending the elbow in mid range 30 to 40 degrees with the forearm resting on the table. Extending the elbow in mid range 30 to 40 degrees while the arm is resting on a table surface (answer B) is correct because muscles with poor minus strength would only be able to move a body part through partial range of motion in a gravity eliminated position. The individual would then need assistance to complete the range of motion while using what strength is available in the body part. Answer A is incorrect because PROM would not utilize the increased strength available since the muscle does not contract. Answers C and D are incorrect because both involve resistive activities and a muscle with poor minus strength would be unable to move against gravity or to take any resistance, even with gravity eliminated. See Reference: Trombly and Radomski. Trombly, CA and Podolski, CR: Assessing abilities and capacities: range of motion, strength, and endurance.

80. (D) To arrive at work on time consistently. Time management skills are based on the ability to "recognize one's values and priorities, structure a daily routine, schedule one's time, and organize tasks efficiently" (p. 467). Answers A, B, and C are ways of coping with being late, not strategies for the time management goal of being on time. See Reference: Early. Psychosocial skills and psychological components.

81. (C) Incorporating simple, familiar activities such as hanging up clothing or catching a ball. Incorporating simple activities would be most effective for gaining active cooperation participation from a person with Alzheimer's. Telling the person to perform repetitions of active exercises (answer A) might not be effective because s/he may not be able to remember to perform repetitions of exercises or may not understand the purpose and become confused. Training in the use of adaptive devices (answer B) would not increase active shoulder motion and could be confusing if cognitive deficits were present. PROM exercises (answer D) would not lead to improvement of active range of motion. See Reference: Hellen. Communication: Understanding and being understood.

82. (A) Improve posture, then improve shoulder stability, then improve grasp. Because the proximal-to-distal approach begins at the center of the body, then proceeds to the extremities, answer A is correct. Postural stability would be developed first, then shoulder stability, and then grasping patterns. Answers B, C, and D are incorrect because they do not follow this order. See Reference: Case-Smith (ed). Exner, CE: Development of hand skills.

83. (D) washing windows. Washing windows (answer D) is a repetitive activity that involves resisted, elevated upper extremity activity. Rests can be taken as needed. Making the bed, peeling potatoes, and polishing furniture (answers A, B, and C) do not provide adequate resistance to achieve upper extremity strengthening. See Reference: Dutton. Introduction to biomechanical frames of reference.

84. (D) Each member will share space while working on a task without disrupting the work of others for 15 minutes. Parallel groups are most appropriate for people who can "...tolerate being with more than one person at a time" (p. 393), but do not have the ability to interact successfully with other group members. Participants in parallel groups are involved in individual tasks that require minimal, if any, interaction. Therefore, appropriate expectations for parallel groups focus on remaining in the group and working alongside others. Experimenting with a new group role (answer A) is a goal consistent with egocentric-cooperative groups. Sharing materials with another group member (answer B) is a project group goal. Expressing feelings within a group (answer C) is consistent with a cooperative group. See Reference: Bruce and Borg. Appendix N.

85. (C) Combine task with additional sensory input (tactile, proprioceptive, and auditory). Answer C is correct because additional sensory input, when combined with a visual memory task, facilitates memory. Answer A is not correct because interest in the task should be high in order to enhance visual memory. Answer B is not correct because visual attention is a prerequisite to visual memory. Answer D is incorrect because serial or varied repetition enhances visual memory. See Reference: Kramer and Hinojosa (eds). Todd, VR: Visual information analysis: Frame of reference for visual perception.

86. (B) Client will draw for 1 hour, taking stretch breaks every 20 minutes. Goals refer to what the therapist anticipates the individual will accomplish and should be functional, measurable, and objective. This answer meets those criteria. Answer A is not measurable. Answers C and D describe what the OT practitioner will do, and would be included in the Plan section of a note. See Reference: Borcherding. Writing functional and measurable goals.

87. (A) Skill building activities with concrete goals, such as time management training. Answer A is correct because "Individuals who display negative symptoms often need highly structured activities with concrete expectations and goals" (p. 157). Answers B, C, and D are all treatment formats which could be used with clients who have schizophrenia, but may present too high a level of challenge at this stage. See Reference: Cara and MacRae (eds). Schizophrenia.

88. (A) the therapist has the child play "sandwich" between heavy mats. The sandwich activity (answer A) provides heavy touch pressure over the body, which can be inhibitory to a child experiencing sensory defensiveness. Answer B is incorrect because use of a feather brush stimulates the light touch system, which is already impaired, and may be extremely uncomfortable for a child with tactile defensiveness. Answer C is not correct because the use of a blindfold, when a child is already reacting to unexpected touch, would most likely create a fearful response, while answer D also might aggravate the child's existing problem due to an unexpected touch from the back. See Reference: Kramer and Hinojosa (eds). Kimball, JG: Sensory integration frame of reference: Theoretical base, function/dysfunction continua and guide to evaluation.

89. (B) Learning proper body mechanics. Learning proper body mechanics (along with achieving a good fitness level) is one of the first steps to reducing the risk of reinjury in a work program. Answer C, work hardening, is appropriate to implement after the physical demands of the job's specific tasks are achieved. Answer D, engaging in vocational counsel-

ing, is appropriate after it is determined that a client cannot return to the same job or employer. Answer A, a prework screening, is typically completed by the practitioner before the employer offers the new employee a job. See Reference: Crepeau, Cohn, and Schell (eds). Fenton, S Gagnon, P and Pitts, DG: Work.

90. (A) Practice preparing a variety of foods using different cooking methods and recipes. Recent findings in motor learning suggest that practicing a variety of tasks in a nonsystematic, but repetitive way (variable practice), can enhance learning retention and transfer of skills, because the novelty introduced into the task engages more cognitive effort. The practice methods identified in answers B, C, and D focus more on systematic or constant practice. This type of practice may result in better performance of different parts of the task, or of one task, but not in improved learning retention and skill transfer. See Reference: Crepeau, Cohn, and Schell (eds). Giuffrida, CG: Motor learning: An emerging frame of reference for occupational performance.

91. (B) Attempt to push the child higher and slightly harder. According to Bundy, Lane, and Murray (2002), "clients who have autism often need to experiment with the intensity, duration, frequency, and rhythm of sensations" (p. 294). Thus, the OT should attempt to push the child slightly higher and harder (answer B) to determine if "pushing the client higher elicited smiles and sounds of pleasure, indicating that more intense input was needed to create a meaningful experience" (p. 294). However, if the more aggressive swinging activity continued to upset the child, then the OT should consider abandoning the activity (answer A). Answer C, asking the child which activity they would prefer to do next, may not be effective, "because many individuals (with autism) cannot communicate verbally" (p. 294). And lastly, determining the child's level of adaptive responses is something that should have been determined prior to the intervention stage. It would be more appropriate to re-evaluate adaptive responses if engagement in SI tasks continues to frustrate the child. See Reference: Bundy, Lane, and Murray (eds). Chapter 12: Creating Direct Intervention from Theory.

92. (C) increase swimming time to 25 minutes or to tolerance. This individual's goal is to maximize strength and endurance. Although ALS is a progressive degenerative disease, improvements in strength and endurance are possible if the individual was not previously functioning at maximum capacity. This individual's performance indicates potential for further improvement. Therefore, the program should be upgraded, not downgraded (answer B). Methods for improving endurance include increasing the frequency, intensity, or duration of the activity. The correct answer (answer C) increases the duration of the activity while recognizing the importance of avoiding fatigue. Answer A continues the program at a maintenance level. Using adaptive equipment (answer D), such as a flotation belt, is an energy saving strategy that would be appropriate if the individual were experiencing fatigue during swimming. See Reference: Dutton. Biomechanical postulates regarding intervention.

93. (A) large, easily interlocking pieces. For the child with fluctuating muscle tone, efforts should be made to provide a means of stabilizing toys and equipment. The interlocking quality of such toys as "bristle blocks" and magnets will provide some stability and assist with controlled release. The large size of the blocks will facilitate a more effective grasp. Small or lightweight blocks (answers B and C) are more difficult to manipulate, and therefore are not recommended for constructive play for a child with coordination difficulties. Colorful blocks (answer D) may stimulate some interest, but have no direct bearing on the child's ability to engage in construction efforts. See Reference: Case-Smith (ed). Morrison, CD and Metzger, P: Play.

94. (B) Explain to the individual and caregiver that one must be "homebound" in order to be eligible for home care services. In order to be eligible for home care services, the individual must be confined to home, a condition referred to as homebound. The individual need not be bedridden, but leaving the residence must require a considerable or taxing effort. Absences from the home are permitted, but must be infrequent in nature, short in duration, or for the purpose of receiving medical treatment. Given that this individual is able to leave the home for a social visit and tolerate riding in a car for 30 minutes, he is not considered homebound. The OT practitioner would first inform and explain this criterion to the individual and caregiver (answer B). After this has been explained, the OT practitioner would communicate with the PT (answer D) and refer the individual for outpatient therapy (answer C). Simply providing a home program and discharging the individual would not meet the individual's needs because he continues to require therapeutic intervention. See Reference: Piersol and Ehrlich (eds). Zahoransky, M. The system and its players.

95. (B) Ask the individual to try some lacing with distant supervision and praise her for what she has been able to do. All of the responses are increments of approaches used for decreasing dependency needs. Answer B is the best next step in this case because it allows the individual to attempt some lacing in the presence of the OT, who in turn offers reassurance that the individual is actually able to do the activity. The step in answer B would be followed by that in answer D. Here the individual is required to attempt some lacing without the benefit of the OT at her side. The OT is nearby, but working with another client. As the individual is able to do more of the activity independently, written instructions (answer A) replace the OT as the instructor. Finally, when the individual is feeling comfortable with self-instruction, asking her to work on the project without OT assistance (answer C) heightens the level of self-responsibility. See Reference: Early. Analyzing, adapting, and grading activities.

96. (C) Provide lateral trunk support. A lateral trunk support in the frontal plane stabilizes the side, helping to maintain correct alignment of the pelvis and trunk in the chair by counteracting the twisting effect of asymmetrical muscle tone. By providing upper extremity support, the lateral trunk support also would prevent improper loading onto an unstable shoulder joint. Using a reclining wheelchair (answer A) is incorrect because doing so would shift the individual's weight to the posterior, but would not prevent the lateral shift of the trunk. An arm trough (answer B) may help maintain a more centered position of the trunk, but the weight of the affected extremity would result in instability and improper alignment of the shoulder, which could lead to shoulder pain. A lateral pelvic support (answer D) would provide stabilization of the pelvis to prevent it from shifting sideways, but this support would be too low to prevent the trunk from moving laterally. See Reference: Pedretti and Early (eds). Gutman, SA: Traumatic brain injury.

97. (B) Brushing her own hair. "The power grasp is often used to control tools or other objects. Oblique object placement in the hand, flexion of the ulnar fingers, less flexion with the radial fingers, and thumb extension and adduction facilitate precision handling with this grasp (e.g., for brushing hair)" (p. 295). Answer A, pegboard activities, would most likely be introduced to facilitate the pincer grasp or tip pinch, while answer C, carrying a briefcase, such as a child's art case, would encourage the hook grasp position. Lastly, the activity of ball-throwing, would most likely be introduced to encourage a spherical grasp position. See Reference: Case-Smith (ed). Exner, C: Development of hand skills.

98. (C) Preparing a frozen dinner. The Rehabilitation Institute of Chicago identified five levels of complexity for meal preparation ranging from easiest (level one) to hardest (level five). Preparing macaroni and cheese, a hot one-dish meal, falls into the fourth level. Because the individual is unable to successfully perform at this level, the task must be downgraded to the next lowest level, i.e., level three, which includes preparation of hot beverages, soups, or frozen dinners. Having the individual prepare a multicourse meal, such as chicken and mashed potatoes (answer A), would be upgrading the activity to level five. Cold meals and foods such as instant pudding and peanut butter and jelly sandwiches (answers B and D) are at level two. Downgrading to this level would be appropriate if the individual had experienced significant difficulty not minimal to moderate as demonstrated here. See Reference: Crepeau, Cohn, and Schell (eds). Culler, KH: Home management.

99. (B) A mobile arm support. A C5 quadriplegic with fair shoulder flexors and abductors, and at least poor minus biceps, upper trapezius, and external rotators, will be able to operate a mobile arm support for self-feeding and facial hygiene activities. A wrist-driven flexor hinge splint (answer A), would be used for a lower level spinal cord injury (C6–C8), in which the individual had functional use of the shoulder and arm muscles, and has fair plus or better wrist extension strength. This splint is indicated for individuals who lack prehension power. An electric self-feeder is indicated for individuals with a higher level of involvement (C4), and who demonstrate poor plus, or weaker, shoulder strength. Built-up utensils may be indicated for individuals with C8 or T1 injuries, because they may lack the strength to tightly grasp regular utensils. See Reference: Trombly and Radomski. Atkins, M: Spinal cord injury.

100. (B) provide a warning tone, such as noisy bracelets on the wrist, or as a reminder to visually scan toward the affected side. Although hazards may be removed from the environment, or padded to prevent injury to an individual, use of these interventions is only feasible in a person's home. It is best to teach the individual visual scanning (attention training through warning tones) of the affected area and the environment, a technique that may be used anywhere. An individual may avoid using sharp tools or extreme water temperature, but this avoidance does not teach him or her how to monitor the affected side visually, because it is a precaution that addresses only the problem with sensation. Noisy bracelets are one technique that may be used to accomplish compensation for both unilateral neglect and absence of sensation. Visual impairments that are not accompanied by sensory or perceptual deficits are more readily overcome with retraining. See Reference: Trombly and Radomski. Quintana, LA: Optimizing vision, visual perception, and praxis abilities.

101. (D) Accept his decision. Individuals with depression are aware they are not performing at their usual level, and recognize when they have not done a good job. It is important to accept his decision and not pursue it further. He will recognize the implied praise (answers B and C) as false, and may be too ashamed or embarrassed to give a poorly executed project as a gift (answer A). See Reference: Early. Responding to symptoms and behaviors.

102. (C) get the shirt all the way on, then line up the buttons and holes, and begin buttoning from the bottom. It is easier to see the buttons and buttonholes at the bottom of the shirt (answer C) than at the top (answer B). Therefore, beginning to button from the bottom is more likely to result in success for the individual with motor or visual-perceptual deficits. Buttoning first (answer A) may result in ripping off the buttons as the shirt is pulled over the head. A buttonhook with a built-up handle (answer D) would be more helpful for an individual with finger weakness or incoordination (e.g., quadriplegia). See Reference: Pedretti and Early (eds). Foti, D: Activities of daily living.

103. (C) adding cabinets with labeled compartments to store items out of sight. For a child with attention deficit disorder to optimize self-organization skills, the environment should provide a minimum of distractions. Placing unused items out of sight reduces visual distraction; labeling compartments (answer C) helps the child retrieve items. Answers A and B add visual distraction, and answer D addresses a limitation in motor function, not self-organization. See Reference: Case-Smith (ed). Cronin, AF: Psychosocial and emotional domains.

104. (B) a tub bench and toilet rails. A tub bench and toilet rails make bathroom transfers easier and safer, and allow the person with a unilateral LE amputation to transfer independently. Lightweight cooking utensils (answer A) are recommended for those individuals with weakness or joint involvement of the upper extremities. Answers C and D are incorrect because long-handled dressing devices and reachers are more likely to be recommended when compensation for hip or trunk flexion is needed, and use of these devices might discourage the normal bending activity in the person with LE amputation.

See Reference: Pedretti and Early (eds). Keenan, DD and Morris PA: Amputations and prosthetics.

105. (B) Raising the handlebars. The correct answer is B because raising the handlebars demands that the arms are raised, thus bringing the child to an upright posture. Answers A and C are not correct because the hips and lower extremities are already positioned correctly. Answer D is not correct because the arms would be lowered, and trunk forward flexion would be increased. See Reference: Kramer and Hinojosa (eds). Colangelo, CA: Biomechanical frame of reference.

106. (A) Discuss issues related to self-concept with the individual. This individual has demonstrated competence in using the cane, but does not seem to want to use it. Her response indicates her discomfort with the cane is related to how it looks, or more likely, how it makes her look. The image of a woman with a cane is not consistent with her self-concept. Discussion about how she feels about using the cane may enable the individual to integrate it more successfully into her self-concept. Memory and time management (answers B, C, and D) appear to be intact, as indicated by her ability to arrive for therapy on time each day. See Reference: Pedretti and Early (eds). Yerxa, EJ: The social and psychological experience of having a disability.

107. (D) use active-listening techniques. Active listening (answer D) is an effective listening response that enables the patient to know that his or her message has been communicated. Behaviors listed in answers A, B, and C can be counterproductive to developing a therapeutic relationship. Answers A and B may be perceived as enhancing a friendship, rather than a therapeutic relationship, and answer C may be considered inappropriate for someone who does not have adequate social skills. See Reference: Sladyk, K and Ryan, SE (eds). Tufano, R: Applied group dynamics and therapeutic use of self.

108. (C) Position the stander at 75 to 80 degrees from the floor. Answer C is correct because by adjusting the prone stander nearest to vertical (the least effect of gravity on the head or posture), the child will be able to tolerate working on head righting. Answer A is not correct because while working on the floor in prone, the head and neck are doing the most work against gravity. Answer D is not correct because the head and neck work the least against gravity in the standing or upright position. See Reference: Kramer and Hinojosa (eds). Colangelo, CA: Biomechanical frame of reference.

109. (A) extend the operated leg forward, reach back for the armrests, then slowly sit. By

extending the operated leg forward, reaching back for the armrests, and slowly sitting, an effective and safe transfer can be accomplished. Answers B, C, and D are all contraindicated transfer training techniques for individuals who must adhere to total hip precautions. These precautions restrict flexing of the hip greater than 80 degrees, hip adduction, and internal rotation. See Reference: Pedretti and Early (eds). Coleman, S: Hip fractures and lower extremity joint replacement.

110. (C) The client independently selected one of six craft designs presented. The notation of the client's response to treatment that contains the most objective information is answer C. The notations that address the client's wants and hostility (answers A and B) are interpretations of behavior versus directly observable responses. The use of the word "appropriate" (answer D) reflects the OT practitioner's judgment. See Reference: Early. Medical records and documentation.

111. (C) Stabilizing the pelvis, hips, and legs. Answer C is correct, because when the pelvis, hips, and legs do not provide a good central base of support, the child resorts to compensatory movements. Stabilizing the trunk (answer A) is not correct because unless the pelvis is stabilized, arm movements may still be compromised. Answer B is not correct, because use of a lap board or chair arms for weight-bearing of the upper extremities will compromise the use of the arms and hands to stabilize the body. Stabilizing the head and neck (answer D) is not correct because the pelvis continues to be unstable, and therefore, is not a good base for arm movements. See Reference: Case-Smith (ed). Nichols, DS: Development of postural control.

112. (D) Recommend hospice OT. OT in hospice or palliative care focuses on role performance, the components of which are quality of life, locus of control, and adaptation. This type of intervention may bring quality and meaning to the individual's remaining days. It is unlikely that this individual, who is depressed about a terminal illness, will actually carry out a home program (answer A). Not all home health OT practitioners (answer B) have the expertise to work with terminally ill patients using a hospice approach. Discontinuing OT services altogether (answer C) would not facilitate continuation role performance. See Reference: Bonder and Wagner (eds). Bye, RA, Llewellyn, GM, and Christl, KE: The end of life.

113. (B) child's writing, dressing, and self-feeding skills. Because the child was being treated for difficulties with fine motor skills, discharge information should focus on fine motor function. Answers A, C, and D describe information that is relevant in overall discharge planning, but is not specifically relevant to the performance problems the child was treated for in OT. See Reference: Case-Smith (ed). Case-Smith, J, Rogers, J, and Johnson, JH: School-based occupational therapy.

114. (A) Stop the activity. Activity should be stopped immediately when symptoms occur during treatment of an acute cardiac patient. Symptoms, including confusion, shortness of breath, profuse sweating, cold skin, clammy skin, chest pain, nausea, and lightheadedness, should be reported to the physician. After the session is over, symptoms should be documented (answer B). Continuing the activity, whether seated or with the patient's permission (answers C and D), is dangerous and may result in further cardiac damage. See Reference: Dutton. Introduction to biomechanical frame of reference.

115. (B) A simple board game of checkers. Answer B is correct because most children between the ages of 3 and 5 "may begin to play simple board games, such as Checkers or Candyland" (Mulligan, 2003, p. 102). Answer A, coloring on paper, is considered to be an activity most appropriate for a 2- to 3-year-old child, while answer C, looking at picture books is more appropriate for 1- to 2-year-old children. Answer D, engaging in an organized sport, is typically initiated with children, not parents, around the age of 5 to 7. See Reference: Mulligan. Typical child development.

116. (B) perform desired activities in a simplified manner to conserve energy. One method used to extend an individual's occupational performance as Parkinson's disease progresses is to introduce task simplification. This allows conservation of energy which can then be expended on desired activities. In a person with long-standing Parkinson's disease, encouragement to "work through" fatigue (answer A) would further deplete available energy. Using pursed-lips breathing is recommended for individuals with pulmonary diagnoses such as COPD (answer C). Recommendations to decrease activity level as much as possible (answer D), also would be detrimental to maintaining occupational performance levels. See Reference: Crepeau, Cohn, and Schell (eds). Pulaski, KH: Adult neurological dysfunction.

117. (A) a can of soup. Grading activities according to complexity is an important part of the therapist's selection of appropriate activities for each individual. Complexity increases as the number of steps, number of different ingredients or tools used, and time to complete the task increases. Answers B, C, and D all require more steps, materials, and time than preparing a can of soup. See Reference: Crepeau, Cohn, and Schell (eds). Culler, KM: Interventions for daily living: home management.

118. (C) Pencil gripper. These are all adaptive devices that can be used with a child who has JRA for various reasons. However, the correct answer is C, because the pencil gripper will probably make grasping the pencil easier and reduce hand grasp fatigue. Because printing and handwriting are common tasks for children this age, it is important to reduce fatigue from hand weakness. The reacher (answer A) frequently requires grasp strength, and is more useful for children who have problems with extended reach. The jar opener (answer B) is a useful tool for individuals with hand weakness, but opening jars is not a task frequently performed by school-age children. The plate guard (answer D) is a useful device for those with incoordination or one-handedness, but is not particularly necessary when hand strength is decreased (adapting the utensil would be more reasonable). See Reference: Case-Smith (ed). Amundson, S: Prewriting and handwriting skills.

119. (D) built-up handles. Built-up handles (answer D), without adding extra weight, allow a comfortable grasp that regular utensils (answer A) do not provide. A weighted handle (answer B) would cause more rapid fatigue and strain to the joints. A person with arthritis most likely has adequate grasp and release with a built-up handle, making it easier to use than a universal cuff (answer C). See Reference: Trombly and Radomski. Yasunda, YL: Rheumatoid arthritis and osteoarthritis.

120. (C) the cultural context and family interaction patterns. Cultural expectations (answer C) may determine behavior standards and the expression of family roles. Continued feeding of a young child with a handicap may be the expression of nurturing and caring. Such an expression may be viewed as more important than the promotion of independence and self-reliance. Answers A, B, and D may be valid issues as well, but should be addressed after the OT practitioner has familiarized himself or herself with the cultural and familial context of the feeding process. See Reference: Case-Smith (ed). Case-Smith, J and Humphry, R: Feeding intervention. Shepherd, J: Self care and adaptations for independent living.

121. (B) have the individual work at the keyboard for 5 minutes. Increasing the duration the individual is able to tolerate working on the computer is the most appropriate way to progress this individual. A heavier mouth stick (answer A) would make the task more difficult than it already is, and yield no benefit. An individual with C4 quadriplegia would not have the potential to use a typing device that inserts into a wrist support (answer C). Teaching the individual how to correctly instruct a caregiver in use of the keyboard (answer D) would be downgrading the activity. See Reference: Crepeau, Cohn, and Schell (eds). O'Mahony: Interventions to improve personal skills and abilities: Strengthening.

122. (B) Incorporate therapeutic activities into family routines. "Suggestions that the family can incorporate into the daily routine are the most successful" (p. 722). Separate "therapeutic activities" (answers A and D) can take up an excessive amount of time and energy, and may interfere with family life. Therefore, long-term follow-through may not be as effective as when activities can be made to fit existing daily routines and develop into habits. Activities provided on an as-needed basis (answer C) will never become habits, and therefore follow-through is less effective. See Reference: Case-Smith (ed). Stephens, LC and Tauber, SK: Early intervention.

123. (C) head erect, chin slightly tucked. "Using a chin tuck position during the swallow may be beneficial in decreasing aspiration in persons who experience a delayed pharyngeal swallow and reduced airway closure...Chin tuck causes the structures of the pharynx to move posteriorly, reducing the size of the opening to the larynx" (p. 529). Full neck flexion (answer D) may make it too difficult to swallow, while slight neck extension (answer A) may increase the likelihood of aspiration. A sitting position is preferable to lying down (answer B). See Reference: Gillen and Burkardt (eds). Avery-Smith, W: Dysphagia management.

124. (A) Begin with activities that have obvious solutions and a high probability of success, and then gradually increase the level of complexity. Beginning with activities that have obvious solutions, that are usually successful, and gradually increase in complexity, is an effective method for developing problem-solving skills. Sensorimotor activities (answer B) in a group can facilitate self-awareness. Increasing the activity time (answer D) facilitates attention span improvement. Activities that require interactions with others (answer C) are useful for developing social conduct and interpersonal skills. See Reference: Early. Analyzing, adapting, and grading activities.

125. (C) use a calm and soothing voice while informing the child about each step of the hair wash prior to doing it. "Even if the child does not yet understand language, each time hair is shampooed and dried, use a soothing voice to repeat what will happen next. The rhythmic repetition of words can be calming. If the child understands the words, knowing what is going to happen next can lessen anxiety" (p. 245). Answers A and B would be inappropriate strategies, because washing the hair with only water or waiting until the child goes to the barber, would not be efficient techniques to maintain proper hygiene in a young child. Answer D, the use of cool water, can actually be contraindicated. Water temperature should be warm, not hot, to increase relaxation. See Reference: Solomon (ed). Jones, LMW and Machover, PZ: Occupational performance areas: Daily living and work and productive activities.

126. (B) use pillows to prop up body parts into the desired position. An individual with low tone may benefit from supportive positioning devices such as pillows, towels, or bolsters that can help to prevent overstretching and fatigue. Slow rocking (answer C) and avoidance of quick stretch (answer D) are both methods for reducing tone and would not be beneficial to an individual having a problem with low tone. A side-lying position (answer A) would be a very difficult position for an individual with lower extremity flaccidity to maintain during sexual activity, but may be preferable for someone requiring energy conservation. See Reference: Pedretti and Early (eds). Burton, GU: Sexuality and physical dysfunction.

127. (B) Incorporate advocacy skill training into the group format. It is essential for individuals with disabilities to have the skills to advocate for themselves. The sense of empowerment that comes with self-advocacy internalizes the locus of control. These same advantages would not be recognized through a stress management group (answer D). Assessing the site for ADA compliance (answer A) is a possible option, and since the OT leading the group can perform the assessment, it would not be necessary to hire an OT. Suing the facility for noncompliance (answer C) would be a last resort after many other attempts to resolve the situation have been made. See Reference: Cottrell (ed). McConchie, SD: Establishing support and advocacy groups.

128. (D) Provide a therapy ball to sit on while the child is playing a game of checkers. Answer D is the most appropriate recommendation because it contributes to the development of postural background movements. This is done by requiring the client to continually adjust to the subtle movements of an unstable surface. Answers A, B, and C provide additional external support (i.e., they provide adaptations using a compensatory approach, rather than facilitating the development of new skills). See Reference: Case-Smith (ed). Nichols, DS: The development of postural control.

129. (D) curved spoon and fork. According to Solomon (2000), "curved utensils can help children who are able to bring their hands close to their mouths, but cannot orient utensils properly" (p. 225), answer D. A child who is unable to reach her mouth due to limitations in shoulder or elbow flexion would benefit from a spoon with an elongated handle (answer A). A child who is unable to hold a spoon because of difficulty with grasp would benefit from a spoon with a built-up handle (answer C). A "spork" (answer B) is helpful for those who need to use one utensil as both fork and spoon. See Reference: Solomon (ed). Jones, LM, and Machover, PZ: Occupational performance areas: Daily living and work and productive activities.

130. (D) hand controls for acceleration and braking. An L4 spinal cord injury would result in paraplegia. Hand controls use hand motions to control the accelerator and brake mechanisms, eliminating the need for any lower extremity function. The palmar cuff and spinner knob (answers A and B) are steering options for individuals who need to steer single-handed and allow constant contact with the steering wheel. Pedal extensions (answer C) can be installed on accelerator and brake pedal for individuals with limited lower extremity reach. See Reference: Pedretti and Early (eds). Lillie, SM: Transportation, community mobility, and driving assessment.

131. (C) Telephone conversations. According to Cook and Hussey, "conversational needs are those that would typically be accomplished using speech if it were available. Examples of these needs are an informal conversation with a friend, a formal oral presentation to a group of people, a telephone conversation [answer C], and a small group discussion" (p. 286). Answers A, B, and D are most representative of graphic communications that typically include pencil and paper, typewriter, and calculator related tasks. See Reference: Cook and Hussey.

132. (D) perform only gentle active range of motion. Gentle active range of motion allows the individual to control the movement and avoid overstretching of inflamed joint tissues. Brisk active range of motion (answer A) and the addition of resistance (answer B) are likely to cause further damage to the joints by increasing stress, which results in increased inflammation. The individual must understand the importance of joint protection during exercise.

Eliminating all range of motion exercise (answer C) would result in further joint stiffness and loss of range of motion. See Reference: Trombly and Radomski. Yasuda, YL: Rheumatoid arthritis and osteoarthritis.

133. (D) A scoop dish. A scoop dish (answer A) is a plate with a high rim that provides a surface against which to push the food. The child would have less difficulty with controlling movement of food because the sides of the scoop dish would provide a shape that aids scooping of food onto the spoon. A swivel spoon (answer A) helps primarily when supination is limited. A nonslip mat (answer B) helps stabilize the plate itself, and a mobile arm support (answer C) positions the arm to help weak shoulder and elbow muscles to position the hand. See Reference: Case-Smith (ed). Case-Smith, J and Humphrey, R: Feeding intervention.

134. (D) any pressure marks or redness from the splint disappears within 20 minutes. A universal and primary concern is that all splints provided to a patient be checked for correct fit, answer D. This is achieved by making adjustments to areas that present with redness or pressure marks after the splint has been removed for 20 minutes. Many types of splints may be made without the fingers flexed or the thumb opposed (answers A and B) as in an antispasticity ball splint or a dynamic extension splint. Most splints are not worn at all times, answer C, but are removed for activities such as self-care or exercise. The OT practitioner should issue a splint wear schedule when the splint is fitted for the patient. See Reference: Crepeau, Cohn, and Schell (eds). Emerson, S and Shafer, A: Splinting and orthotics.

135. (C) avoid opposing the client or arguing for change. The correct answer is C, avoid opposing the client or arguing for change. This is an important client-centered technique within motivational enhance therapy (MET), where the therapist attempts to "roll with it" rather than oppose resistance directly. "Resistance is the client's signal that the therapist needs to act differently in responding to the client" (p. 463). When the resistance is decreased, then the therapist can explore the client's feelings toward change and help the client to find answers and solutions to problems. Answers A and B would be confrontational methods and answer D would be the therapist, rather than the client, providing solutions to problems. Answers A, B, or C would not be desirable responses when using the motivational interviewing approach where the goal is to change the client's capacity to change, rather than to change the client directly. See Reference: Cara and MacRae (eds). Stoffel, VC and Moyers, PA: Occupational therapy and substance use disorders.

136. (B) Help the child develop cognitive strategies for anxiety-producing activities. Children with innate temperament problems need cognitive strategies (answer B) to help them overcome anxiety in order to approach and participate in activities. Parents need to understand the innate temperament problem and the discomfort the child feels during activities, and limit-setting (answer A) will not promote understanding. Children find a predictable routine helpful rather than an unpredictable routine so answer C is incorrect. Answer D is incorrect because the parent and child need to learn mutual play in an environment that promotes positive engagement. See Reference: Kramer and Hinojosa (eds). Olson, LJ: Psychosocial frame of reference.

137. (C) Hand-over-hand assistance. In this method, the caregiver places one hand over the resident's hand and provides assistance while guiding the resident's hand through the steps of the task, in this case, guiding the resident's hand from the food into the mouth. This method provides maximum assistance while still allowing the resident to feel involved and connected to the task. Given the resident's attention span deficits, the use of demonstration (answer A), verbal feedback (answer B), and even chaining (answer C) would be insufficient to sustain the resident's active participation. See Reference: Hellen. Daily life care activities.

138. (A) Ask group members to discuss how they feel about taking their medications. "Any effort to help a client manage medication independently should begin with a discussion of his or her feelings about it" (p. 421). Also, clients can often benefit from hearing about the experiences of others. Using diaries (answer B), timers (answer C), lists, and other environmental supports also can increase success in independent medication management. Knowledge of the medication schedule is critical, but the first action the OT should take is leading the discussion on feelings about taking medications. See Reference: Early. Activities of daily living.

139. (C) multisensory input. Each of the possible four answers describes appropriate treatment interventions for infants in the NICU. However, an infant approaching full term or post term is now equipped with a maturing sensory system tolerant and in demand of a multisensory diet including oral stimulation, vestibular input, and auditory and visual orientation, to assist with age-appropriate motor and behavioral skill acquisition. Often these very premature infants get limited amounts of social interaction

and appropriate sensory stimuli, because of necessary medical equipment and procedures (e.g., ventilators, IV catheters, isolettes, warmers, bililights, and nasogastric tubing). Therefore, stable, growing post-term premature infants would most benefit from a multisensory diet (answer C) to best meet the demands of their maturing sensory system and to capitalize on their socialization skills. Answers A, B, and D are all possible treatments for the 32- to 35-week-old infant who responds best to unimodal sensory input and minimal direct intervention, e.g., ROM and positioning, because of immature sensory systems and compromised respiratory systems. See Reference: Case-Smith (ed). Hunter, JG: Neonatal Intensive Care Unit.

140. (B) A key guard. A key guard is a device that covers computer keys and provides a guide for a finger or stick without punching extra keys. A moisture guard (answer A) is a flexible plastic cover that protects the keys from drool, moisture, or dirt. An autorepeat defeat mechanism (answer C) stops repetition of letters or numbers caused by overlong or involuntary depression of keys. One-finger-access software (answer D) allows the user to lock out keys such as "shift" or "enter." This enables an individual who uses only one finger or a stick to type capital letters or perform other keyboard functions that require simultaneous depression of more than one key. See Reference: Cook and Hussey. Control interfaces for assistive technology.

141. (A) Monitor the individual's response to activities to prevent him from performing at activity levels that are too high and unsafe. "Denial is common among patients with cardiac disease. Patients in denial must be closely monitored during the acute phase of recovery. Persons in denial may ignore all precautions and could stress and further damage their cardiovascular systems" (p. 970). This individual, because of his denial, is unlikely to be willing to learn or apply energy conservation techniques (answer B), which can benefit him. The OT should attempt to understand and modify the individual's behavior through collaborative goal setting. The OT, along with the patient and his family should engage in educational sessions prior to referring for psychological services. See Reference: Pedretti and Early (eds). Matthews, MM: Cardiac and pulmonary diseases.

142. (C) righting reactions. Righting reactions develop after the integration of primitive reflex patterns, which are thought to be necessary for survival in the normal newborn. Righting reactions allow children to right their heads against gravity and to realign their bodies around the movement of the head in that process. Prehensile reactions refer to grasping patterns and reach, which differentiate humans from other primates. Equilibrium reactions develop after righting reactions and allow the child to maintain a standing and walking posture. See Reference: Crepeau, Cohn, and Schell (eds). Kohlmeyer, K: Sensory and neuromuscular function.

143. (B) Use heavy utensils, pots, and pans. Using heavy kitchen items (answer B) increases stability for individuals with incoordination. Other suggestions include using prepared foods, nonskid mats, easy open containers, serrated knives, and tongs. Built-up handles (answer A) are useful for individuals with limited grasp. A high stool (answer C) benefits those who fatigue easily. Placing the most commonly used items on shelves just above and below the counter (answer D) is a useful way to adapt the environment for individuals with limited reach. See Reference: Pedretti and Early (eds). Foti, D: Activities of daily living.

144. (A) 2 degrees of flexion. Carpal tunnel syndrome is a condition that results from compression of the median nerve at the wrist. Wrist splints should position the wrist in neutral (2 degrees of flexion and 3 degrees of ulnar deviation) to minimize intratunnel pressure and alleviate symptoms. See Reference: Mackin, Callahan, Skirven, Schneider, and Osterman (eds). Evans, RB: Therapist's management of carpal tunnel syndrome.

145. (D) flushing and perspiration. These responses (answer D) are autonomic nervous system signs of sensory overload. Answers A, B, and C are not correct because they do not describe autonomic responses to the activity. See Reference: Case-Smith (ed). Parham, LD, and Mailloux, Z: Sensory integration.

146. (C) Altered task method. "When the task method is altered, the same task objects are used in the same environment, but the method of performing the task is altered to make the task feasible given the clients impairments" (p. 501). An example would be substituting one-handed techniques for someone who previously used both hands (i.e., one-handed shoelace tying for an individual who recently had an above elbow amputation). Problem-solving (answer A) is the ability to organize information from several levels to generate a solution to a problem. Retraining (answer B) teaches the same skills of an activity to the individual who previously had mastery of those skills (e.g., having an individual with hand weakness practice tying knots). Compensation (answer D) would be avoiding performance of the activity entirely by using an alternative piece of equipment or method. See Reference: Crepeau,

Cohn, and Schell (eds). Holm, MB, Rogers, JC, and James, AB: Interventions for activities of daily living.

147. (D) Add a thickening agent to liquids. Individuals with swallowing problems usually have more difficulty with thin liquids than with thicker ones. A straw (answer A) is useful for individuals who are unable to lift a cup or glass to their mouth. "Sippy cups" (answer B) benefit individuals who tend to spill when they are drinking. It may be important to monitor fluid intake (answer C) for individuals who drink too much or do not drink enough. See Reference: Crepeau, Cohn, and Schell (eds). Holm, MB, Rogers, JC, and James, AB: Interventions for daily living.

148. (A) 2 inches wider than the widest point across the child's hips with the brace on. Measuring the child with the brace on and adding 2 inches (answer A), allows the child to easily get in and out of the chair, while preventing pressure to the child's sides. Answer B measures only the hips and would not allow enough room for the child to sit or move easily in the chair while wearing the brace. Answers C and D are both incorrect measurements for seat length, because both would have the seat too deep for the individual's leg length. The correct length of the seat should be 2 inches shorter than the distance from the back of the bent knee to the back of the buttocks. See Reference: Pedretti and Early (eds). Adler, C and Tipton-Burton, M: Wheelchair assessment and transfers.

149. (C) swimming in a cool water pool. Swimming is an excellent activity for promoting physical fitness, and the cool water pool (temperature under 84 degrees) will prevent the overheating that is contraindicated for individuals with MS. Jogging and volleyball (answers A and D) are both likely to result in overheating, and volleyball would probably also fatigue weak hand muscles. Painting (answer B) is a lightweight activity that would probably appeal to an artist, but would do very little to promote physical fitness. See Reference: Pedretti and Early (eds). Schultz-Krohn, W, Foti, D, and Glogoski, C: Degenerative diseases of the central nervous system.

150. (A) Instruct the individual to wear clothes for 2 days and to then launder those items. Teaching the individual to recognize and judge when clothing needs to be laundered has been unsuccessful, indicating that the individual may not have the capacity to learn this skill. If the OT practitioner determines that the individual can usually wear clothes for 2 days before they need to be laundered, then providing a rigid schedule based on this average removes the need for judgment, and provides an environmental compensation—a schedule that will result in the individual wearing clean clothes most of the time, if not always. Assessment of the individual's clothing management capabilities (answer B), would have been performed before the implementation of the initial intervention. Taking the clothes to the dry cleaner (answer C), would be cost prohibitive and would still require judgment to determine when they needed to be cleaned. Turning the responsibility over to the staff (answer D), would not promote independence in clothing management. See Reference: Bruce and Borg. Cognitive disability frame of reference-acknowledging limitations.

151. (C) have the individual repeatedly squeeze with the hand against increasing amounts of resistance. The biomechanical approach is a treatment approach used when a person has a deficit in strength, endurance, or range of motion, but has voluntary muscle control during performance of activities. The biomechanical approach focuses on decreasing the deficit area to improve the person's performance of daily activities. Eliciting functional grasp using reflex inhibiting postures (answer A) is a neurophysiological approach, which emphasizes an understanding of the nervous system in a person with brain damage, and how to elicit a desired response from that person. Muscles can be stimulated through a variety of neurodevelopmental techniques (answer B) using an understanding of the nervous system to elicit a response in a developmental sequence. Building up utensils (answer D) is an example of the rehabilitative approach, which teaches a person how to compensate for a deficit on either a temporary or permanent basis. See Reference: Trombly and Radomski. Jackson, J, Gray, JM, and Zemke, R: Optimizing abilities and capacities: Range of motion, strength, and endurance.

152. (A) in the individual's home. Because individuals who require task-specific training are unable to generalize learning to other situations (including other garments and other environments), it is important to train the individual in the environment where the task will be performed. This type of training should take place at least five times a week. See Reference: Crepeau, Cohn, and Schell (eds). Toglia, JP: Cognitive-perceptual retraining and rehabilitation.

153. (B) continue the same positioning and splinting program that was indicated before discharge. It is necessary to continue positioning and splinting after discharge because active scar development continues for many weeks, depending on the severity of the burn. The same positioning and splinting devices used at the hospital are used at home, with changes made as needed during follow-up visits. Individuals stay in the hospital until their conditions can be managed at home, with outpatient visits to maintain status. Individuals are not kept in the hospital until they are completely healed, which would be the only situation in which a home program would not be necessary (answer A). If an individual follows the home program only as he or she deems appropriate during the day or night (answers C and D), instead of as scheduled by the therapist, the position time may not be sufficient to prevent deformity from occurring. See Reference: Trombly and Radomski. Pessina, M and Orroth, A: Burn injuries.

154. (A) position the switch to facilitate easy access and reposition as needed. The OT should determine a position in which the switch can be easily accessed to increase independence and self-efficacy of the child (answer A). Answer B addresses a limitation in range of motion; answer C is a strategy for dealing with a visual impairment; and answer D pertains to behavioral and cognitive issues, none of which were mentioned as concerns for this child. See Reference: Case-Smith (ed). Exner, CE: Development of hand skills.

155. (A) Store the most frequently used items on shelves just above or below the counter. When an individual experiences difficulty reaching because of limited range of motion, convenient placement of commonly used items will facilitate home management. Using the largest joint available (answer B) is an important principle of joint protection, and although it may be an appropriate suggestion if this individual has arthritis, it would not address the specific problem of reaching high shelves. Although it is possible that range-of-motion exercises and reaching for high shelves (answers C and D) may eventually improve this individual's shoulder function, neither provides a home management solution. See Reference: Pedretti and Early (eds). Foti, D: Activities of daily living.

156. (B) (1) position shirt on lap; (2) place left hand into sleeve and pull up sleeve past elbow; (3) place right hand into sleeve and pull up sleeve; (4) pull shirt up over head. Answer B would be the best sequence because positioning the shirt first on the lap may provide cues for patients with unilateral neglect. Also, starting with the left side allows the unaffected right hand to perform the first part of the task successfully, and requires the eyes to then scan to the left to locate the left arm. Answers A, C, and D are all examples of sequences that are less likely to be successful. See Reference: Pedretti and Early (eds). Foti, D: Activities of daily living.

157. (B) give praise for completed dressing; do not help the child get dressed. Since the child has achieved dressing independence, he does not need assistance (answer A), clothing adaptations (answer C), or verbal prompts (answer D) to complete the task. In fact, assisting him now may cause him to lose his independence and regress to relying on his parents again. According to Shepherd (2001), "the social environment, family and other caregivers...provide encouragement and support self-care independence. They also hold certain expectations regarding the child's self-care occupations" (p. 492). While it is desirable to have the child maintain their level of independence, it also is important to be aware of social, cultural, and physical routines/expectations. See Reference: Case-Smith (ed). Shepherd, J: Self-care and adaptations for independent living.

158. (B) Patient's ability to work at the computer has increased from 10 minutes to 3 hours with stretch breaks every 30 minutes. The objective section of a discharge summary should summarize the patient's condition upon discharge from the facility and "summarize the patient's stay" (p. 49). Some facilities compare initial and final evaluations, while others only address progress from the time of the previous note. Answers A and D are subjective reports. Answer C is an example of a statement that belongs in the assessment section of a discharge summary. See Reference: Borcherding. Writing the "O"-objective.

159. (C) Making a checklist of steps in the process, then consulting the list while doing laundry in the actual setting. Making a checklist and having the individual use the checklist during the activity, would provide an external memory aid during practice of the functional activity. This would provide compensation for cognitive deficits during task training in the specific context where it will be performed. Answers A, B, and D are methods that require an individual to be able to transfer learning of skills from one context to another. See Reference: Trombly and Radomski. Radomski, MV and Davis, ES: Optimizing cognitive abilities.

160. (D) have the child climb up onto her lap. All answers describe the use of good body mechanics. Answer D, having the child climb onto her lap, is preferable, though, because it minimizes the amount of bending and lifting required. See Reference: Trombly and Radomski. Bear-Lehman, J: Orthopaedic conditions.

161. (D) Assist clients in the selection of simple, short-term tasks. The skills required at the parallel level are the "ability to work and play in the presence of others comfortably and with an awareness of their presence" (p. 295). At this level, the OT must be available to provide support, encouragement and assistance when indicated. Parallel group members (answer D) typically work on individual tasks within the group. Therefore, it would not be expected that the OT encourage experimentation (answer A), because this level would require the client to be working at the project group level. This level focuses on the client working with another group member while encouraging trust. Answer C, the OT participating as an active member also is inappropriate. This level of assistance typically occurs during the mature group level, where individuals take on the roles necessary to achieve a balance between meeting the group task, and the emotional needs of the group. Answer B also would be an incorrect selection because the OT must act as an authority figure in the parallel group in order to set limits, encourage interaction, and assist the patient in feeling safe. See Reference: Early. Group concepts and techniques.

162. (C) increase the management of texture by slowly increasing texture of food with a baby food grinder. This method (answer C) offers a gradual increase in texture that encourages chewing. Answer A is not correct because scraping off food from a spoon with the child's teeth does not encourage any voluntary oral motor control. Answer B is incorrect because it combines liquid with pieces of food (soft and chewy), and this combination of textures will be too unpredictable for a child who is having difficulty organizing oral motor skills to manage food. Answer D is incorrect because a raisin is too large of a step from pureed food in terms of texture. See Reference: Case-Smith (ed). Case-Smith, J and Humphry, R: Feeding intervention.

163. (C) keeping the knees bent. Keeping the knees bent is the only correct choice. All of the other answers could potentially contribute to injury. For prevention, the OT practitioner should stand close to the individual, keep the back in a neutral position, and maintain a wide base of support. See Reference: Pedretti and Early (eds). Creel, TA, Adler, C, and Tipton-Burton, M and Lillie, SM: Mobility.

164. (D) A center for independent living. According to Shamberg, "centers for independent living are unique community-based nonprofit non-residential programs that are substantially controlled by consumers with disabilities" (p. 784). Cradle-to-grave homes (answer A) are houses designed and built with accessibility in mind. If a resident of a cradle-to-grave home begins to use a wheelchair later in life, the home will already be wheelchair accessible. Transitional living centers (answer B) are temporary living arrangements for individuals who are in between a hospital or institution and living independently in the community. Adult day programs (answer C) are rehabilitation-oriented day programs for individuals who live in the community; they are not residential. See Reference: Trombly and Radomski. Shamberg, S: Optimizing access to home, community, and work environments.

165. (C) Coping strategies for continuing medication compliance. Medication noncompliance (answer C) is a primary factor related to frequent readmissions for individuals with psychiatric conditions. Each of the other topics (answers A, B, and D) listed is important in preparing for transition to the community, but none is as significant a risk factor for rehospitalization as not continuing to use medications consistently. See Reference: Early. Activities of daily living.

166. (C) all children with disabilities before they receive special education services. The federal government requires that an individualized educational program be developed before special education services begin. This plan, prepared once a year, is completed by all members of the team involved in a child's education. Continuing education plans (answer A) vary according to the requirements of the practitioner's professional organization, employer, and state licensure board. Some state licensure boards require CEUs (continuing education units) at the time of licensure renewal. As a component of the rehabilitation program for adults with head injury (answer B), the rehabilitation team produces a document known as the treatment plan or plan of care. OT practitioners usually involve the family of the patient in family training before the patient's discharge from the rehabilitation unit. The OTR or COTA documents these training sessions, and provides an assessment of the family's ability to follow discharge plans, but this documentation (answer D) is not referred to as an individualized education program. See Reference: Case-Smith (ed). Case-Smith, J, Rogers, J, and Johnson, JH: School-based occupational therapy.

167. (C) Provide a transfer tub bench and install grab bars. The best adaptation to achieve access to the tub would be providing the individual with a transfer tub bench, which is recommended for individuals who cannot step over the edge of the tub. Bathroom grab bars also should be installed to provide stability during the move into the tub. Tearing out the original tub and installing a walk-in shower (answer A) would be an unreasonable expense when answer C is an option. Shower doors (answer B) would make it very difficult to transfer into the tub using a transfer bench, which is the safest option. Nonskid decals and mats are primarily safety measures to prevent slipping and falling (answer D). See Reference: Pedretti and Early (eds). Smith, P: Americans with Disabilities Act: Accommodating persons with disabilities.

168. (A) Individuals write fears and concerns on index cards and then the therapist collects and reads the cards to the group for discussion. This method allows for anonymity by having each patient write down their concerns without including their names, thereby eliminating any fear of embarrassment. Answers B and C require the individuals to make public their concerns, which might prevent complete openness when attempting to express their concerns and fears. Although there are certain concerns that might be common to many in the group, and having a team member address these concerns in general would be helpful (answer D), this approach would not address the specific concerns of the patients in this group. See Reference: Early. Group concepts and techniques.

169. (C) the side-lying position. The side-lying position reduces the influence of reflexes, extensor tone, and gravity, all of which make protraction of the shoulders and forward reach difficult. Answer A is incorrect because the standing position will not reduce extensor tone. Moreover, it encourages shoulder retraction and makes forward reaching of both arms to midline more difficult. Answer B also is incorrect because in the prone position the upper extremities are involved in weight-bearing. However, this position may help facilitate forward reach by developing shoulder protraction. Answer D is not correct because in the quadruped position, the upper extremities are involved in weight-bearing. However, if the position is attainable, shoulder protraction and forward reach may be facilitated. See Reference: Kramer and Hinojosa (eds). Colangelo, CA: Biomechanical frame of reference.

170. (B) Teach the child to dress her hemiparetic extremities first. Occupational therapy practitioners, "help children compensate for delays or deficits in performance by adapting activities or applying assistive technology...A child with hemiparesis is taught to dress his or her affected extremities first" (p. 10). Answer A (dressing in bed) also is considered to be an adapted technique, but would be most appropriate for an individual with poor balance. While answer C, educating the child's mother regarding dressing, is something the OT would do at some point in the occupational therapy process dependent upon the child's age, it is not something the OT would do to encourage independent dressing skills for an 8-year-old child. Finally, answer D, teaching the child to dress her non-hemiparetic extremities first, is not considered an adaptive skill since this technique will typically interfere with independent dressing skill development. See Reference: Case-Smith (ed). Case-Smith, J: An overview of occupational therapy for children.

171. (B) the potential for noncompliance, apathy, and depression. The potential for noncompliance, apathy, and depression may be seen once individuals with burns are discharged as they are "...faced with the overwhelming task of becoming responsible and self-reliant while dealing with the aggravation of developing scars." (p. 914). Answer A, the possibility of decreased range of motion and sensation, is a physical response to a burn. Answers C and D are psychological reactions typically associated with the early and intermediate stages of recovery. See Reference: Pedretti and Early (eds). Reeves, SU: Burns and burn rehabilitation.

172. (A) Vinyl floor. Vinyl floors are the easiest and least expensive surface over which to maneuver a wheelchair. Although it is possible to find inexpensive short pile carpeting (answer B), a smooth, uncarpeted surface is still the easiest to maneuver over. The friction provided by deep pile carpets (answer C) makes them difficult to push a wheelchair across, and wheeling over the edge of an area rug (answer D) also increases the level of difficulty for wheelchair users. See Reference: Christiansen and Matuska (eds). Christenson, MA: Environmental adaptations: Foundation for daily living.

173. (D) hold the child firmly when dressing him. Holding the child firmly (answer D) inhibits responses to light touch, which are usually uncomfortable for children with tactile defensiveness. Tickling (answer A) and light stroking (answer C) also are uncomfortable or intolerable for a child with tactile defensiveness. A strong stimulus such as loud music (answer B) causes further discomfort during a time when the child is extremely vulnerable to the sensation of light touch (i.e., when clothing is being removed). See Reference: Case-Smith (ed). Parham, LD and Mailloux, Z: Sensory integration.

174. (C) ask another person for assistance. It is often necessary to get assistance when transferring obese individuals. Trying to attempt this transfer alone could result in injury to the patient and/or the therapist, even if proper body mechanics are used (answer A). Asking someone else to do a diffi-

cult task (answer B) is not professional. If the patient needs to be transferred, not transferring him (answer D) is not an option. See Reference: Pedretti and Early (eds). Adler, C and Tipton-Burton, M: Wheelchair assessment and transfers.

175. (B) environmental hazard analysis and fall risk during performance of ADL. On a team, each member provides assessment and recommendations in his/her special knowledge and skill areas (p. 909). For example, statistical analysis of data (answer A) might be performed by risk management or human resources personnel. Answer C, evaluation of gait and mobility device use, is an area of specialized expertise for the physical therapist. Medical and/or pharmacology personnel (such as the nurse, physician, or pharmacist) would most likely assess the impact of medication on fall incidence (answer D). Assessment of environmental hazards and evaluation of fall risk during occupational activities is an area of special expertise for the occupational therapist (p. 75). See reference: Crepeau, Cohn, and Schell (eds). Cohn, ES: Interdisciplinary communication and supervision of personnel. See reference: Pedretti and Early (eds). Harlowe, D: Occupational therapy for prevention of injury and physical dysfunction.

176. (A) A game of rhythmic exercises performed to music. Rhythmic activities facilitate motor performance in individuals with Parkinson's disease, especially when performed to music. Time capsules (answer B) are a meaningful activity for those who are approaching the end of life, but the description of the activity provides no rationale for why it would benefit the motor skills of those individuals with Parkinson's disease. Races (answer C) are generally not a good idea for this population because of the difficulty they often have stopping during ambulation. Reading out loud (answer D) is an effective intervention for addressing the communication, not motor deficits, frequently experienced by these individuals. Group activities are particularly beneficial because of the added advantage of social interaction. See Reference: Pedretti and Early (eds). Schultz-Krohn, W: Degenerative diseases of the central nervous system Section 5: Parkinson's Disease.

177. (A) motor performance. Motor performance in schools is typically identified through daily activities performed within the school environment. According to Case-Smith, "children in school are expected to independently travel within the school and move safely within the classroom, playground, and hallways. They must manipulate their schoolbooks, writing, and cutting tools" (p. 764), answer

A. Answer B would be related to the assessment of sensory skills and sensory integration (i.e., the student not tolerating the "feel" of scissors), while answer C, perception, is typically assessed through visual-perception tasks. Answer D, cognition, would most likely be identified through problem-solving and organizational skill assessment. See Reference: Case-Smith (ed). Case-Smith, J., Rogers, J., and Johnson, J.H.: School-based occupational therapy.

178. (B) increasing overall physical activity levels and fitness. Wellness programs focus on developing personal control of behaviors through educational approaches and active participation in activities that promote health, such as increasing levels of physical activity to improve physical fitness. Answers A, C, and D reflect traditional occupational therapy therapeutic interventions to improve performance in specific deficit areas, rather than promoting general good health. See Reference: Cottrell (ed). Swarbrick, P: A wellness model for an acute psychiatric setting.

179. (B) nonspecific job-simulated work tasks. Nonspecific job-simulated work tasks such as carrying, pushing, and pulling are appropriate examples of work conditioning that will improve skills needed for a variety of physical labor jobs and also increase physical endurance. Answer C, job-specific work tasks, are tasks that relate to developing skills to prepare for a determined job and is representative of a work-hardening program. Performing adapted work activities, answer A, is an example of work hardening that is implemented after the clients achieve work-conditioning goals. Answer D, performing range of motion and strengthening exercises, would not provide task-specific endurance training. See Reference: Crepeau, Cohn, and Schell (eds). Fenton, S, Gagnon, Pitts, DG: Intervention to promote participation Section I: Work.

180. (D) Meeting the vocational instructor weekly to discuss adaptations to work tasks. Effective consultation involves ongoing communication that helps team members problem-solve more effectively. Answers A and B are activities typically done by the vocational teacher. A vocational instructor should already be able to perform assessments (answer C). See Reference: Case-Smith (ed). Spencer, K: Transition services: From school to adult life.

181. (B) Improved verbal and nonverbal communication skills. Improved verbal and nonverbal communication skills would be the most relevant behavioral outcome indicating program effectiveness in the area of social skills development. Answers A, C, and D may all indirectly benefit as a result of improved social and communication skills, but these would not directly reflect positive outcomes for measuring effectiveness of social skill training programs. See Reference: Cottrell (ed). Salo-Chydenius, S: Changing helplessness to coping: An exploratory study of social skills training with individuals with long-term mental illness.

182. (B) Leather lacing change purses from kits. All of the choices are good leisure group activities. However, activities that can be completed in one session, that are structured for success, and that yield a tangible end product (such as a kit) are very likely to turn out well regardless of the individual's skill level. They are best for promoting a sense of competence and mastery over the environment. Collages (answer A) are useful for expressing thoughts or feelings about a particular theme, such as nutritional foods or leisure activities one enjoys participating in; however, the end product is not always predictable. Going to the movies (answer C) can incorporate goals related to community mobility and money management; however, there is no tangible end product. Putting on a resident talent show (answer D) can promote self-esteem and self-expression; however, it usually requires more than one session to prepare. See Reference: Cottrell (ed). Kearney, PC: Occupational therapy intervention with homeless women.

183. (A) Activities that promote home and community safety. The "Well Elderly Study," conducted at the University of Southern California, demonstrated that individuals who participated in an occupation-based program that included the relationship between activity and health, joint protection, and energy conservation education, use of adaptive equipment, use of public transportation, and home and community safety, experienced significant health benefits compared to those who participated in a socialization intervention (answer B) or no intervention. A physical therapy program would be more likely to focus on balance and ambulation activities (answer C). While caregiver training (answer D) is important, it would not be the emphasis of a health promotion program. See Reference: Scaffa, ME (ed). Scaffa, ME, Desmond, S, and Brownson, CA: Public health, community health, and occupational therapy.

184. (B) walking as part of a walking club. Walking as part of a walking club throughout a facility can provide an outlet for the movement needs of some people with dementia. Walking in a structured way can be calming, provide an activity of exploration, and help to refocus the resident. Answers A,

C, and D are good activities, but would not provide the element of movement to the same degree. See Reference: Hellen. Meaningful activities: Daily life stuff.

185. (C) Remove the threshold altogether.
Removing the threshold altogether would be the simplest and safest solution. Door thresholds may have a maximum height greater than 0.5", and these must be beveled; keeping it as it is (answer A) would provide a barrier to wheelchair accessibility and a safety hazard for people with visual deficits. Placing a throw rug to cover the threshold (answer B) would not improve accessibility and would present a slipping hazard. Because the threshold height is more than half an inch, placing a ramp over the threshold (answer D) would be required if the threshold could not be removed. The best solution would still be to remove the threshold altogether to provide the most accessible surface. See Reference: Pedretti and Early (eds). ADA Accessibility Guidelines.

186. (C) determine how frequently falls occur, how many individuals are affected, and how the problem is currently being addressed. The first step in program development is to profile the community. This includes collecting demographic information about the target population and information about the characteristics of the problem (frequency of occurrence, number of individuals involved, factors contributing to the problem, etc.). Next, the consultant should perform a needs assessment by collecting data from individuals with a variety of viewpoints, including staff, administration (answer B) and the population. Goals are established and recommendations (answer D) are made once the needs assessment is complete and goals have been established, and may include evaluation of individual residents (answer A). See Reference: Fazio. Profiling the community, targeting population, and assessing need for services.

187. (C) prosthetist. Prosthetists are professionals trained to make and fit artificial limbs. The physiatrist (answer A) is a physician with specialized training in physical medicine. The orthotist (answer B) specializes in fitting and fabricating permanent splints and braces. The physical therapist (answer D) is a rehabilitation professional trained to administer exercise and physical modalities to restore function and prevent disability. See Reference: Case-Smith (ed). Rogers, L, Gordon, CY, Schanzenbacher, KE, and Case-Smith, J: Common diagnoses in pediatric occupational therapy practice.

188. (C) Use the handout only as a resource while developing the presentation. According to

Hansen, "all professional documentation must be accurate and complete. This means, of course, keeping accurate and complete patient records and billing correctly. It also requires accuracy in our professional resumes, professional presentations, and scholarly writing" (p. 957). The options presented in answers A, B, and D do not give the necessary credit to the author for his or her contribution. See Reference: Crepeau, Cohn, and Schell (eds). Hansen, RA: Ethics in occupational therapy.

189. (D) reinforcement and enhancement of performance. The emphasis of OT is on performance, specifically, performance of work, play, or activities of daily living. As OTs, the focus has been on reinforcing and enhancing the execution of these occupations and the activities that are part of the occupations. Answers A, B, and C are incorrect because skill acquisition, compensation, and environmental adaptation are methods used to achieve the goal of improving performance, and therefore are not the primary emphasis of the profession. See Reference: Christiansen and Baum (eds). Baum, C, and Christiansen, C: The occupational therapy context: Philosophy—principles—practice.

190. (C) Advanced supervision. Advanced levels of supervision occur on an as-needed basis. Individuals being supervised at this level have demonstrated skill and expertise in the area of OT in which they are working. They also may serve as a resource person and assist in continuing education or research as it relates to their expertise. Answer A describes close supervision, which is direct daily contact between the supervisor and the employee. This form of supervision is recommended for entry-level therapists and therapists reentering the OT profession. Answers B and D describe routine supervision and general supervision. These forms of supervision are for the therapist who can function independently and have mastered basic role functions of OT. See Reference: AOTA: Guidelines for Supervision, roles, and responsibilities during the delivery of occupational therapy services.

191. (A) DRGs. Diagnostic related groups (answer A) were created in order to establish the level of payment per diagnosis. The intent of the government was to impose constraints on health-care spending for the beneficiaries of Medicare. PPS (prospective payment system) is a reform implemented by the U.S. government regarding a transformation from a retrospective to a prospective payment system. PAMs, answer C, represents physical agent modalities, while cost shifting (answer D) is what occurs when a hospital increases its prices to all customers in order to make up for the shortfall of reimbursement by a few providers. See Reference: Crepeau, Cohn, and Schell (eds). Evanofski, M: Occupational therapy reimbursement, regulation, and the evolving scope of practice.

192. (B) Universal precautions. Health-care personnel should follow universal precautions (answer B) when blood or body fluids are present regardless of diagnosis. Suicide, escape, and medical precautions (answers A, C, and D) are guidelines developed for individuals identified with risks that are not noted in this question. See Reference: Early. Safety techniques.

193. (C) Make a report to appropriate authorities. OT practitioners, as health professionals, are in the position of being a "mandated reporter" and must make a report if there is any reason to believe a child has been abused. A report of the injury should be made to appropriate authorities. Answers A, B, and D delay or prevent proper assistance to a family involved in the occurrence of child abuse. All agencies serving children have policies and procedures for reporting injury in these situations. See Reference: Crepeau, Cohn, and Schell (eds). Davidson, DA: Child abuse and neglect.

194. (C) unacceptable because it violates the Code of Ethics. Whether or not an alternate date has been arranged (answer A) or the agency the practitioner works for allows it (answer B), stating services were provided on a day when they, in actuality, were not, is falsification of documentation and violates the OT Code of Ethics. The individual's inability to participate in therapy the next day because of illness (answer D) would only serve to further complicate an already compromised situation; however, this is not the reason why the action is unacceptable. See Reference: Crepeau, Cohn, and Schell (eds). Hansen, RA: Ethics in occupational therapy.

195. (D) the OT problem-solves with the teacher. Answer D is correct because the consultation relationship in the school is based on a shared relationship with the school staff for whom the OT is hired to consult. Answer A is incorrect as the teaching role is usually associated with monitoring type of service. Answer B is incorrect as a provision of therapy is direct service. Answer C is incorrect because it describes an authoritarian approach, which would take away the teacher's commitment to solving the problems of mainstreaming a child with a disability. Answer D reflects one of the essential tenets of consultation—that the consultee, by sharing in problem solution, will become committed to a child's pro-

gram. See Reference: Case-Smith (ed). Case-Smith, J, Rogers, J, and Johnson, JH: School-based occupational therapy.

196. (C) Probation. Probation is the period of time a practitioner is given to retain the counseling or education required for maintaining certification. Answer A, a reprimand, is a formal written expression of disapproval against a practitioner's conduct, which is retained in the NBCOT files. Answer B, a censure, is a formal disapproval of the conduct of an OT practitioner that is made public. Answer D, revocation, is permanent loss of NBCOT certification. See Reference: Crepeau, Cohn, and Schell (eds). Hansen, RA: Ethics in occupational therapy.

197. (C) Help place food on the spoon for a patient practicing the use of a universal cuff in the patient's room at lunchtime, while the OT supervisor runs a lunch group in the dining room. An aide may be delegated client-related tasks when (a) the outcome of the task being delegated is predictable; (b) the situation of the client and the environment is stable and will not require that judgment, interpretations, or adaptations be made by the aide; (c) the client has demonstrated some previous performance ability in executing the task; (d) the task routine and process have been clearly established. The aide also must be trained and demonstrate service competency while carrying out certain tasks, as well as be aware of signs and symptoms that would indicate the assistance of an OTR or COTA. When these conditions are met, answers A, B, and D are all acceptable. Answer C states that the patient is "learning" to use a universal cuff. This would indicate that changes may still be in progress that could require the judgment and skill of an OT practitioner. See Reference: AOTA: Guidelines for Supervision, roles, and responsibilities during the delivery of occupational therapy services.

198. (B) Withhold treatment, but gather information on the course of events for documentation and consultation with the treatment team. The treatment plan may need to be revised as a result of the change in the individual's status. According to AOTA's Standards of Practice (1998), "a registered occupational therapist modifies the intervention process to reflect changes in client status, desires, and response to intervention." The OT must modify the intervention process to reflect changes in status; therefore, answer C is incorrect. Treatment cannot continue as originally planned (answer A), because of the change in status. Waiting for the OT director to return and collect information about the change in status (answer D) could delay resumption of treatment. See Reference: AOTA: Standards of practice for occupational therapy.

199. (C) ease the child to a lying position, remove or pad nearby objects, and loosen clothing. The most important action to take is to protect the child during the seizure by preventing injuries that can occur from falling or hitting objects during movements. Other protective measures include loosening clothing that is restrictive, and placing a blanket or cushion underneath the child if possible. Answer A is incorrect because checking breathing would not be done until the seizure has stopped. Answer B is incorrect because any attempt to restrain the child could result in injury. While it is important to let the seizure end without any interference, Answer D, taking no action except observation, would not help to protect the child from environmental hazards. See Reference: Case-Smith (ed). Rogers, SL, Gordon, CY, Schanzenbacher, KE, and Case-Smith, J: Common diagnosis in pediatric occupational therapy practice.

200. (B) beneficence. According to Hansen, beneficence (answer B) is "the act or attitude of doing good or causing good to happen for others; the duty to try to do what is best for another person" (p. 954). Prudence (answer A) "is the ability to govern and discipline oneself through the use of reason," while justice (answer C) "places value on the upholding of such moral and legal principles as fairness, equity, truthfulness, and objectivity" (p. 956). Fidelity (answer D) is "the duty to be faithful to another person and to that individual's best interests; included is the idea of holding information about that person in confidence" (p. 954). See Reference: Crepeau, Cohn, and Schell (eds). Hansen, RA: Ethics in occupational therapy.

Simulation Examination 4

Directions: Circle the correct answer to the following questions. When you have completed this examination, check your answers against the answer key that follows. As you will see, an explanation is given for each answer along with a reference for further study. The book author is listed as well as the chapter author. See the bibliography for complete references. Study the areas in which your comprehension was low.

■ PEDIATRICS

1. A teenager with fine motor incoordination reports difficulty with self-care. Which of the following options would this individual find MOST beneficial?
- A. Wash mitt
- B. Spray deodorant
- C. Toothpaste with a flip-open cap
- D. Toothbrush with a built-up handle

2. A child diagnosed with autism demonstrates a craving for tactile stimulation, rubbing objects on his arms and legs. He also avoids being touched by others. This behavior MOST likely indicates a sensory integration problem related to:
- A. poor modulation of tactile input.
- B. hypersensitivity to tactile input.
- C. hyposensitivity to tactile input.
- D. poor modulation of proprioceptive input.

3. An OT practitioner has provided a "nosey cup" to a school-aged child with dysphagia and explains to the family that the purpose of the cut-out in the nosey cup is to:
- A. slow the drinking process.
- B. allow the chin to remain tucked when drinking.
- C. allow the caregiver to control the flow of liquid.
- D. minimize biting reflexes when the cup is placed in the mouth.

4. A child has considerable difficulty with problem-solving when playing with Lego blocks, becomes frustrated and gives up easily. This MOST likely indicates a problem in which area of play?
- A. Sensorimotor
- B. Imaginary
- C. Constructional
- D. Game

5. The OT practitioner is instructing the parents of a child with strong lower extremity extensor tone in dressing techniques. What would be the BEST way to position the child in order to make putting shoes and socks on less difficult?
- A. Extend the child's hips and knees.
- B. Flex the child's hips and knees.
- C. Extend the child's shoulders.
- D. Dorsiflex the child's ankles.

6. Evaluation of a school-age child diagnosed with moderate mental retardation should generally focus on:
- A. positioning and communication skills.
- B. communication, self-care, and social skills.
- C. ADLs and IADLs.
- D. feeding and personal hygiene.

7. An OT practitioner is working with the family of a 3-year-old child who lacks sitting balance in the bathtub. The child seems to enjoy submersing herself in the warm bathtub water, but their insurance does not cover durable medical equipment costs. Which should the OT recommend?
- A. Place a foam-lined plastic laundry basket in the tub.
- B. Place a horseshoe-shaped inflatable bath collar around the child's neck while bathing.
- C. Utilize a bath hammock in the tub while bathing.
- D. Suggest that the child shower in a standing position instead of bathing in the tub.

8. **An OT practitioner is working with a 3-year-old child who has spastic diplegia. The mobility device that would be MOST appropriate to use in assisting this child to explore space would be a(n):**
   A. body-length prone scooter.
   B. airplane mobility device.
   C. tricycle.
   D. power wheelchair.

9. **An OT observes a child with autism flapping his right hand in front of his eyes repeatedly in an apparently purposeless manner. This behavior MOST likely indicates:**
   A. the child is able to focus his eyes at close range.
   B. pain in the right hand.
   C. right hand dominance.
   D. the presence of self-regulatory functions.

10. **A child with limited pincer grasp wishes to zip his own pants in school, because he gets embarrassed that he has to ask his teacher for assistance after using the bathroom. Which should the OT recommend the child try FIRST?**
   A. A large key ring
   B. Oversized fasteners
   C. Colored zippers
   D. Velcro fasteners

11. **When selecting activities for an 8-year-old child with Duchenne's muscular dystrophy, which of the following developmental issues is MOST important to consider?**
   A. Establishment of basic trust
   B. Freedom to use his initiative
   C. Development of self-identity
   D. Reinforcement of competence

12. **The goal of a work program for homeless youths is to develop job skills that will improve housing status. Which of the following must occur FIRST?**
   A. Help clients feel safe and supported, and explore the meaning of the worker role.
   B. Develop work skills, habits, and appropriate interpersonal and work behaviors.
   C. Emphasize quality and productivity and identify realistic work interests.
   D. Evaluate participants' performance strengths and weaknesses.

13. **A child has difficulty controlling food in her mouth when swallowing. In helping the parents plan snacks, the OT would MOST likely recommend:**
   A. chicken noodle soup.
   B. peanut butter.
   C. carrot sticks.
   D. pudding.

14. **When an OT practitioner selects a standardized test to assess a child, the practitioner can assume that the test:**
   A. is valid.
   B. has normative data.
   C. has a standard format.
   D. is reliable.

15. **An OT practitioner is working with a 4-year-old child who has significant hearing loss. The child also demonstrates decreased fine motor coordination for her age. Which of the following activities would the OT MOST likely implement to address these needs?**
   A. Parachute activities to increase gross motor and sensory input.
   B. Visually color-code the child's right and left shoes to compensate for decreased reception of verbal cues.
   C. Introduce the child to other children via socialization groups to increase social interaction and game playing.
   D. Digging in "Play Doh" to search for various coins and then placing them in a piggy bank.

16. **While observing a child for the first time, the OT practitioner notes that the child responds to a loud noise by abducting and extending the arms. The response observed in this child is documented by the OT as a:**
   A. rooting reflex.
   B. Moro reflex.
   C. flexor withdrawal reflex.
   D. neck righting reaction.

17. **When preparing a home program with the goal of independent toileting for a young child with postural instability, the MOST important adaptation the OT practitioner can recommend is:**
   A. replacing zippers and buttons on clothes with Velcro closures.
   B. mounting a safety rail next to the toilet.
   C. introducing toilet paper tongs.
   D. placing a colorful "target" in the toilet bowl.

18. A young child has been wearing a left upper extremity prosthesis for 3 weeks. The MOST important activity recommendation that the OTR gives to the child's preschool teacher is to:

    A. offer toys that the child can manipulate with one hand.

    B. stress bilateral play and school activities incorporating the prosthesis.

    C. teach the child one-handed manipulation techniques.

    D. involve the child in activities that do not require manipulation.

19. Through the evaluation process, the OT practitioner may consider many possibilities for intervention, however, the specific plan for implementation of intervention is MOST often developed at which point in the OT process?

    A. After observation or screening

    B. After the interview

    C. After the evaluation

    D. After the development of the goals and objectives

20. The OT plans to use a top-down approach for evaluating a child's self-feeding performance skills. The OT will MOST likely assess the child's:

    A. seating and positioning needs.

    B. ability to feed herself a snack.

    C. use of assistive devices.

    D. performance component limitations.

21. The OT practitioner is working with the parents of a 4-year-old boy who demonstrates a strong tonic bite reflex when eating. What type of utensils will the OT MOST likely recommend to the child's parents?

    A. Pediatric weighted universal grips

    B. Curved utensils

    C. Swivel utensils

    D. Rubber-coated spoons

22. A child has poor independent sitting skills as a result of inadequate postural reactions. The FIRST activity the OTR would use to promote the development of independent sitting is:

    A. swinging on a playground swing with a bucket seat.

    B. wide-base sitting on the floor while reaching for a suspended balloon.

    C. straddling a bolster swing while batting a ball.

    D. riding a "hippity-hop" while using only one hand for support.

23. A student is unable to focus on a blackboard 20 feet away and then refocus on the book on her desk to copy a mathematics problem. This MOST likely indicates a problem with:

    A. ocular motility.

    B. binocular vision.

    C. convergence.

    D. accommodation.

24. An OT practitioner consulting to a community center is developing a club for youth at risk for violence with the primary goal of engaging the children in meaningful occupations designed to protect and build the community. Which one of the following activities is MOST consistent with this goal?

    A. Develop a community-based chess competition.

    B. Provide a psychoeducational intervention on anger management.

    C. Plant flower seeds in small pots to be taken home once they sprout.

    D. Convert an empty lot filled with trash into a garden.

25. A child with developmental delay has just developed the strength and stability in his right hand to hold scissors properly and make snips in paper. Which activity would help the child to develop the next level of scissor skills?

    A. Cut cardboard and cloth.

    B. Cut along curved lines to cut out a circle.

    C. Cut along straight lines to cut out a triangle.

    D. Cut the paper in two following a straight line.

26. Which of the following is the BEST position for promoting isolated head control in a child with very limited postural control and significant upper and lower extremity weakness?

    A. Standing in a standing frame with knee and hip support

    B. Quadruped with chest supported in a sling

    C. Prone over a wedge

    D. Sitting on a therapy ball with hips supported by the therapist

27. A 9-year-old child with a diagnosis of mental retardation has achieved independence in dressing and feeding, and is now being discharged from OT. The BEST advice for the OT to give his parents in order to maintain the child's independence in dressing at home is:

A. give assistance when the child asks for it to provide a successful experience.

B. give praise for completed dressing, but do not help the child get dressed.

C. give him oversized clothing with Velcro closures and large snaps.

D. give him verbal prompts when needed, and help with closures only.

28. During an initial evaluation, the OT practitioner suspects that a child has dyspraxia. The MOST relevant activity to elicit performance level skills would be to determine the child's ability to:

A. print or write.

B. read.

C. calculate mathematics.

D. plan new motor tasks.

29. An OT practitioner is attempting to order a wheelchair for a child with severe cerebral palsy who will most likely never ambulate. The child has no cognitive limitations and frequently expresses the desire to be independent in mobility, especially within the school setting. The OT will MOST likely recommend that the family order a:

A. power wheelchair.

B. standard wheelchair.

C. caster cart.

D. powered scooter.

30. Upon arrival to an infant's therapy session in the neonatal intensive care unit, the OT practitioner finds the infant's parents present. Of the following, which is the OPTIMAL intervention to pursue in order to assist the parents in responding to their infant's behaviors?

A. Review the chart to complete birth history information and speak to the infant's primary nurse.

B. Introduce yourself as their child's OT practitioner, explain your role in their child's developmental care, and excuse yourself from the situation secondary to limited availability for intervention.

C. Issue written positioning and state regulation and readiness information for the parents to review.

D. Review appropriate behavioral and developmental positioning techniques with parental observation and interaction.

31. Following initial evaluation of a 1-year-old child requiring early intervention services, the OT should:

A. independently develop an IEP.

B. collaboratively develop an IEP.

C. independently develop an IFSP.

D. collaboratively develop an IFSP.

32. A child with motor delays is being evaluated to determine how he performs self-care activities. Which of the following is MOST likely to provide relevant information about self-care function?

A. Standardized tests of motor development

B. Review of the medical record

C. A developmental screening test

D. Home observation and parent interview

33. A 13-year-old child with paraplegia wants to take a bath without assistance from his mother. The OT would MOST likely recommend:

A. A tub seat with a handheld shower attached to the faucet

B. A hydraulic lift with a sling seat

C. An inflatable tub

D. A wheeled shower chair

34. A 3-year-old child demonstrates the ability to use the toilet independently except for wiping and readjusting clothing afterward. This behavior indicates the child is performing at which of the following levels?

A. Significantly below age level

B. Slightly below age level

C. At age level

D. Above age level

35. A sixth grader with a diagnosis of athetoid cerebral palsy needs an adapted computer for communication. Her upper extremity control is poor because of fluctuating muscle tone. The OT practitioner suggests that the BEST way for her to operate her computer is to use a:

A. single pressure switch, firmly mounted within easy reach.

B. lightweight keyboard placed at midline.

C. low-resistance mouse and pad.

D. mercury switch headband set to respond to minimal movement.

36. An OT practitioner is providing an informational session for parents with children with disabilities who believe that their children could benefit from OT consultation at school. A key piece of information, which needs to be included in the presentation, is that a specific form must be completed in order for a school-age child to receive OT services within a school system. This form is called:

- A. UB-82.
- B. FIM.
- C. IEP.
- D. CMS-1500.

37. An 8-year-old boy with conduct disorder is disruptive, uncooperative, and occasionally combative during therapy. From a behavioral point of view, the MOST appropriate strategy to use to address the child's conduct would be to:

- A. allow the child to express his anger without restraint for a short period to vent his frustration.
- B. ignore the behavior and continue with therapy with or without the child's cooperation.
- C. attempt to reason with the child to get his cooperation.
- D. set clear expectations for behavior and enforce consequences, such as a time-out, if the child loses control.

38. Of the following, the MOST important aspect of administering a standardized test for an OT practitioner is the use of:

- A. subjective judgment to determine how best to administer the test.
- B. previous experience as a way to gauge test results.
- C. specific instructions for administration and scoring.
- D. practice to learn the best way to administer and score the test.

39. A child with poor sitting balance is unable to put on and remove lower extremity clothing. Which of the following approaches would BEST address this functional issue?

- A. Teach the child to dress in a side-lying position.
- B. Add loops to the waistbands of pants and skirts.
- C. Use Velcro fasteners in place of zippers.
- D. Teach the child to dress in a standing position.

40. A school-age child with multiple handicaps is beginning to develop some controlled movement in the upper extremities. It would be MOST appropriate to introduce switch-operated assistive technology when the child:

- A. develops tolerance of an upright sitting posture.
- B. can reach and point with accuracy.
- C. demonstrates any reliable, controlled movement.
- D. develops isolated finger control.

41. The OTR has written the following statement: "Continue social skills training program and encourage client to attend one new after-school club activity within the next week." The MOST appropriate section of a SOAP note in which to place this statement is the:

- A. subjective section.
- B. objective section.
- C. assessment section.
- D. plan section.

42. A second-grade child has a diagnosis of muscular dystrophy. The child operates a manual wheelchair, but his mobility is slow because of muscle weakness. The OT practitioner should consider a powered wheelchair when the:

- A. child starts junior high school and will be expected to switch classrooms several times daily.
- B. child's speed over long distances becomes less than that of a walking person.
- C. child's home can be made accessible for a power wheelchair.
- D. child becomes unable to propel a manual wheelchair.

43. The BEST way to utilize sensory stimulation for a child with tactile defensiveness is to:

- A. apply intense light touch stimulation, such as tickling on the abdomen, for desensitization.
- B. avoid all forms of tactile stimulation to accommodate the child's preferences.
- C. allow the child to self-apply tactile stimuli to maximize the child's tolerance.
- D. avoid all deep pressure tactile stimuli to decrease defensiveness.

44. An OT practitioner is administering a standardized test to a child who suddenly becomes uncooperative and complains that the test is "too hard." The MOST appropriate response would be to:

A. switch to easier items to improve the child's self-esteem.

B. terminate the session and schedule another session to administer the remainder of the test.

C. follow administration instructions and note changes in behavior.

D. adapt the remaining test items to ensure success.

45. A child with CP demonstrates fair sitting stability and good head control with fluctuating lower extremity extensor tone. The OT would MOST likely position the child during feeding in a:

A. prone stander with lateral trunk supports.

B. Rifton child's chair with a padded abductor post.

C. wedge that positions the hips in 115 degrees of flexion when the child is supine.

D. beanbag chair.

46. A child is lacing a series of geometric beads by copying from a stimulus card and is unable to identify a moon-shaped bead when it is turned sideways on the table. This MOST likely indicates difficulty with:

A. figure-ground perception.

B. form constancy perception.

C. position in space perception.

D. visual sequencing.

47. An OT practitioner is formulating a home program of play activities for the parents of a 4-year-old child with developmental delay. The type of activities that would be BEST for development of symbolic play skills would be:

A. building blocks.

B. board games.

C. craft kits.

D. a doll house and dress-up clothes.

48. Which of the following BEST represents the integrated therapy model within a school-based setting?

A. The OT provides treatment in a clinic outside of the classroom in order to avoid distraction from peers.

B. The OT provides individualized treatment in collaboration with the child's teacher in a quiet room away from the traditional classroom setting.

C. The OT pulls the child out of the classroom to work on activities in the hallway.

D. The OT provides intervention in the classroom setting with the child's peers present.

49. A sixth grade student has a diagnosis of juvenile rheumatoid arthritis. Which of the following leisure activities would BEST suit this child for helping him maintain range of motion?

A. Swimming

B. Basketball

C. Soccer

D. Aerobics

50. When developing a self-care program for a 3-year-old child with significant visual impairment, the home care OT would MOST likely implement which of the following?

A. Create a reliable route to the bathroom, encouraging the child to familiarize herself with the smells and sounds of the bathroom.

B. Have the child practice various obstacle courses at a local playground to improve body image/awareness.

C. Practice handwriting and fine motor skills with a "Lite Brite" activity board.

D. Introduce the child to other children who have visual impairments.

51. In order to develop letter recognition skills in a preschool child, the OT would MOST likely encourage the child to:

A. use flash cards.

B. form letters out of clay.

C. match cut-out letters to a sample.

D. color large letter outlines.

52. During assessment of a 10-month-old child with Down syndrome, the OT practitioner notes hyperextensibility of all joints, which MOST likely reflects:

- A. increased muscle tone.
- B. decreased muscle tone.
- C. anterior horn cell disease.
- D. muscle and joint disease.

53. When instructing the parents of a toddler in the use and care of a hand splint, the OT should place MOST emphasis on:

- A. checking for irritation and pressure problems.
- B. avoiding excessive heat exposure.
- C. cleansing the splint regularly.
- D. adhering strictly to the wearing schedule.

54. An OT practitioner learns that a young child receiving OT is easily aroused because of a sensory-processing disorder. Which of the following describes the MOST effective environmental adaptation for assisting the child to fall asleep?

- A. A mini-trampoline in the bedroom to tire the child out before going to bed
- B. A noise machine producing white noise at bedtime
- C. A lightweight, fuzzy blanket providing light touch
- D. Shutters on the windows to produce total darkness

55. An OT practitioner is working with a group of children in an early intervention program. All of the children in the group are able to sit independently on the floor except for one child with cerebral palsy. The child has told the OT that he wishes to sit on the floor like his peers and not in his wheelchair. The OT would MOST likely recommend that the child use a(n):

- A. hammock.
- B. floor sitter.
- C. adapted wheelchair insert.
- D. prone stander.

56. An 11-month-old child who was born 3 months prematurely is being evaluated at an OT outpatient clinic. The MOST accurate assessment profile can be obtained if the OT practitioner compares this child's abilities with those of a typically developing child aged:

- A. 11 months.
- B. 14 months.
- C. 8 months.
- D. 10 months.

57. An OT practitioner is evaluating developmental stages in a 10-month-old baby who is beginning to "cruise" while holding onto furniture. The OT would MOST likely document this as:

- A. dysfunctional mobility.
- B. advanced development.
- C. normal development.
- D. delayed development.

58. A child with cerebral palsy has tongue thrust. Prior to feeding, the OT practitioner should do which of the following FIRST?

- A. Position the child's trunk, head, neck, and shoulders in proper alignment.
- B. Hyperextend the child's head.
- C. Place his digits directly under the child's chin, facilitating tongue retraction.
- D. Provide upward pressure under the child's lower jaw prior to chewing.

59. A treatment plan for a child with a visual discrimination problem would MOST likely include which of the following adaptations of visual materials?

- A. Low contrast and defined borders
- B. High contrast and defined borders
- C. High contrast and unclear borders
- D. Low contrast and unclear borders

60. During an infant's OT session, the mother reports she has observed that her baby has difficulty with swallowing and frequently chokes. The OT can position the infant to MOST effectively reduce the risk of aspiration and facilitate swallowing by keeping the head:

- A. in a neutral position.
- B. slightly flexed.
- C. slightly extended.
- D. rotated toward the feeder.

61. A 2-year-old child has hypotonia, extremely poor head control, and the inability to maintain a sitting position. The BEST method for the OT to use during the FIRST pre-sitting activity is to provide stability for the child as needed and then move the child:

- A. forward and backward on a ball with the child in a prone position.
- B. forward and side-to-side with the child sitting on the therapist's lap.
- C. to a sitting position by pulling the child up from a supine position on a mat.
- D. forward and side-to-side on a tilting board with the child in a quadruped position.

■ MENTAL HEALTH/ COGNITION

62. An individual diagnosed with substance abuse has recently begun attending a partial hospitalization program, and the OT has received a request to evaluate the individual's leisure performance. Which of the following methods would MOST effectively evaluate how this individual spends his leisure time?

    A. Administer an interest checklist.
    B. Administer a time-use assessment.
    C. Assess his ability to play a sport.
    D. Observe him playing a game.

63. An extremely withdrawn individual has developed the ability to tolerate interaction with one other group member while glazing slip molds in an ongoing ceramics group. Which of the following steps should be taken NEXT in order to develop this individual's ability to interact with others?

    A. Involve the individual in a three-member task group.
    B. Progress the individual from glazing slip molds to building coil pots.
    C. Instruct the individual in how to pour the molds in addition to glazing them.
    D. Encourage the individual to choose his own project and glazes.

64. An OT practitioner is using a sensory integration approach with a group of residents of a mental health setting who display very low energy level, hyposensitivity to stimuli, and poor visual and tactile perception. The activity that would be BEST for beginning a session with these individuals, who can tolerate no more than a half-hour session, would be to:

    A. go around the circle and ask each patient to introduce himself or herself.
    B. pass around a scent box and ask each patient to smell the contents.
    C. ask each patient to select a favorite poem and read it.
    D. discuss the lunch menu and healthy eating habits.

65. An individual with mental illness attends group on a regular basis, but interrupts others, grabs tools and supplies, and bosses others around at almost every group session. What is the BEST way to respond to this disruptive behavior?

    A. Have the individual contribute to a discussion identifying the "rules" for the group.
    B. Tell the individual he may not return to the group until he is able to treat others with respect.
    C. Ignore the behavior during the group and speak to him about it afterward.
    D. Explain to him that this type of behavior is unacceptable.

66. A woman being interviewed by an OT practitioner experienced repeated sexual abuse by her father as a child and states that his actions were due to the stress of being fired from his job. In the evaluation report, the OT practitioner should identify the use of this defense mechanism as:

    A. identification.
    B. projection.
    C. denial.
    D. rationalization.

67. An OT practitioner in a residential community mental health setting is developing a psychoeducational program to promote healthier eating habits among the residents of the setting. To accomplish the group's goals using this approach, the practitioner would be MOST likely to:

    A. have each client make a healthy food collage.
    B. have the group plan and shop for a meal.
    C. designate 1 day a week for the residents to be responsible for cooking dinner.
    D. show a video about nutrition and keep a meal diary for a week.

68. A new mother recently returned to her job and reports that she has difficulty concentrating at work because she keeps thinking about the baby, and that when she's at home, she is distracted because she feels she should be at work. This MOST likely suggests the need to help this individual work on:

    A. parenting skills.
    B. attention span.
    C. assertiveness.
    D. role performance.

69. An OT practitioner is using leather stamping as part of a group activity for individuals with neurological deficits and needs to increase the degree of problem-solving demand within the group. The BEST approach for encouraging problem-solving in a craft media group is to:

A. begin with activities that have obvious solutions and high probabilities of success, and then gradually increase the complexity.

B. begin with activities that require gross motor responses and progress to activities that require fine motor responses.

C. structure the number and kinds of choices available.

D. gradually increase the time used in the activity by 15-minute increments.

70. An OT practitioner conducts assessments of individuals with MR living in a supervised community environment and finds that most can perform work tasks involving repetitive processes and social interaction. The MOST appropriate service delivery model for the therapist to recommend would be:

A. an adult activity center.

B. supported employment.

C. volunteer work.

D. a sheltered workshop.

71. An OT practitioner is working with an individual who has orientation deficits resulting from a head injury. The MOST appropriate compensatory intervention to facilitate awareness of person, place, and time would be to:

A. provide verbal cues, external aids, such as calendars, and opportunities to practice using the aids.

B. reduce the number of distractions by moving the individual to a quiet room when reviewing information.

C. present information about the environment in short units, spaced with time between each segment.

D. connect new orientation information to previously learned knowledge.

72. An OT practitioner is working with an individual in a psychosocial partial hospitalization program who is having difficulty making decisions. The practitioner has suggested a baking activity, but the individual is unsure if she wants to do this activity. The OT practitioner's response that would BEST facilitate decision-making is:

A. "I think baking would be a helpful activity to try. Baking something you like offers you several choices and decisions. You wanted to bake cookies today, didn't you?"

B. "I think baking would be a helpful activity to try. Baking something you like offers you several choices and decisions. What do you want to bake?"

C. "I think baking would be a helpful activity to try. Baking something you like offers you several choices and decisions. These choices and decisions can help you feel more positive about making other decisions. You can choose a cake mix or a cookie mix. Which would you like?"

D. "I think baking would be a helpful activity to try. Baking something you like offers you several choices and decisions. These choices and decisions can help you feel more positive about making other decisions. Do you want to bake cookies?"

73. An individual with borderline personality disorder has been referred to occupational therapy. Which of the following would be MOST important to evaluate?

A. Activities of daily living

B. Instrumental ADLs

C. Relationships with others

D. Sensorimotor skills

74. An individual with moderate cognitive limitations lives in a group home and has difficulty telling the difference between his toothbrush and everyone else's. This individual will benefit MOST from:

A. using an electric toothbrush.

B. having the only red toothbrush.

C. putting a built-up handle on his toothbrush.

D. having a caregiver brush his teeth twice a day for him.

75. An OT practitioner is working with a patient who demonstrates unilateral neglect. Of the following, which would be the MOST effective strategy for increasing attention to the left?

A. Encouraging participation in bilateral activities

B. Encouraging any available hemiplegic limb movements before or during a task

C. Participation in tasks that do not cross the midline

D. Participation in tasks placed on the uninvolved side

76. The OT practitioner asks an individual with schizophrenia to describe what brought him to the hospital for admission. The individual responds by saying, "I took a cab." The OT practitioner is MOST likely to identify this response as:

A. delusional thinking.

B. a distractible response.

C. a concrete response.

D. an insightful response.

77. An OT practitioner realizes that an adult worker with a developmental disability is having difficulty learning an assembly sequence during packaging a game box and decides to use backward chaining. The OT practitioner can BEST implement this technique by:

A. encouraging the individual to reverse the packaging sequence.

B. having the worker put only the last piece into the game package.

C. putting only the pencil or the pad into the game box.

D. having the therapist demonstrate and repeat the correct sequence before each of the worker's attempts.

78. An OT practitioner is working in a psychosocial setting with individuals who are classified as being at risk for suicide. In selecting craft media, the activity that would MOST likely be the safest is a:

A. leather checkbook cover with single cordovan lacing.

B. macramé plant hanger.

C. ceramic ashtray.

D. stenciling project on poster board.

79. An individual who is functioning at Allen's Cognitive Level 4 has difficulty remembering to take his medication twice daily. Which of the following is the MOST appropriate recommendation?

A. Instruct the client to take medication at 9 a.m. and 9 p.m.

B. Instruct the client to take "one white and one blue pill" with the morning and evening meals.

C. Instruct the caregiver to remind the client to take medication twice daily.

D. Instruct the caregiver to place pills into client's hands at the designated times.

80. In a psychiatric hospital, an OT practitioner is developing a transition program for individuals with mental illness who have experienced long-term hospitalization and do not feel ready for discharge. Which of the following program elements should come FIRST in this type of predischarge program?

A. Visits to the day program the individuals will be attending with introductions to the other clients and staff.

B. Collaboration with clients on developing goals they need to achieve in order to live in the community successfully.

C. Introduce and discuss concepts of community living, and give clients an opportunity to voice their concerns.

D. Evaluate skills related to community living such as money management, personal safety, and self-care.

81. During a self-care evaluation of an individual who recently sustained a head injury, the OT practitioner asks the person to comb his hair right after he washes his face. The individual washes his face quickly, but when the therapist must give him several reminders to comb his hair, the therapist is MOST likely to identify this as a deficit in:

A. short-term recall.

B. judgment.

C. hearing.

D. abstraction.

82. A mother of two children is about to be discharged to home following a brief hospitalization for substance abuse. Her husband asks the OT practitioner what he "should do with her" for her first weekend at home. Which of the following suggestions is MOST appropriate?

A. Throw a party for some close friends.

B. Take her to see her favorite band.

C. Take her and the kids on a mini-vacation.

D. Attend an AA meeting.

83. A homeless individual with mental illness has recently begun coming to a shelter. Which type of group is MOST likely to engage this individual?

A. Highly structured craft group

B. Volunteer activity group, such as stuffing envelopes

C. Simple meal preparation group

D. Social skills group

84. A member of a discussion group frequently monopolizes the discussion and interrupts others. The OT practitioner has tried to give the client various indirect cues to decrease the individual's behavior, but the client continues to monopolize discussion. Which direct intervention should the OT implement NEXT to modify the individual's behavior?

A. Sit beside the individual who is monopolizing the discussion and touch his or her hand or arm as a reminder not to interrupt others who are talking.

B. Confront the individual's behavior and ask, "Are you aware that your frequent interruptions prevent others from having a chance to contribute?"

C. Redirect the individual and say, "Now let's hear what others have to say about this."

D. Restructure the task by selecting a group activity that requires sequential turn taking.

85. An OT practitioner is scheduled to interview an individual with a head injury about her home environment and family and child care responsibilities. Knowing the individual has an attention span of 10 to 15 minutes, which of the following should the therapist do FIRST?

A. Schedule a 30-minute treatment session.

B. Obtain as much information as possible from the chart.

C. Interview the individual using appropriate verbal and nonverbal communication.

D. Perform the interview in an environment where distractions can be minimized.

86. An individual was unable to achieve the goal "the client will initiate two requests to other group members for sharing materials within a 1-week period." The BEST revised goal is:

A. the client will initiate two requests to other group members for sharing group materials within a 2-week period.

B. the client will initiate one request to one other group member for sharing group materials within a 1-week period.

C. the client will initiate two requests to each of the five group members for sharing one group tool within 2 weeks.

D. the client will say "hello" to the group leader at the start of each group session.

87. An OT practitioner needs to identify why an individual who attends a day program for adults with developmental disabilities has difficulty participating in group activities. The BEST way to determine whether the individual is experiencing anxiety during group sessions would be to:

A. observe the individual's body language during group sessions.

B. ask the individual to complete a questionnaire rating her anxiety level after each session.

C. have group members provide feedback to the individual and OT about her anxiety level.

D. allow the individual to select two other clients she feels she'd be comfortable with in a small group.

88. An individual with Alzheimer's disease becomes confused with multiple-step instructions during self-care activities. Which is the MOST effective method that the OT practitioner can recommend to the caregiver for giving directions to the individual with Alzheimer's disease at home?

A. Give simple, step-by-step instructions, and physical guidance.

B. Provide three-step instructions with gestures for demonstration.

C. Write instructions down for the individual that are over three steps.

D. Have individual verbally repeat instructions after the therapist gives them.

89. Which goal would BEST address an individual's need to communicate feelings and attitudes appropriately in a social situation in order to improve conversational skills?

A. The client will identify and pursue activities that are pleasurable to the self.

B. The client will use facial expressions and gestures that are consistent with stated emotions during assertive, passive, and aggressive role-play situations.

C. The client will recognize his or her own behavior and possible negative and positive consequences.

D. The client will identify his or her own assets and limitations after an art or movement group.

90. An OT practitioner has been hired as a program manager to develop a community-based program for individuals with chronic mental illness. The FIRST step in the process that the practitioner must complete is:

A. program planning.

B. program implementation.

C. needs assessment.

D. program evaluation.

91. In a community mental health facility, an OT practitioner is working on improving stress management skills with a group of patients with schizophrenia who have histories of psychotic behavior. Which of the following stress management strategies would be MOST appropriate for this group?

A. The use of visual imagery as a relaxation method

B. Discussing one's problems with an empathetic listener

C. Engaging in a new, challenging activity

D. Progressive relaxation of muscles

92. An OT practitioner is developing a program of self-awareness activities for a group of individuals with substance abuse problems. Which of the following is MOST important to grade over time to improve self-awareness with this group?

A. Activities that emphasize the importance of self-awareness

B. Activities that encourage self-reflection and feedback

C. Activities that encourage problem-solving skills

D. Activities that allow for increasing social interaction

93. An individual diagnosed with borderline personality disorder tells an OT practitioner that she is the only one she can trust. The next day she accuses the therapist of lying to her. The best way for the therapist to respond is to:

A. tell the individual her feelings have been hurt.

B. remain matter of fact and consistent in approach.

C. ask the individual how she has felt when lied to in the past.

D. apologize and try to determine how the misunderstanding occurred.

94. Which of the following activities would MOST effectively evaluate group interaction skills during an OT session?

A. The clients make individual collages, sharing a set of magazines to complete the activity.

B. All group members construct one tower that incorporates all of the pieces provided in a set of constructional materials (e.g., Legos or Erector set).

C. All group members work together to make pizza and salad for their lunch that day.

D. Each client selects a short-term craft activity from four available samples.

95. After attending several OT group sessions, a young man with a history of low self-esteem is showing more self-confidence and asks the OT practitioner for her phone number because "you're so nice to me." The MOST appropriate response is to:

A. give him her phone number and tell him to call when he is feeling depressed.

B. ignore the request, but remind him he's doing a good job.

C. tell him she has a boyfriend.

D. in private, explain the nature of the client-therapist relationship.

96. A patient who is asked to show the path she would take to get from her room to the therapy clinic at the other end of the corridor becomes easily confused and makes several wrong turns. This behavior MOST likely indicates:

A. spatial relations disorders.

B. figure-ground discrimination deficits.

C. topographical disorientation.

D. form discrimination deficits.

97. In a long-term care facility, an elderly resident with dementia repeatedly asks for her mother and becomes increasingly upset. The strategy that will BEST communicate understanding and reassurance for this individual's concerns is to:

A. use reality orientation by explaining that her mother has been dead for a long time.

B. set limits by firmly telling her to stop asking for her mother.

C. use therapeutic "fibbing" by telling the resident that her mother will be coming shortly.

D. respond to the emotional tone expressed by the words and provide extra attention and reassurance.

98. During lunch, an OT observes one individual who grabs the ketchup away from her neighbor, chews with her mouth open, and does not make eye contact with those around her while others seem to be trying to avoid her. The behaviors exhibited by this individual MOST likely indicate a deficit in which of the following?

A. Social relations skills

B. Physicality in communication

C. Self-control

D. Coping skills

99. An OT practitioner in a residential community mental health setting is planning activities for clients within a psychodynamic frame of reference. Which of the following types of activities would the practitioner would be MOST likely to use?

A. Activities exploring one's perceptions of past, current, and future events and how they are connected

B. Activities matched to the specific cognitive level of group members

C. Activities that can serve as reinforcers for desired behaviors

D. Activities that can teach the use of problem-solving strategies

100. An 8-week stress management program directed toward either a well or disabled population should include in the first session:

A. a physical activity such as yoga or tai chi.

B. diaphragmatic breathing or progressive relaxation techniques.

C. information on the definition and physiological signs of stress.

D. role playing stressful situations.

101. The occupational therapy treatment approach that will MOST likely meet the overall needs experienced by individuals with substance abuse problems is to:

A. assist with skill development in the areas of life skills, leisure, and self-expression.

B. educate the family members about making safety modifications to the home to prevent accidents.

C. encourage Alcoholics Anonymous involvement, address personal appearance, and social relationships.

D. provide time-management and budgeting training.

102. An individual with depression is ready to return to the job held before taking a leave of absence. Which of the following is the FIRST action the OT practitioner should take?

A. Perform a job analysis.

B. Request reasonable accommodation.

C. Emphasize activities that promote a sense of self-efficacy.

D. Encourage the individual to participate in a weekly support group.

103. An OT practitioner is running a group for individuals who have difficulty coping with chronic pain. Based on a cognitive-behavioral frame of reference, which of the following steps would the therapist BEGIN with?

A. Providing the individuals with information on activity pacing

B. Developing awareness about how thoughts and behaviors affect one's perceptions of and ability to cope with pain

C. Practicing meditation and relaxation techniques to be used when the individual recognizes he is experiencing stress

D. Setting up a method for individuals to monitor and report on how successful their use of recommended techniques was at home

104. When conducting a structured interview, it is MOST important for the OT practitioner to:

A. rephrase the interview questions in his or her own words.

B. ask questions the therapist thinks are pertinent to this patient.

C. ask the questions as they are stated on the interview sheet.

D. ask additional questions (other than those listed) to gain further insight into the patient.

105. An OT practitioner is working with an individual who had a TBI and demonstrates deficits in sequencing and problem-solving. The first meal preparation activity the therapist should have the individual prepare is:

    A. brownies.

    B. a cheese sandwich.

    C. a casserole.

    D. a spaghetti dinner with salad and garlic bread.

106. An individual with a traumatic brain injury is impulsive during self-feeding, which is exemplified by placing too much food in his mouth at one time. What method would MOST effectively develop safer eating habits?

    A. Cut the food into smaller pieces.

    B. Have the individual count to 10 between bites of food.

    C. Have the individual set down the utensil until the mouth is cleared.

    D. Serve the food in separate containers on the meal tray.

107. An OT practitioner wants to use an activity that will allow the individuals in the group to experience success after making a mess, and one that will delay gratification (requiring self-control). The activity process that BEST provides this experience is:

    A. having a discussion about mosaic tile crafts.

    B. selecting the design pattern for a tile trivet.

    C. applying grout to a tile trivet and waiting for it to dry.

    D. encouraging the individual to clean off the table at the end of the group.

108. When evaluating an individual in the early stages of dementia, the OT practitioner will MOST likely expect deficits in which of the following areas?

    A. Short-term memory

    B. Fine and gross motor skills

    C. Social skills

    D. Dressing skills

109. An individual with major depressive disorder is withdrawn and exhibiting a low energy level. Which would be the MOST appropriate type of intervention activities for the OT practitioner to present in the initial stages of treatment for this patient, given that the client has expressed willingness to perform the activity?

    A. Selecting a leisure activity of interest and identifying materials needed

    B. Performing a clerical task such as sorting papers

    C. Practicing meditation

    D. Writing suggestions for coping with daily life stresses

110. An individual with memory and attention deficits exhibits poor table manners and is working to address this in an ADL group. Which type of intervention would be MOST appropriate to plan for this individual?

    A. Use role plays that include practicing good table manners.

    B. Reward the individual with dessert when he uses good manners.

    C. Instruct group members to remind him when he forgets his good manners.

    D. Reinforce use of good manners with praise and rewards.

111. An OT practitioner observes that when an individual with neurological deficits reaches for her brush in her bathroom cabinet, she becomes very distracted by the other items on the shelf. Which of the following activities does the practitioner use with the individual to address the underlying cognitive problem?

    A. Playing a simple, repetitive card game in a quiet environment

    B. Measuring ingredients for a recipe while there is music playing

    C. Referring to a catalog and filling out a catalog form

    D. Walking and bouncing a ball simultaneously

112. An OT practitioner wishes to identify how a patient spends his leisure time, which leisure activities he especially enjoys, and which others he has participated in that he would be interested in renewing. The MOST appropriate tool for this purpose is a(n):

    A. evaluation of living skills.

    B. interest checklist.

    C. activity configuration.

    D. self-care evaluation.

■ PHYSICAL DISABILITIES

113. A long-term goal for an individual with progressive weakness is for the family to carry out his feeding program. Which statement is the MOST appropriate short-term goal?

    A. Patient will participate in feeding program.

    B. Patient will feed himself with moderate assistance.

    C. Family will feed patient safely and independently 100% of the time.

    D. Family will demonstrate independence in current positioning and feeding techniques 50% of the time.

114. An individual is recovering from a hand injury and complains of pain when any sensation is felt on the affected hand. When implementing a program of desensitization training for the patient, the MOST appropriate sequence for grading the sensory stimuli that will be applied to the patient's hand is from:

A. soft to hard to rough.
B. tap to rub to touch.
C. light to medium to heavy.
D. rough to hard to soft.

115. The goal for an individual in the later stages of Parkinson's disease is to dress independently. The BEST adaptation to compensate for this person's physical deficits would be:

A. Velcro closures on front opening clothing.
B. large buttons on front opening clothing.
C. larger clothing slipped on over the head with no fasteners.
D. stretchy fabric clothing with tie closures in the back.

116. A homemaker with weak grip strength wishes to prepare a muffin mix but cannot open the bag. Which of the following would the OT MOST likely recommend?

A. A hand-powered mixer
B. Looped handle scissors
C. An electric knife
D. Prepare slice cookies instead of muffins

117. An individual with ALS and mild dysphagia becomes extremely fatigued at meals. Which is the FIRST intervention the OT practitioner should consider recommending?

A. Speak with the physician about tube feedings.
B. Sit in a semi-reclined position during meals.
C. Eat six small meals a day.
D. Substitute pureed foods for liquids.

118. An individual with COPD has identified a long-term goal of being able to shop independently for groceries. Which statement is the BEST short-term goal for this individual?

A. Individual will purchase 10 items at the supermarket with supervision.
B. Individual will cook a one-dish meal with items purchased at the supermarket.
C. Individual will identify food items needed for developing a shopping list.
D. Instruct individual in energy conservation techniques that apply to grocery shopping.

119. An individual who is s/p traumatic brain injury exhibits good strength, but demonstrates ataxia in both upper extremities. The writing adaptation that would be MOST appropriate in compensating for this individual's deficit areas would be:

A. using a keyboard.
B. a universal cuff with pencil holder attachment.
C. using a balanced forearm orthosis with built-up felt-tip pen.
D. a weighted pen and weighted wrists.

120. Which type of data would be MOST useful for an OT practitioner consultant in an adult day care facility for the purpose of identifying the overall needs of the adult day-care population at the site?

A. ADL and IADL performance-based tests results
B. Leisure and recreational checklists filled out by clients
C. Data about overall occupational performance, activity needs, and health issues of clients
D. Results of standardized cognitive level assessments for each client

121. An OT practitioner is evaluating assistive technology vocational needs for an adult with severe motor limitations. The OT will MOST likely:

A. make recommendations for ways of operating the technology.
B. assist with vocational goals.
C. seek job placement for the client.
D. solve mechanical or software problems.

122. An individual with hemiplegia and her spouse need to learn how to perform transfers. The MOST important transfer(s) to learn would be to:

A. the unaffected side of the individual's body.
B. the affected side of the individual's body.
C. both sides of the individual's body.
D. the side of the body from which the individual will be approaching the transfer.

123. An individual with paraplegia is learning to perform wheelchair-to-car transfers. What is the highest level of independence this individual is likely to achieve?

A. Minimal to moderate assistance
B. Independent transfer unrealistic; recommend public transportation
C. Independent with use of a sliding board
D. Independent using tenodesis functions

124. An individual is beginning to demonstrate return in the right upper extremity following a CVA, but has mildly impaired sensation in the right hand, which results in the inability to identify objects. Which would be the BEST method to help improve stereognosis?

A. The OT practitioner verbally describes how a object looks prior to touching it.

B. The individual looks at the object before touching it.

C. The individual works with "theraputty" to strengthen her hand.

D. The individual attempts to find coins in a pocket while occluding vision.

125. When evaluating an individual with dysphagia for MOTOR problems associated with swallowing, the OT practitioner should look for:

A. coughing or choking.

B. disorientation or confusion.

C. pain while swallowing.

D. decreased smell and taste.

126. An OT practitioner is instructing an individual with left hemiplegia how to remove a pullover shirt. The correct sequence is:

A. (1) remove shirt from unaffected arm; (2) remove shirt from affected arm; (3) gather shirt up at the back of the neck; and (4) pull gathered back fabric off over head.

B. (1) remove shirt from affected arm; (2) remove shirt from unaffected arm; (3) gather shirt up at the back of the neck; and (4) pull gathered back fabric off over head.

C. (1) gather shirt up at the back of the neck; (2) pull gathered back fabric off over head; (3) remove shirt from affected arm; and (4) remove shirt from unaffected arm.

D. (1) gather shirt up at the back of the neck; (2) pull gathered back fabric off over head; (3) remove shirt from unaffected arm; and (4) remove shirt from affected arm.

127. An individual with complete C7 quadriplegia demonstrates fair plus (3+) strength in the wrist extensors. Which of the following interventions would the OT practitioner introduce to MOST effectively increase strength in the wrist extensors?

A. A craft activity using increasingly heavy hand tools

B. Mildly resistive activities that are halted as soon as the individual begins to fatigue

C. Electric stimulation to the wrist extensors

D. Mild resistance during AROM to the wrist

128. An OT practitioner is working with an individual who sustained a BKA (below-the-knee amputation) 1 year ago and is still experiencing stump hypersensitivity. Which of the following pain management techniques should the therapist implement to decrease chronic pain in the residual limb?

A. Proper body mechanics

B. Rubbing, tapping, or applying pressure

C. Work simulation activities

D. Passive range of motion and immobilization

129. In order to ascertain oxygen saturation levels during an ADL evaluation, the OTR should:

A. count respirations.

B. measure heart rate.

C. read the pulse oximeter.

D. note the individual's breathing pattern.

130. An individual is about to be discharged to home following a hip arthroplasty. The individual is able to ambulate with a quad cane, but balance remains slightly impaired. Which is the MOST important safety recommendation for the OT practitioner to make?

A. Remove all throw or scatter rugs.

B. Place lever handles on faucets.

C. Install a ramp if steps exist.

D. Install a handheld shower.

131. During an evaluation of shower safety following a knee replacement, the individual begins to fall toward the operated leg. The OT practitioner determines that the individual is demonstrating:

A. unilateral neglect.

B. lower extremity weakness.

C. impaired balance.

D. impaired gross motor coordination.

132. A patient who had a CVA has difficulty using his left upper extremity for reaching activities because of fluctuating muscle tone. According to the Neurodevelopmental Treatment approach, one of the MOST effective ways to teach a person to normalize high muscle tone in affected extremities prior to functional activities is by:

A. placing a weighted cuff on the extremity.

B. weight-bearing through the extremity in sitting or standing.

C. using the unaffected arm for all reaching activities.

D. "forced use" of the affected extremity.

133. An OT practitioner is instructing an individual with a total hip replacement (posterolateral approach) how to perform a passenger side car transfer. Which of the following is the BEST method for entering the car?

   A. Stand the body parallel to the car, hold onto a stable section of the car, lift and place the involved leg into the car, and slowly sit and follow with opposite leg.

   B. Back up the body to the passenger seat, hold onto a stable section of the car, extend the involved leg, and slowly sit in the car.

   C. Back up the body to the passenger seat, hold onto a stable section of the car, flex both legs simultaneously, and slowly sit in the car.

   D. Back up the body to the passenger seat, hold onto a stable section of the car, flex the involved leg, and slowly sit in the car.

134. The FIRST step an OT practitioner should take in screening visual problems with a developmentally disabled adult would be to:

   A. assess and adapt lighting in the client's living environment.

   B. administer formal visual assessments of acuity and visual fields.

   C. refer the client to an ophthalmologist or eye care professional.

   D. observe for signs of visual deficits during daily living activities.

135. An individual with low endurance complains of becoming too fatigued during sexual activity to enjoy it. The BEST strategy for the OT practitioner to recommend is for the individual to:

   A. time sex for the end of the day.

   B. take the top, prone position.

   C. take the bottom, supine position.

   D. experiment with a variety of positions.

136. One of the key positioning strategies an OT practitioner plans to provide for a patient with a hip replacement while the patient is sitting or supine is to:

   A. place pillows on the lateral side of the hips.

   B. elevate the foot on the side of the hip surgery.

   C. place a foam wedge between the legs of the patient.

   D. place a roll under the patient's knees.

137. An OT practitioner is teaching several elderly individuals with COPD energy conservation techniques in home management skills. Following learning principles for older adults, the MOST effective way to present the information would be to:

   A. present all the important principles to be covered together in a single presentation.

   B. keep the presentation loosely structured, rather than highly organized.

   C. attempt to persuade individuals about the importance of those points on which they do not seem to agree.

   D. present important principles in small units that are spaced at a slower than normal pace.

138. While evaluating an individual with arthritis, the OT observes PIP joint hyperextension and DIP joint flexion in the digits. The OTR will MOST LIKELY document this as a:

   A. boutonnière deformity.

   B. mallet finger deformity.

   C. congenital deformity.

   D. swan neck deformity.

139. An individual with Guillain-Barré syndrome demonstrates poor to fair strength throughout the upper extremities. Which is the most appropriate approach for the OT practitioner to use when planning treatment for the EARLY stages?

   A. Gentle, nonresistive activities

   B. Progressive resistive exercise

   C. Fine motor activities

   D. Active range of motion against moderate resistance

140. An OT practitioner has been asked to perform an ergonomic evaluation and provide ergonomic interventions to a job site where the rate of cumulative trauma disorders is unusually high. Which of the following actions BEST addresses this request?

   A. Introduce relaxation seminars for employees to decrease stress while on the job.

   B. Treat corporate clients for cumulative trauma disorders.

   C. Provide work-simulation activities.

   D. Suggest furniture and accessories that promote better positioning at work.

141. An individual with Parkinson's disease is at risk for aspiration. When instructing the primary caregiver in proper positioning during feeding, the OT practitioner should recommend:

A. feeding the individual in bed in a supine position.

B. seating the individual upright on a firm surface with the chin slightly tucked.

C. positioning the individual in a semi-reclined position in a reclining chair.

D. feeding the individual in bed in a side-lying position.

142. The PRIMARY reason for providing adaptive equipment to an individual with arthritis is to:

A. decrease joint stress and pain.

B. correct deformity.

C. simplify work.

D. decrease independence.

143. An individual with chronic pain avoids household chores because certain actions increase pain. An OT practitioner would be MOST likely to document this individual's MOTOR response to pain as:

A. inability to concentrate on tasks because of pain.

B. frequent complaints of aching pain.

C. repeated protecting of the joints while moving.

D. refusal to partake in certain ADL to prevent the accompanying pain.

144. The strategy that will enable the HIGHEST level of independence in feeding for an individual with a C3 spinal cord injury is for the individual to:

A. clearly direct a caregiver in preferred head position, food portion size, and choice of food to eat.

B. use a mobile arm support.

C. use a wrist support with a utensil inserted into the cuff.

D. use a universal cuff with a utensil inserted into the cuff.

145. An individual newly diagnosed with Parkinson's disease exhibits hand tremors, slight rigidity of the upper extremities, and decreased endurance. Which type of intervention would BEST address the individual's goal to prepare for work in the mornings as independently and efficiently as possible?

A. Recommend showering in the morning to decrease joint stiffness.

B. Train the spouse in how to assist the individual with tub transfers.

C. Precede morning activities with a series of exercises to maintain range of motion of trunk and extremities.

D. Suggest clothing modifications such as slip-on shoes, zipper pull, and pullover shirts.

146. An OT practitioner is working on sitting balance with an individual with C6 quadriplegia. The BEST position for the individual's hands to be in when using them for support is to have the fingers:

A. extended and adducted.

B. flexed at all joints.

C. extended and abducted.

D. adducted and flexed only at the metacarpalphalangeal joints.

147. An individual complains of perspiration, which is causing his resting hand splint to be uncomfortable. The BEST action for the OT practitioner to take is to:

A. recommend putting talcum powder in the splint.

B. line the splint with moleskin.

C. fabricate a new resting hand splint with perforated material.

D. provide a stockinette sleeve for the individual to wear inside the splint.

148. An OT practitioner is introducing dressing techniques to an individual with an L5 spinal cord injury. Which of the following would be MOST beneficial?

A. A buttonhook zipper pull device

B. A clip-on tie

C. Adapted shoes

D. Loose-fitting clothing

149. An individual with amyotrophic lateral sclerosis has asked how to maintain strength in weak (fair plus) wrist extensors. Which is the MOST appropriate intervention for the OT to recommend?

A. A cock-up wrist support

B. Playing Velcro checkers to tolerance

C. Active range of motion of the wrist daily without resistance

D. Wrist extension exercises several times a day against maximal resistance

150. Which pieces of adaptive dressing equipment would an OT practitioner MOST likely recommend to a young adult who presents with a complete T10 to L1 spinal cord injury?

A. Reacher, sock aid, and dressing stick

B. Sock aid and dressing stick

C. Dressing stick

D. No equipment

151. An individual's PIP joint appears flexed, and the DIP joint appears hyperextended. The OT can BEST document this condition as a:

A. mallet deformity.

B. boutonnière deformity.

C. subluxation deformity.

D. swan neck deformity.

152. An OT practitioner is evaluating an individual who sustained a complete T8 spinal cord injury. Which level of independence in bathing, dressing, and transfers would the practitioner MOST likely expect this individual to achieve?

A. Complete independence with self-care and transfers

B. Independence with self-care and minimal assistance with transfers

C. Minimal assistance with self-care and moderate assistance with transfers

D. Dependence with both self-care and transfers

153. A 60-year-old auto-mechanic with diabetes and impaired sensation in the residual lower limb has been referred to OT following an above-knee amputation. The FIRST item the OT practitioner should address is:

A. skin inspection.

B. grooming techniques (shaving, trimming toe-nails, etc.).

C. retirement planning.

D. returning to work.

154. After wearing a new splint for 20 minutes, an individual develops a reddened area along the ulnar styloid process. The FIRST modification the OT practitioner should make to correct the splint is to:

A. line the splint with moleskin.

B. line the splint with adhesive backed foam.

C. flange the area around the ulnar styloid.

D. reheat and refabricate the entire splint.

155. The MOST appropriate assessment instrument for the OT practitioner to use for measuring range of motion of the hand is a(n):

A. goniometer.

B. dynamometer.

C. pinch meter.

D. aesthesiometer.

156. An individual is bedridden, and flexion contractures have begun to develop in the right hand. Which of the following would the OT practitioner MOST likely fabricate for this individual?

A. Dorsal wrist splint

B. Functional-position resting splint

C. Volar wrist cock-up splint

D. Dynamic finger-extension splint

157. Which of the following interventions is MOST appropriate for an individual who has recently been diagnosed with rheumatoid arthritis and is in the acute stage of the disease?

A. Strengthening with resistive exercises

B. Positioning, adaptive equipment, and patient education

C. Discharge planning

D. Preparing the patient for surgical intervention

158. A nonspeaking person who uses a wheelchair is suddenly making many errors on the augmentative communication device, but experienced no difficulty the previous day. Which of the following is the FIRST step the OT practitioner should take in responding to this problem?

A. Refer the person to a physician for evaluation.

B. Reposition the person in the wheelchair to allow optimal positioning.

C. Reassess the person's communication abilities.

D. Replace the communication device.

159. An OT practitioner is evaluating a young cabinetmaker who complains of sensory changes over the dorsal thumb and proximal phalanx of the index, long, and half of the ring finger. The practitioner will MOST likely suspect involvement of the:

A. ulnar nerve.
B. median nerve.
C. radial nerve.
D. brachial plexus.

160. An OT practitioner is developing a lifestyle redesign program at the hospital where she works for adults with obesity. In order to obtain information on the perceived needs of the population, the OT practitioner should:

A. collect information concerning the incidence of obesity in the community and factors that contribute to the problem.
B. interview a hospital administrator about what the hospital is already doing to meet the needs of this population.
C. survey doctors from the internal medicine department of the hospital.
D. run a focus group comprising obese adults from the local community.

161. During an ADL evaluation of an individual with a stroke, the OT practitioner notes that the individual is unable to find the buttons on a shirt with printed fabric. This observation would MOST likely lead the practitioner to perform more in-depth evaluation of which area of perception?

A. Position in space
B. Figure-ground discrimination
C. Body image
D. Visual closure

162. A person with peripheral neuropathy exhibits loss of pinprick, light touch, pressure, and temperature sensation resulting in an absence of protective sensation. The MOST appropriate form of intervention to address this type of sensory loss would be a program emphasizing:

A. sensory reeducation.
B. desensitization.
C. sensory bombardment.
D. compensation.

163. An individual with MS is independent with bathtub transfers using a grab bar. The MOST important self-care recommendation the OT practitioner can make regarding bathing is to:

A. use cool water.
B. use moderately heated water.
C. take showers and avoid bathing.
D. bathe at the sink with a basin.

164. As part of an initial evaluation of an individual with carpal tunnel syndrome, the OT practitioner evaluates light touch sensation using a cotton ball. When the individual returns for reevaluation after two weeks, the MOST appropriate method for re-evaluation of light touch is:

A. a cotton ball.
B. an aesthesiometer.
C. Semmes-Weinstein monofilaments.
D. a pin or straightened paper clip.

165. When administering an evaluation of upper extremity function to a newly admitted patient with Guillain-Barré syndrome, it is MOST important to:

A. test proximal muscle strength first.
B. perform the evaluation over several sessions.
C. include sensory testing.
D. evaluate range of motion.

166. An OT practitioner applies weights to the wrists of an individual who is making a macramé planter to improve shoulder strength. The therapist is MOST likely implementing which of the following treatment approaches?

A. Neurophysiological
B. Neurodevelopmental
C. Biomechanical
D. Rehabilitative

167. While observing an individual who has just been admitted to the rehabilitation unit after a right CVA with left hemiplegia, the OT practitioner notices that the individual's left arm lies limply by his side. This MOST likely indicates:

A. normal upper extremity function.
B. flaccidity.
C. subluxation.
D. spasticity.

168. During a functional assessment of strength, the OT observes that the individual can move the arm through the full range of motion to reach a high bathroom shelf, but can lift and place nothing heavier than a can of spray deodorant on the shelf. The strength according to the manual muscle test (MMT) would be documented as:

A. fair minus (3−).
B. fair (3−).
C. fair plus (3+).
D. good minus (4−).

169. An individual has been instructed to place towels, one at a time, on a high shelf in order to improve shoulder function. The individual is able to easily place 10 towels. Which of the following modifications would MOST effectively improve endurance in the shoulder flexors?

A. Place the towels on a higher shelf.
B. Increase the number of towels from 10 to 20.
C. Place the towels on a lower shelf.
D. Add a 1 pound weight to each arm.

170. The technique of stabilizing a person's forearm on the table when writing would MOST likely be used if the individual exhibited:

A. decreased vision.
B. poor endurance.
C. impaired fine motor performance.
D. incoordination.

171. An OT practitioner is treating an individual who developed a severe PIP joint contracture in the third digit 2 months after a burn injury. Which of the following static splinting techniques would BEST address the needs of this individual?

A. Plaster cylindrical splint
B. Dynamic outrigger splint
C. Blocking splint
D. PIP-DIP splint

172. What is the best position for the OT practitioner to assume when performing a stand/pivot transfer with an individual from a wheelchair to a car?

A. Move slowly, twisting from the trunk.
B. Keep feet shoulder width apart, lifting with the arms.
C. Keep knees bent and feet planted when moving.
D. Maintain a neutral spine, slowly shifting feet as the turn is completed.

173. An individual who has been receiving treatment for an overuse syndrome is about to be discharged. Which of the following is the BEST example of the assessment section of a discharge summary?

A. "Pt. can work for up to 3 hours at the computer using periodic stretch breaks."
B. "Pt. will take stretch breaks every 30 minutes when working at the computer."
C. "Pt. reports being able to work at the computer much longer and more comfortably than initially."
D. "Pt. has improved significantly in his ability to work at the computer by using periodic stretch breaks."

174. An individual is working on prehension skills in order to return to work as an automobile mechanic. Which of the following activities would BEST provide the opportunity to practice prehension?

A. Loosening nuts and bolts by hand
B. Removing an air filter using a screwdriver
C. Cranking a car jack
D. Grasping a hammer

175. The OT practitioner observes an individual being treated for low back pain engaging in poor body mechanics when lifting a box from the floor. The MOST appropriate instruction to give the individual about lifting is to:

A. keep both knees straight, flex the back, and keep the object an arm's length away from the body.
B. bend both knees, keep the back straight, and bring the object close to the body.
C. keep both knees and back straight, and bring object close to the body.
D. bend one knee while keeping the other leg straight, and keep the object an arm's length away from the body.

176. When evaluating an individual with a brachial plexus injury (Erb's Palsy), the OT practitioner should specifically assess:

A. strength in the deltoid, brachialis, biceps, and brachioradialis muscles.
B. sensation in both the radial and ulnar aspects of the hand.
C. static and dynamic sitting balance.
D. fine motor coordination.

177. A medically stable, elderly individual is being discharged from an acute care setting following a car accident. The individual requires assistance with all ADLs, and would benefit from additional OT to maximize functional independence and eventually return home alone. The individual is weak and tolerates only brief periods of therapy. The MOST appropriate disposition for this individual would be:

A. acute rehabilitation.
B. to remain in acute care hospital.
C. a subacute facility.
D. to return home with home health-care services.

178. Which of the following interventions would be MOST appropriate for instructing an individual with chronic neck pain to use pain management techniques?

A. Biofeedback, distraction, and relaxation techniques
B. Specific skill training
C. Strength and endurance building techniques
D. Cognitive retraining techniques

179. Which of the following actions should the OT practitioner instruct a patient to perform FIRST when initiating a safe wheelchair transfer?

A. Have the patient scoot forward to the front of the seat.
B. Position foot plates in the up position.
C. Swing away the leg rests.
D. Lock the brakes.

180. A local branch of the Arthritis Association has hired an OT practitioner to develop programming to promote socialization, joint flexibility, and overall physical fitness in individuals with rheumatoid arthritis. The intervention that would BEST satisfy these requirements is:

A. a weightlifting program.
B. providing adaptive equipment.
C. an aquatic therapy class.
D. educational programming in joint protection and energy conservation.

181. The key symptoms to assess when evaluating an individual with suspected complex regional pain syndrome (formerly called "reflex sympathetic dystrophy") are:

A. night pain and tingling of thumb, index, and middle fingers.
B. pain, edema, skin temperature, and skin color.
C. ability to pinch a piece of paper between thumb and index finger
D. decreased range of motion and strength.

182. An OT practitioner is helping a family plan a wheelchair ramp to the front door of their home. The minimum amount of space needed in front of the door to allow easy wheelchair access is:

A. 3 feet by 5 feet.
B. 4 feet by 4 feet.
C. 4.5 feet by 3 feet.
D. 5 feet by 5 feet.

183. When an OT practitioner plans a work-hardening program for a homemaker with severe back pain, the expected outcome is that the client will:

A. acquire a part-time job out of the home.
B. resume previous leisure activities.
C. experience decreased pain levels.
D. resume the homemaker role.

184. What wheelchair feature would be MOST appropriate to recommend for an individual who will be traveling by car with family members to community outings and bringing a wheelchair?

A. A frame with crossbar folding construction
B. A one-arm drive
C. An amputee frame
D. A reclining backrest

185. A computer programmer arrives at an OT clinic complaining of upper extremity pain while on the job. Which of the following are MOST likely to be considered work-related injuries specifically linked to the age of technology?

A. Systemic diseases
B. Edema and paresthesias
C. Burns and electrocution
D. Carpal tunnel and chronic cervical tension

186. In administering an assessment of fingertip pinch strength, the OT practitioner would instruct the individual being tested to place his thumb against the:

A. tip of the index finger.

B. side of the index finger.

C. tips of the index and middle fingers.

D. tips of all the fingers at once.

■ SERVICE MANAGEMENT AND PROFESSIONAL PRACTICE

187. An instructor from a local nursing school has asked an OT practitioner to speak about OT to a class of first year nursing students. The practitioner feels uncertain about giving the lecture because of a lack of resources. The MOST appropriate action to take is to:

A. recommend that the nursing course instructor call AOTA and obtain public relations information to share with the nursing students.

B. decline to do the in-service, but send information to the instructor.

C. decline to do the in-service and try to find another OT to do the lecture.

D. use brochures, posters, videotapes, and films available from the AOTA to enhance the presentation.

188. When an experienced OT uses a standardized assessment to determine a client's performance level and then asks the supervising OT to perform the same assessment on the same client 1 week later, the OT practitioner is MOST likely seeking:

A. supervisory feedback.

B. evidence of competence.

C. instrument reliability.

D. evidence of incompetence.

189. Many COTAs are employed in long-term care facilities and perform many functions. The function that the OTR MUST perform in this setting is:

A. activity programming, environmental adaptations, and caregiver and staff education.

B. ADL training, and running feeding and leisure activity groups.

C. interpreting results of assessments for the purposes of treatment planning.

D. positioning, providing adaptive devices, and instructing in use of splints.

190. A patient who has had surgery for a malignant tumor was seen once by OT and is now being discharged home. The patient is weak, requires moderate assistance with ambulation, and needs to receive IV chemotherapy with a home health nurse. The MOST appropriate recommendation the OT could make regarding the continuation of OT services would be to:

A. obtain services from a home health OT.

B. stay in the hospital a little longer.

C. go to a rehabilitation center.

D. come back for outpatient OT.

191. An OT practitioner is offered a job upon completion of fieldwork and accepts the position even though she had not yet applied for her temporary license. What would be the BEST action for this therapist to take under the circumstances?

A. Schedule an immediate start date and send for a temporary license.

B. Confide in the Rehab director and follow her recommendation to start as scheduled.

C. Decline the current offer, ask if company can wait to hire, and apply for a temporary license.

D. Start the job knowing that no one with the company will ask to see her license.

192. A client refuses to be treated by a level II fieldwork student, stating he would only participate in OT "with someone who's qualified." What action should the supervising OT take FIRST under these circumstances?

A. Attempt to persuade the client to participate with the student.

B. Cancel the session for that day and document that the client refused OT.

C. Consult with the supervising OTR.

D. Treat the client with the student observing the session.

193. An OT manager is attempting to find a way to have financial success in the department while ensuring patient satisfaction. Which of the following is MOST likely to be implemented to assess patient flow, develop critical pathways, and cut costs?

A. Quality improvement

B. Peer review teams

C. Cost accounting

D. Interdisciplinary care improvement teams

194. A hospital-based multidisciplinary team meets bimonthly to monitor their services in regard to the creation of an environment that meets or exceeds consumer needs. This model is MOST appropriately called:

    A. total quality management.

    B. cost accounting.

    C. employee empowerment.

    D. horizontal structuring.

195. A COTA working in outpatient rehabilitation teaches herself how to use paraffin by reading books on physical agent modalities (PAMs), carefully reading the instructions that came with the paraffin bath unit, and practicing on herself for several weeks. Is it now acceptable for this COTA to provide paraffin treatments?

    A. No, COTAs may not administer PAMs.

    B. No, it violates the AOTA's Position Paper on modalities.

    C. Yes, she has demonstrated service competency.

    D. Yes, only when an OTR is on duty in the facility.

196. At a team planning meeting for a 2-year-old child with multiple handicaps, it is decided that the OT will fulfill the roles of other therapies needed as well. This decision requires a "role release" from the teacher, PT, and speech therapist. Which of the following team approaches for young children does this method describe?

    A. Unidisciplinary

    B. Multidisciplinary

    C. Interdisciplinary

    D. Transdisciplinary

197. An OT practitioner is asked by administration to complete billing paperwork early by projecting therapy time for patients that have yet to be seen. One of these patients later refuses therapy because of medical illness. What is the BEST course of action to take?

    A. Contact administration to let them know of the unforeseen change in service delivery and make appropriate adjustments to billing.

    B. Leave the billing "as is" and document that services were attempted, but not provided.

    C. Strongly encourage the patient to attempt to participate in treatment and consider the associated time and effort as billable activity.

    D. Make no changes to billing, but try to make the time up during subsequent treatment sessions.

198. An OT manager in a large department is trying to determine which staff will be able to supervise level-II fieldwork students in the upcoming months. OT practitioners may only be selected to be primary student supervisors if they:

    A. are certified OT practitioners with at least 6 months of experience.

    B. have at least 1 year of experience as a certified OT practitioner.

    C. are certified by the NBCOT.

    D. have supervised a level-I student before the level-II student.

199. The program that funds health care for poor and medically indigent individuals is referred to as:

    A. Medicare.

    B. Medicaid.

    C. Workers' Compensation.

    D. the Education for All Handicapped Children Act.

200. A supervising OT asks an experienced COTA to complete a portion of an assessment. The portion that is MOST appropriate for the COTA to complete independently would be:

    A. collecting chart review information.

    B. analyzing and interpreting assessment information.

    C. establishing the treatment goals.

    D. establishing the treatment plan.

Answers for Simulation Examination 4

1. (C) Toothpaste with a flip-open cap. An individual with fine motor incoordination would be able to manage a toothpaste cap that flips open much more easily than a cap that must be removed completely from the tube. Also, toothpaste tubes with flip-open caps are larger in diameter, which make them easier to manage. A wash mitt (answer A) and a toothbrush with a built-up handle (answer D) are good options for those with weak grasp. Spray deodorant (answer B) has a small button to push, which would be difficult to operate for someone with incoordination. See Reference: Pedretti and Early (eds). Foti, D: Activities of daily living.

2. (A) poor modulation of tactile input. This is the only answer that describes both his hypersensitive and hyposensitive responses to tactile input. The child with autism may be unpredictable in terms of response to sensory stimuli, both avoiding and craving stimulation at various times. Answers B and C are incorrect because they describe only one part of the problem. Answer D is wrong because he appears to be craving deep pressure or proprioceptive input in order to modulate the tactile system. See Reference: Case-Smith (ed). Parham, LD, and Mailloux, Z: Sensory integration.

3. (B) allow the chin to remain tucked when drinking. Tucking the chin toward the chest maximizes airway protection for individuals with dysphagia (answer B). Methods the caregiver can use to control or slow the rate of liquid intake for individuals who demonstrate poor judgment or impulsivity (answers A and C) include using a drinking spout with a small opening, pinching a straw, or using a vacuum feeding cup with a control button. Plastic cups and plastic-coated utensils are best for individuals with a bite reflex (answer D) to prevent damage to their oral structures. See Reference: Trombly and Radomski. Avery-Smith, W: Dysphagia.

4. (C) Constructional. Constructional play involves building and creating things. It is in this area of play that children develop a sense of mastery and problem-solving skills. Sensorimotor play (answer A) generally develops a child's body awareness and sensory experience. Imaginary play (answer B) involves manipulating people and objects in fantasy as a prelude to dealing with reality. Game play (answer D) requires the ability to learn and apply rules in play. See Reference: Kramer and Hinojosa (eds). Luebben, AJ, Hinojosa, J, and Kramer, P: Legitimate tools of pediatric occupational therapy.

5. (B) Flex the child's hips and knees. Answer B is correct because flexing the hips and knees inhibits ankle plantarflexion (which makes the task very difficult) through the key point of the hip. Answer A is not correct, because hip and knee extension would contribute to, not inhibit, plantarflexion of the ankle. Answer C is not correct, because shoulder extension would probably have more influence on hip and knee flexion than on ankle plantarflexion. Answer D is not correct, primarily because the abnormal pattern at the ankle is usually influenced by inhibition from the key point of the hip. See Reference: Case-Smith (ed). Shepherd, J: Self-care and adaptations for independent living.

6. (B) communication, self-care, and social skills. Children with moderate mental retardation are likely to have deficits in the areas of academic performance, communication, self-care, and social skills (answer B). Individuals with profound mental retardation are dependent on others for nearly all their needs, and often have neuromuscular, orthopedic, or behavioral deficits. Evaluation of these individuals should focus on positioning and communication skills (answer A). Individuals with mild mental retardation have the potential for independence in ADLs and IADLs (answer C), and may achieve academic performance at the third to seventh grade level, and may eventually obtain employment. Individuals with severe mental retardation may be able to learn habitual activities, such as feeding and personal hygiene (answer D). They may learn to communicate verbally or nonverbally, and will require significant support to engage in most tasks. See Reference: Solomon (ed). Newman, D: Mental retardation.

7. (A) Place a foam-lined plastic laundry basket in the tub. Answer A, a laundry basket with a foam-lined bottom, would be the most appropriate item for the OT to recommend because this piece of equipment addresses both cost and positioning concerns. The laundry basket also will permit the child to continue to submerse herself in the tub, an activity that was stated as enjoyable to the child. Answer B, a horseshoe-shaped bath collar, would be indicated for a child with "severe motor limitations who is lying supine in shallow water" (p. 516). Whereas, answer C, a bath hammock, might be considered as an alternative choice for this child, because "bath hammocks fully hold the body and enable the parent to wash the child thoroughly" (p. 516), this type of equipment would not be as cost effective as the laundry basket. Answer D, suggesting that the child stand in the shower versus showering, does not address the parent or child's immediate needs of bathing in the bathtub. If the child lacks sitting balance, it is likely that they also will lack standing balance, thus indicating the need for durable medical equipment, such as a shower bench and/or grab bars. See Reference: Case-Smith (ed). Shepherd, J: Self-care adaptations for independent living.

8. (A) a body-length prone scooter. Spastic diplegia is defined as abnormal tone affecting all four extremities, but with primary involvement of the lower extremities. Therefore, the child may use his upper extremities to propel himself through space while having his lower extremities positioned on a scooter (answer A). The airplane mobility device (answer B) is designed for children with good lower extremity function who need support in the upper body. A tricycle (answer C) requires good lower extremity control, including reciprocal movement. A power wheelchair (answer D) is designed for individuals with limited upper and lower extremity function. See Reference: Case-Smith (ed). Wright-Ott, C and Egilson, S: Mobility.

9. (D) the presence of self-regulatory functions. Self-regulatory functions are often seen in autistic children and frequently interfere with function. The other answers are less relevant in terms of essential data for intervention planning. An autistic child may be normal in terms of his or her ability to focus at close range, answer A, while answers B and C, pain and hand dominance, are most likely not the reason for the hand flapping. See Reference: Miller-Kuhaneck. The pervasive developmental disorders: A holistic view.

10. (A) A large key ring. According to Solomon, "a large key ring or a piece of fishing line make inexpensive zipping aids for children with limited grasping ability, ROM, strength, or coordination" (p. 236). Answer B, oversized fasteners, would not address the child's need to become independent in zipping, unless all of the zippers were removed from the child's pants and replaced with fasteners. Colored zippers, answer C, would mostly be helpful for a child with visual discrimination problems. Velcro fasteners, answer D, are something the OT may recommend if the more convenient and less expensive key ring adaptation does not assist the child in meeting his goals. See Reference: Solomon (ed). Jones, LMW and Machover, PZ: Occupational performance areas: Daily living and work and productive activities.

11. (D) Reinforcement of competence. According to Erikson, an 8-year-old child is usually at the stage of industry versus inferiority, during which time he or she develops a sense of competency. For a client who is expected to lose motor function gradually, a treatment plan that will provide an ongoing sense of competence (possibly in other areas) is especially relevant. Answers A, B, and C describe other developmental issues identified by Erikson that are typically achieved at other ages: basic trust (answer A) in infancy; initiative (answer B) during the toddler years; and self-identity (answer C) during adolescence. See Reference: Case-Smith (ed). Law, M, Missiuna, C, Pollock, N, and Stewart, D: Foundations of occupational therapy practice with children.

12. (D) Evaluate participants' performance strengths and weaknesses. The first step in any intervention is almost always evaluation. The next step in this process, which is based on a developmental model because of the age and backgrounds of the clients, is developing trust and exploration (answer A). This is followed by skill development (answer B). Once basic skills are in place, greater emphasis is placed on work quantity and quality (answer C). See Reference: Cottrell (ed). Kannenberg, K and Boyer, D: Occupational therapy evaluation and intervention in an employment program for homeless youths.

13. (D) pudding. Foods with even consistency, uniform texture, and increased density such as pudding (answer D) are the easiest to control and swallow. Foods with multiple textures like chicken noodle soup (answer A), sticky foods like peanut butter (answer B), and foods that are fibrous or break up in the mouth like carrot sticks (answer C), should be avoided. See Reference: Case-Smith (ed). Case-Smith, J and Humphry, R: Feeding intervention.

14. (C) has a standard format. Standardization of a test means that the test is administered in a prescribed manner and that scoring and interpretation of scores also are completed in a prescribed way. The presence of data concerning the test's "norms" and the establishment of reliability and validity (answers A, B, and D) may be, and often are, provided with standardized tests, but are not assumed to be part of the test unless this information is included. The aspects of standardized tests that are always assumed are the specific and standardized method of administration, scoring, and interpretation. See Reference: Case-Smith (ed). Richardson, PK: Use of standardized tests in pediatric practice.

15. (D) Digging in "Play Doh" to search for various coins and then placing them in a piggy bank. The most appropriate selection the OT can make is to encourage the child to work on fine motor skills since this child will most likely rely on signing as a way to communicate. "The movements of the hands of a fluent signer require opposition, finger and thumb flexion and extension, and finger and thumb abduction and adduction. The hand's coordination seems to be related to its sensory abilities, particularly tactile discrimination" (thus introducing the "Play Doh") (p. 784). "The therapist can enhance kinesthetic, tactile, and visual processing through multi-sensory activities" (p. 783). Answer A, parachute activities, are indicated for gross motor and/or kinesthetic needs, but are not necessarily related to the child's fine motor limitations. Answer B, visually coding the child's shoes, is an appropriate choice when attempting to encourage self-care skills. "Adapting techniques or assistive devices may be needed. At times, self-care skills involve concrete concepts that require concrete cues for the child to learn" (p. 784). While answer C, introducing the child to socialization groups, would be appropriate to address because many children with hearing impairments feel isolated from the hearing community, the goal of the OT in this scenario is to address the child's fine motor limitations. See Reference: Case-Smith (ed). Snow-Russel, E: Services for children with visual or auditory impairments.

16. (B) Moro reflex. The Moro reflex (answer B) is characterized by abduction, extension, and external rotation of the arms. The rooting reflex (answer A) is the turning of the head toward tactile stimulation near the mouth. The flexor withdrawal reflex (answer C) is characterized by flexion of an extremity in response to a painful stimulus. The neck righting reaction (answer D) involves body alignment in rotation after turning of the head. Only the Moro reflex causes an extension movement. See Reference: Crepeau, Cohn, and Schell (eds). Kohlmeyer, K: Evaluation of performance skills and client factors.

17. (B) mounting a safety rail next to the toilet. In order to sit independently on the toilet and relax sufficiently to control muscles needed for elimination, the child has to feel posturally secure. Safety rails next to the toilet, low toilets that allow the child to put both feet on the ground, and reducer rings to decrease the size of a toilet seat, all help to provide maximal stability for the child with unstable posture. Answers A, C, and D describe adaptations used for other deficits. Replacing zippers and buttons with Velcro closures (answer A) is helpful for a child with reduced strength or fine motor coordination. Introducing toilet paper tongs (answer C) helps increase reach in a child with limited range of motion. Placing a colorful "target" (answer D) helps boys aim into the bowl, a difficulty associated with perceptual or cognitive limitations. See Reference: Case-Smith (ed). Shepherd, J: Self care and adaptations for independent living.

18. (B) stress bilateral play and school activities incorporating the prosthesis. Two-handed activi-

ties for play, school, and self-care (answer B) should be used to incorporate the prosthesis into the child's body image and to help develop bilateral skills. Activities that avoid the use of the prosthesis, as in answers A, C, and D, would not help the child to integrate the prosthesis into normal patterns of use. See Reference: Case-Smith (ed). Rogers, SL, Gordon, CY, Schanzenbacher, KE, and Case-Smith, J: Common diagnoses is pediatric occupational therapy practice.

19. (D) After the development of the goals and objectives. The initial evaluation may incorporate observation, screening, interviews, and evaluations (answers A, B, and C). Goals and objectives are developed following evaluation. "Once short- and long-term goals have been agreed upon, an implementation plan must be made regarding how to provide services to meet these goals most effectively" (p. 256). See Reference: Case-Smith (ed). Richardson, PK and Schultz-Krohn, W: Planning and implementing services.

20. (B) ability to feed herself a snack. According to Cohn, Schell, and Neistadt (2003), "to use a top-down approach, therapists first focus on clients' occupational performance rather than beginning the evaluation with an emphasis on potential underlying performance component limitations" (p. 282). Answer B, focusing on the child's ability to self-feed is representative of a top-down approach, whereas answers A, C, and D are considered to be centered around client limitations. See Reference: Crepeau, Cohn, and Schell (eds). Cohn, E, Schell, B, and Neistadt, M: Introduction to evaluation and interviewing.

21. (D) Rubber-coated spoons. "Children who have a strong tonic bite reflex can use rubber coated, plastic, or rubber spoons" (p. 225). This will allow the parent and/or child to more easily remove the utensil from the child's mouth. Rubber-coated spoons provide a smoother surface than that of a regular stainless-steel utensil. Answers A, B, and C would not be recommended for a child with a strong tonic reflex, but for other limitations such as incoordination, tremors, and apraxia. See Reference: Solomon (ed). Jones, LMW and Machover, PZ: Occupational performance areas: Daily living and work and productive activities.

22. (B) wide-base sitting on the floor while reaching for a suspended balloon. The child first practices skills in unsupported sitting on a stable surface, using a wide base of support (answer B). As skills improve, the wide base is reduced to a more narrow one. Reaching activities are used to promote postural reactions, because they involve displacement of the center of gravity and weight shifting. Answers A, C, and D are activities involving unstable support surfaces, typical of more advanced skills. See Reference: Case-Smith (ed). Nichols, DS: The development of postural control.

23. (D) accommodation. Visual accommodation (answer D) is the ability to focus efficiently from near to far distance, and vice versa. Answer A, ocular motility, refers to the ability to pursue an object visually in an efficient and smooth manner. Answer B, binocular vision, is the ability to focus the eyes on an object at varying distances and on seeing a single object clearly. Answer C, convergence, is the ability to move the eyes inward or outward with continued focus on the object. See Reference: Kramer and Hinojosa (eds). Todd, VR: Visual information analysis: Frames of reference for visual perception.

24. (D) Convert an empty lot filled with trash into a garden. Activities based on the concepts of building and creating and that result in one shared outcome are more effective for team building than those involving competition (answer A) or individual reward (answer C). Anger management skills are important for children at risk for violent behavior, however, a psychoeducational format (answer B) will not contribute to protecting or building the community. See Reference: Fazio. Programming examples within the community of clubs.

25. (D) Cut the paper in two following a straight line. Scissor skills develop from first cutting snips to cutting a single straight line (answer D). The ability to cut heavier materials such as cardboard and cloth (answer A) develops last in the sequence of scissor skills. The ability to cut along curved lines (answer B) develops after the ability to cut a straight line. The ability to cut along straight lines with enough control to cut out a triangle (answer C), develops after the ability to cut a single straight line, and before the ability to cut a curved line. See Reference: Case-Smith (ed). Exner, CE: Development of hand skills.

26. (C) Prone over a wedge. Considering the information given, answer C offers the best position because head control is isolated with the trunk supported. The child does not have adequate control to stand in a standing frame (answer A). Answer B is not correct because, although the chest is supported by a sling, the child's shoulders, arms, and hips must be able to control the position. Sitting on a therapy ball (answer D) would require both head and trunk control. See Reference: Case-Smith (ed). Nichols, DS: Development of postural control.

27. (B) give praise for completed dressing, but do not help the child get dressed. According to

Case-Smith (2001), "as the child learns new tasks, he or she develops a sense of accomplishment and pride in his or her own abilities...the increasing independence also gives the parents, teachers, siblings, and other caregivers more time and energy for other tasks" (p. 490). Since the child has achieved dressing independence, he does not need assistance (answer A), clothing adaptations (answer C), or verbal prompts (answer D) to complete the task. In fact, assisting him now may cause him to lose his independence and regress to relying on his parents again. See Reference: Case-Smith (ed). Shepherd, J: Self-care and adaptations for independent living.

28. (D) plan new motor tasks. Dyspraxia refers to difficulty planning new motor tasks (answer D). Inability to print or write (answer A) is termed "dysgraphia." The term "dyslexia" (answer B) literally means dysfunction in reading. Inability to perform mathematics (answer C) is known as "dyscalcula." See Reference: Case-Smith (ed). Rogers, SL, Gordon, CY, Schanzenbacher, KE, and Case-Smith, J: Common diagnoses in pediatric occupational therapy practice.

29. (A) power wheelchair. A power wheelchair would be the most appropriate choice in this situation. According to Hays, "children without locomotion (i.e., the ability to move their body from one place to another)" (p. 340) can be placed in a specific functional group. One of these groups is that of "children who will never ambulate and need a power wheelchair, such as children who have severe cerebral palsy or spinal muscle atrophy" (p. 340). Answer B, a standard wheelchair, may be something the family would like to purchase in addition to the power wheelchair. Standard wheelchairs tend to be less expensive, lightweight, and portable. They also are convenient when a power wheelchair is in for repairs. Answers C and D (a caster cart and powered scooter) are not considered appropriate for the child with severe cerebral palsy, because adequate upper extremity function is required for use of the caster cart and scooter. See Reference: Solomon (ed). Clayton, KS and Mathena, CT: Assistive technology.

30. (D) Review appropriate behavioral and developmental positioning techniques with parental observation and interaction. The NICU environment can often undermine the importance of the family. Therefore, implementing and integrating parental involvement with daily neonatal care becomes of primary importance for the carryover of learned techniques to best promote developmental acquisition. Answers B, C, and D are all family-centered strategies and are recommended for NICU intervention. However, answer D is clearly the optimal strategy for fostering parental observation and interpretation skills, building positional and handling skills, and responding to their infant's behaviors. Initial chart review and updating with nursing staff (answer A) are essential assessment steps made prior to initial contact with the infant and family, and are the least optimal intervention strategy to pursue with the family present. See Reference: Case-Smith (ed). Hunter, JG: Neonatal Intensive Care Unit.

31. (D) collaboratively develop an IFSP. The service plan required by federal law (IDEA, 99 to 457, Part H) and provided through early intervention programs is called an individual family service plan (answer D). Answers A and B refer to the IEP (individual education plan), a service plan required for school-aged children. Answer C is not correct because the IFSP must be developed collaboratively with other team members. See Reference: Case-Smith (ed). Stephens, LC, and Tauber, SK: Early intervention.

32. (D) Home observation and parent interview. "Observation of children in familiar settings and routines allows more characteristic views of their abilities and may be actually more reflective of how children can be expected to perform" (Case-Smith, p. 207). Parent interviews provide information about the child's abilities from the parent's point of view and can identify the priorities of the child's caregiver. Answers A, B, and C provide necessary information about performance components, development, and other parameters, but are not as effective in helping the evaluator learn about the child's self-care functioning. See Reference: Case-Smith (ed). Stewart, KB: Purposes, processes, and methods of evaluation.

33. (A) A tub seat with a handheld shower attached to the faucet. Answer A would be the most appropriate choice, because an individual with paraplegia would most likely be able to transfer himself out of the wheelchair and onto a tub seat. Because the child will not have use of his legs, a handheld shower would permit the child to wash without having to adjust the faucet overhead. Answer B, a hydraulic lift, would be indicated for an obese individual or for someone who has very limited function of both the upper and lower extremities. Answer C also would be used for an individual with limited function, in that the child can be rolled onto the tub prior to its inflation. Answer D, a wheeled shower chair, would be a choice made for washing in a shower, not a tub. The chair can simply be rolled into a stall. See Reference: Solomon (ed). Jones, LMW and Machover, PZ: Occupational performance areas: Daily living and work and productive activities.

34. (C) At age level. At 3 years of age, a child is expected to know when he or she has to use the toilet and be able to get on and off the toilet. Three-year-old children may need assistance to cleanse themselves effectively and to manage fasteners or difficult clothing. Complete independence in using the toilet (answer D) is usually achieved by the age of 4 to 5 years. By the age of 2 years (answer B), most children have daytime control over elimination, with occasional accidents, so they still need to be reminded to go to the toilet. One-year-old infants (answer A) typically indicate discomfort when wet or soiled. See Reference: Case-Smith (ed). Shepherd, J: Self care and adaptations for independent living.

35. (A) single pressure switch, firmly mounted within easy reach. A child with fluctuating muscle tone lacks stability and demonstrates extraneous movement, therefore, deliberate motor action is most effectively executed on a securely mounted device using simple movement patterns. Answers B, C, and D involve devices that would respond to slight touch, and therefore would not be effective for a person with extraneous movement and difficulty grading motor action. See Reference: Case-Smith (ed). Swinth, Y: Assistive technology: Computers and augmentative communication.

36. (C) IEP. The individual education plan (answer C) is a form that must be completed for children receiving services in the school system. This documentation standard was defined in the Education of the Handicapped Act (1975 and 1986). The UB-82 form (answer A) is used to process insurance claims. FIM (answer B), which stands for "functional independence measure," is a method used on rehabilitation units to measure an individual's level of independence. The CMS-1500 form (answer D) is used to bill Medicare and other insurance carriers for health-care services. See Reference: Crepeau, Cohn, and Schell (eds). Perinchief, JM: Documentation and management of occupational therapy services.

37. (D) set clear expectations for behavior and enforce consequences, such as a time-out, if the child loses control. The behavioral frame of reference can be useful in helping children with maladaptive behavior to learn to modify their behaviors and to learn new more adaptive behaviors through the principle of reinforcement. To use this effectively, the child must clearly understand the expectations for behavior (or rules), and that there will be consistent consequences for behaviors that break the rules. Answers A and B, allowing the child to express his anger and ignoring the behaviors, would not help the child to learn new behaviors and could cause an increased loss of control. A child who is out of con-

trol and responding to impulses is not able to respond to an insight-based approach such as reasoning. See Reference: Sladyk, K and Ryan, SE (eds).
Florey, L: A second-grader with conduct disorder.

**38. (C) specific instructions for administration
and scoring.** In standardized assessments, the instructions to the examiner are detailed and fixed so
that procedures are followed consistently each time
the test is administered. Following these instructions
assures the highest level of reliability and validity
possible. Subjective judgment (answer A) and previous experience (answer B) may be factors in administration of nonstandardized tests, which depend
on the skill and judgment of the OT practitioner
administering them, but not in the administration
and scoring of standardized tests. While practice of
a test (answer D) can help to develop competence
in the use of the test, it would not influence how to
administer and score the test. See Reference: Pedretti
and Early (eds). Occupational therapy evaluation and
assessment of physical dysfunction.

**39. (A) Teach the child to dress in a side-lying
position.** The side-lying position (answer A) eliminates the need for the child to maintain balance in
order to dress the lower extremities. Answer B is not
correct because the primary purpose of putting loops
on waistbands is to help a child with limited grasp
strength to pull on garments. Answer C is not correct because using Velcro in place of zippers also is
an adaptation designed to help children with limited
ability to grasp and pull, whereas answer D, teaching
the child to dress in a standing position, is considered
to be more difficult than dressing in a sitting position. See Reference: Case-Smith (ed). Shepherd, J:
Self-care and adaptations for independent living.

**40. (C) demonstrates any reliable, controlled
movement.** As long as the child can produce any
reliable, controlled movement, switches can be
adapted to meet positioning and mobility needs.
Accurate reach and pointing (answer B) or isolated finger control (answer D) are not necessary
to use simple pressure switches. An upright sitting
position (answer A) would not be required if the
child needed to be positioned in a reclining or
side-lying position. See Reference: Case-Smith (ed).
Swinth, Y: Assistive technology: Computers and
augmentative communication.

41. (D) plan section. The plan section of a SOAP
note (answer D) includes statements related to continuing treatment; the frequency and duration of
the treatment; suggestions for additional activities
or treatment techniques; the need for further evaluations; and when needed, recommendations for new
goals. The subjective portion of a SOAP note (answer

A) refers to an individual's or caregiver's comments
about the treatment or their condition. The objective portion of the SOAP note (answer B) focuses
on measurable and/or observable data obtained
by the OT practitioner through specific evaluations, observations, or use of therapeutic activities.
The assessment part of a SOAP note (answer C)
refers to the effectiveness of the treatment and
any changes needed, the status of the goals, and
any justification for continuing OT treatment. See
Reference: Borcherding. Writing the "P"-Plan.

**42. (B) child's speed over long distances
becomes less than that of a walking person.** A
child should be considered for a power wheelchair
when the current means of locomotion proves less
efficient and slower than locomotion by walking
(answer B). Because the child will be experiencing
progressive muscle weakness, energy conservation
is of primary importance. Answers A and C address
valid environmental considerations to be made after
determining the general need for a powered chair.
Waiting until the child becomes unable to propel
the wheelchair (answer D), would make the transition more difficult and prevent the child from getting around independently in the meantime. See
Reference: Case-Smith (ed). Wright-Ott, C and
Egilson, S: Mobility.

**43. (C) allow the child to self-apply tactile
stimuli to maximize the child's tolerance.** Tactile
defensiveness is an overreaction or negative reaction
to sensations of touch. Answer C is correct because
"generally, tactile stimuli that are actively self-applied
by the child are tolerated much better than stimuli
that are passively received, as when being touched
by another person" (p. 352). Answer A is incorrect
because light touch sensations are particularly disturbing for children with tactile defensiveness,
and may create overwhelming feelings of anxiety.
Answer B is not correct because avoiding all forms
of tactile sensation is virtually impossible, and such
complete avoidance would not help the child to
develop coping skills. Answer D also is incorrect
because deep touch stimuli is often comfortable for
children with tactile defensiveness; however, it may
possibly provide "relief from irritating stimuli when
deep pressure is applied over the involved skin
areas" (p. 350). See Reference: Case-Smith (ed).
Parham, LD and Mailloux, Z: Sensory integration.

**44. (C) follow administration instructions and
note changes in behavior.** Although the tester
may not deviate from the protocol, changes in behavior represent important test data and should be
recorded. The responses described in answers A, B,
and D may make the test results invalid by altering

the sequence of test items, the grouping of items, or the actual test item itself. These may not be changed unless it is specified in the test manual. See Reference: Case-Smith (ed). Richardson, PK: Use of standardized tests in pediatric practice.

45. (B) Rifton child's chair with a padded abductor post. A Rifton child's chair "places the child in a completely upright position and requires good head control.... a pelvic abductor pad can be added to the system" (p. 481). The abductor post keeps the legs separated when or if extensor tone increases. The prone stander (answer A) would place the child in a standing or extended position, which would reinforce undesirable extensor tone. A supine position (answer C) is not appropriate for eating if other positions are available. The child would not benefit from a beanbag chair (answer D) "since a beanbag is particularly inappropriate for children with extensor posturing because it does not successfully inhibit these postures" (p. 469). See Reference: Case-Smith (ed). Case-Smith, J and Humphry, R: Feeding intervention.

46. (B) form constancy perception. Form constancy perception (answer B) is the ability to match similar shapes regardless of change in their orientation in space. Figure-ground perception (answer A) is the ability to distinguish the bead from the background. Position in space perception (answer C) is the ability to determine the spatial relationships of the beads to each other. Visual sequencing (answer D) is an activity that requires the ability to copy the same sequence of beads. Although these abilities are all required for this bead stringing task, the error described refers to a form constancy error. See Reference: Pedretti and Early (eds). Wheatley, CJ: Evaluation and treatment of perceptual and perceptual motor deficits.

47. (D) a doll house and dress-up clothes. To encourage symbolic play, the child should be exposed to toys offering imaginative, open-ended play opportunities, encouraging formulation of ideas and feelings. Answers A, B, and C are not only representative of the younger (answer A) or older child (answers B and C), but they also encourage more defined, closed-ended play with predictable results. See Reference: Case-Smith (ed). Morrison, CD and Metzger, P: Play.

48. (D) The OT provides intervention the classroom setting with the child's peers present. According to Case-Smith, "in an integrated therapy model, the practitioner provides intervention within the classroom, emphasizing nonintrusive methods" (p. 769), answer D. Answers A, B, and C are most representative of "pull out" services where

the child is removed from the classroom and treated in another area within the school. See Reference: Case-Smith (ed). Case-Smith, J, Rogers, J, and Johnson, JH: School-based occupational therapy.

49. (A) Swimming. Swimming (answer A) provides active movement through wide ranges of motion with minimal impact on the joints. Other activities recommended for individuals with JRA include creative dance and bicycle riding. The sports in answers B, C, and D involve bouncing, jumping, and kicking, which place additional stress on the joints and would be contraindicated. See Reference: Reed. Arthritis—Juvenile rheumatoid.

50. (A) Create a reliable route to the bathroom, encouraging the child to familiarize herself with the smells and sounds of the bathroom. A primary goal for the OT working with a child with visual impairments is to address the development of self-care skills at an age appropriate level. By creating a reliable route to the bathroom, encouraging the child to focus on tactile and olfactory cues (answer A), the OT can establish compensatory techniques for the visual deficit. Having the child practice with obstacle courses (answer B) would be appropriate for the development of movement in space and body image/awareness, but would not be considered part of a daily self-care routine. Answer C, practicing handwriting and fine motor skills, would be more closely related to the development of hand manipulation skills. Introducing the child to other children with similar impairments would be an appropriate socialization activity for the child, but is not directly related to a self-care program. See Reference: Case-Smith (ed). Snow-Russel, E: Services for children with visual or auditory impairments.

51. (B) form letters out of clay. Preschoolers learn best using a multisensory approach. Making letters out of such materials as clay, bread dough, pudding, or sandpaper (answer B) uses the child's tactile, kinesthetic, and in some cases, gustatory senses, as well as vision. In this way, new learning is reinforced through a variety of sensory channels. Flash cards (answer A), matching to sample (answer C), and coloring (answer D), are methods that rely primarily on visual processing, and cognitive skills and are better suited for strengthening existing skills in older children. See Reference: Case-Smith (ed). Schneck, CM: Visual perception.

52. (B) decreased muscle tone. Decreased muscle tone (answer B) is usually characterized by joints that are lax and hyperextensible. Low muscle tone and joint hyperextensibility also are common characteristics of Down syndrome. Answer A is incorrect because loss of range of motion would be the joint characteristic of increased muscle tone. Answers C and D are incorrect because they are diagnoses that cannot be made on the basis of joint laxness, even though instability at the joint may occur with either of these conditions. The observation of joint hyper-extensibility is merely an indication of below normal muscle tone and not necessarily the indication of a specific condition or disease process. See Reference: Kramer and Hinojosa (eds). Colangelo, CA: Biomechanical frame of reference.

53. (A) checking for irritation and pressure problems. Because a toddler cannot always articulate discomfort effectively, skin irritation may go unnoticed. Therefore, a young child is at higher risk for developing skin and pressure problems than an older, more verbal one. Although answers B, C, and D describe important factors in splint care, primary emphasis for the young child should be placed on answer A. See Reference: Case-Smith (ed). Exner, CE: Development of hand skills.

54. (B) A noise machine producing white noise at bedtime. For a child who is easily aroused, a constant, monotonous auditory input can be calming enough to induce sleep. The other answers may actually increase arousal. Quick repetitive proprioceptive input, as experienced when jumping on a trampoline (answer A), and light touch provided by a fuzzy blanket (answer C), are types of sensory input that have direct arousing effect on the nervous system. Blocking out all light (answer D) may produce arousal as a result of fear generated by total darkness. See Reference: Case-Smith (ed). Cronin, AF: Psychosocial and emotional domains of behavior.

55. (B) floor sitter. "A floor sitter may enable the child with cerebral palsy to play on the floor near his or her typically developing peers" (p. 725). Occupational therapy practitioners can recommend and provide appropriate adapted equipment and positioning devices when working in an early intervention setting. A hammock (answer A) would not allow the child to feel as if he "fits in." The child verbalized the desire to sit on the floor like his peers, whereas the hammock may make the child feel even more different than when he sits in his wheelchair. Hammocks are typically utilized in therapy to provide sensori-motor/vestibular input, and would not be indicated in this situation unless no other viable options were available. Introducing an adapted wheelchair insert and a prone stander (answers C and D), would be ignoring the child's desire to sit on the floor with his peers. Wheelchair inserts are often used for positioning a child in a wheelchair to permit increased trunk support and stability, thus allowing for more independent use of the upper extremities. A prone stander would allow a child to assume a standing or weight-bearing position, but would not assist with positioning the child while sitting on a mat. See Reference: Case-Smith (ed). Stephens, LC and Tauber, SK: Early intervention.

56. (C) 8 months. Answer C is correct, because 3 months (number of months premature) are subtracted from the child's chronological age to adjust for prematurity. This child is then given the benefit of time lost because of a shorter gestation period. See Reference: Case-Smith (ed). Hunter, JG: Neonatal intensive care unit.

57. (C) normal development. Answer C is correct because according to Mulligan (2003), children between the ages of 10 and 12 months "may take first steps; walk with one hand held or behind a push toy" (p. 127). Children 10 to 12 months old typically begin to cruise (walking sideways while holding onto furniture), thus making answers A, B, and D incorrect. See Reference: Mulligan. Chapter three: Typical Child Development.

58. (A) Position the child's trunk, head, neck, and shoulders in proper alignment. Proper positioning is the first thing the OT must address prior to feeding the child. "Proper positioning is vital for tongue control. The trunk, head, neck, and shoulders need to be stable and aligned" (p. 224). Answer B, hyperextending the child's head, would be contraindicated, because "abnormal tongue movements tend to occur more frequently when the head is hyperextended" (p. 224). Answers C and D are techniques commonly utilized to facilitate proper feeding techniques, but they should not be initiated until after the child is appropriately positioned. See Reference: Solomon (ed). Jones, LMW and Machover, PZ: Occupational performance areas: Daily living and work and productive activities.

59. (B) High contrast and defined borders. Visual material that is adapted as in answer B, high contrast and defined borders, provides the only combination of features that assist children with visual discrimination problems. High contrast of the stimuli (shape, letter, number, and so on) in relation to the background, and defining important areas of the stimuli with a border, attract the eye, and provide clear input. Answer A is incorrect because low contrast of the stimuli, such as blue ditto lettering, is difficult for the eyes to discriminate. Answer C, undefined borders around the important stimuli, make for less clear input. In answer D, both low contrast and unclear borders, would make visual discrimination difficult. See Reference: Kramer and Hinojosa (eds). Todd, VR: Visual information analysis: Frame of reference for visual perception.

60. (B) slightly flexed. Postural alignment is important in promoting oral motor function. The spine and pelvis should be in a neutral position. Normally, the head should be in a position that is neutral or slightly flexed (answer A). When a child has difficulty swallowing, however, tucking the chin slightly can reduce the risk of aspiration and can facilitate swallowing. Positioning the infant with the head in extension (answer C) can increase the risk of choking. Rotating the head (answer D) does not facilitate swallowing. See Reference: Case-Smith (ed). Case-Smith, J and Humphry, R: Feeding intervention.

61. (B) forward and side-to-side with the child sitting on the therapist's lap. Answer B is correct because the position of the child requires the least resistance to gravity. By tilting the child in this position, the OT controls how much the child will work against gravitational pull and ensures that the child is well supported. Answers A and D are incorrect because they would require the child to lift his or her head directly against gravity. Answer C also is incorrect because the child's head is positioned against gravity in the quadruped position and a child with extremely poor head control probably could not hold this position. See Reference: Case-Smith (ed). Nichols, DS: Development of postural control.

■ MENTAL HEALTH/ COGNITION

62. (B) Administer a time-use assessment. Time-use assessments (e.g., the Barth Time Construction) examine how individuals spend their time in work, leisure, and self-care activities. The individual records all activities engaged in each day on a chart, often for a full week. The OTR also may want to obtain information on the individual's feelings about the various activities. As with all self-report assessments, the value of the assessment is dependent on the individual's ability and willingness to be honest and accurate. Interest checklists (answer A) typically assess the individual's level of interest and perceived skill in various leisure activities, but not how time is actually utilized. Actual skill in leisure activities would best be evaluated through direct observation (answers C and D), but this method would not provide useful information about how the individual actually spends his time. See Reference: Early. Data collection and evaluation.

63. (A) Involve the individual in a three-member task group. Adding an additional group member to the experience is the most appropriate way to upgrade this activity when addressing the goal of social interaction. Progressing from slip molds to coil pots (answer B) may be a way of providing an outlet for creativity or self-expression. Adding the responsibility of pouring the molds in addition to glazing them (answer C) may progress the individual toward more independent performance of ceramics activities. Decision-making skills can be enhanced by providing opportunities for the individual to make choices about his project (answer D). See Reference: Early. Analyzing, adapting, and grading activities.

64. (B) pass around a scent box and ask each patient to smell the contents. Sensory integration theory holds that individuals can learn by receiving, processing, and responding to sensory stimulation. Starting a group for regressed individuals with sensory stimuli such as touch and smell helps to get an individual's attention and arouse interest. Asking individuals in this type of a group to introduce themselves (answer A) can be confusing and time consuming, especially when dealing with regressed individuals with limited attention spans. Reading favorite poems (answer C) and discussing lunch menus (answer D) are activities more suited to patients functioning on higher levels than the group described here. See Reference: Early. Group concepts and techniques.

65. (A) Have the individual contribute to a discussion identifying the "rules" for the group. This approach is most likely to elicit cooperation and to heighten the individual's awareness regarding his behavior. Rules such as showing respect for others, asking permission to borrow tools and supplies, and waiting for another person to finish speaking, are more likely to be respected when the individual contributes to the development of these rules. Ignoring his inappropriate behavior during group (answer C) disregards the needs of other group members. This individual may not have the skills or insight to treat others with respect at this time, and explaining that the behavior is unacceptable (answer D) may not be enough. Denying him access to groups (answer B) may be a last resort only after all other options have been exhausted. See Reference: Early. Psychosocial skills and psychological components.

66. (D) rationalization. Making excuses for, or justifying, the behavior of others that is generally considered to be unacceptable is called rationalization. Identification (answer A) occurs when one takes on the characteristics of another person. Projection (answer B) is the blaming of other people for performing the behaviors. Denial (answer C) is refusing to acknowledge that the behavior occurred. See

Reference: Christiansen and Baum (eds). Bonder, B: Coping with psychological and emotional challenges.

67. (D) show a video about nutrition and keep a meal diary for a week. The psychoeducational model utilizes a teacher-student format as opposed to a learning-by-doing approach. It often includes a homework component. Answers A, B, and C can all be used to promote healthier eating; however, they all involve learning through occupation-based activities rather than psychoeducational activities. See Reference: Cottrell (ed). Crist, PH: Community living skills: A psychoeducational community-based program.

68. (D) role performance. Role performance is "identifying, maintaining, and balancing functions one assumes or acquires in society (e.g., worker, student, parent, friend, religious participant)" (p. 462). This individual is having difficulty balancing the roles of worker and mother, and is feeling stressed and conflicted. This stress may result in difficulty maintaining attention (answer B). Evaluation by an OT could include assessment of parenting and assertiveness skills (answers A and C) to determine if these are areas of need, and if so, interventions could be designed to address these areas to support successful role performance. See Reference: Early. Psychosocial skills and psychological components.

69. (A) begin with activities that have obvious solutions and high probabilities of success, and then gradually increase the complexity. This strategy is effective in developing problem-solving skills. Gross and fine motor activities (answer B) can heighten awareness of self and develop coordination. Increasing the time spent on the activity (answer D) helps development of attention span. Structuring the number and kinds of choices (answer C) is a method for developing decision-making skills. See Reference: Creek (ed). Finlay, L: Groupwork.

70. (B) supported employment. Answer B, supported employment, provides a structure for persons with developmental disabilities to work in actual job sites while also offering assistance from a job coach and would be more appropriate for an individual living in the community. Answer A focuses on leisure, rather work possibilities. Volunteer work, answer C, could be a useful form of activity, but would not address employment needs. Answer D, sheltered workshops, are designed to help individuals master basic work skills, but have been criticized for "creating dependency and not preparing workers for real life employment" (p. 306), and few such programs now exist outside of the institutional facilities. See Reference: Scaffa, ME (ed). Scheinholz, MK: Community-based mental health services.

71. (A) provide verbal cues, external aids, such as calendars, and opportunities to practice using the aids. Verbal cues, external aids, and opportunities to practice using the external aids (answer A) would be most appropriate for clients with deficits in orientation. Answer B, reducing distractions, and answer C, presenting information in short units, would be adaptive strategies to promote attention and information processing. Answer D, connecting new information to previously held knowledge and skills, is a technique to aid retrieval of information and improve memory. See Reference: Unsworth (ed). Schwarzberg, S: Clinical reasoning with groups.

72. (C) "I think baking would be a helpful activity to try. Baking something you like offers you several choices and decisions. These choices and decisions can help you feel more positive about making other decisions. You can choose a cake mix or a cookie mix. Which would you like?" Answer C is correct because it offers some limited options and provides the rationale for the choices. "A program to help someone improve the ability to make decisions must logically include many opportunities to face real choices and decide among them" (p. 486). Answer A is a leading question that really offers only one choice. Answer B does not provide any options. Answer D is a closed question, offering no real choice for the individual. See Reference: Early. Nelson, DL: Analyzing, adapting and grading activities.

73. (C) Relationships with others. The primary problem area for most individuals with a personality disorder is their inability to interact with others. Specific personality disorder categories indicate that there is some variation among the types of relationships that are impacted. For example, authority relationships seem particularly dysfunctional in those with antisocial personality disorders, and difficulty in establishing relationships is linked to avoidant personality disorders. Answers A and B (ADLs) are often problems for individuals with mood and thought disorders. Answer D is often a problem in those with schizophrenia. See Reference: Early. Understanding psychiatric diagnosis: The DSM-IV.

74. (B) having the only red toothbrush. This is an environmental adaptation, and does not require new learning that may be beyond the individual's ability. The color red is easily recognizable, and if it is the only red one (answer B), he will not get it mixed up with others. Switching to an electric toothbrush (answer A) requires a new set of skills and this individual is likely to have difficulty with new learning. A built-up handle (answer C) is appropriate for individuals who have difficulty grasping the handle of a toothbrush. Having the individual's teeth brushed by a caregiver (answer D) is not desirable if the individual is able to do it himself. See Reference: Crepeau, Cohn, and Schell (eds). Holm, MB, Rogers, JC, and James, AB: Interventions for daily living.

75. (B) Encouraging any available hemiplegic limb movements before or during a task. Any contralesional limb movement (even shoulder elevation) will activate additional motor units, which will then increase attention to the left. Bilateral activities (answer A) may reduce attention to the left by inhibiting function of the affected hemisphere. Activities that do not cross the midline (answer C), and activities that focus on the uninvolved side of the body (answer D) only reinforce neglect of the involved side of the body. See Reference: Unsworth (ed). Corben, L and Unsworth, C: Evaluation and intervention with unilateral neglect.

76. (C) a concrete response. Literal responses to general inquiries reflect the type of "overly concrete thinking" (p. 856) that persons with schizophrenia may exhibit. Difficulty in understanding questions with several possible meanings also suggests disorganized thought processes seen in persons with schizophrenia. Delusional responses (answer A) would most likely be completely off topic. A distractible response (answer B) would change the topic or stop in the middle of responding. An insightful response (answer D) would include reasons that led up to being hospitalized. See Reference: Crepeau, Cohn, and Schell (eds). Ward, J: Adults with mental illness. Section I: Psychiatric diagnoses and related intervention issues.

77. (B) having the worker put only the last piece into the game package. Working backward from the last successful step of a sequence is known as "backward chaining." Answer A represents the opposite of backward chaining. Answer C is more descriptive of shaping behaviors, and answer D is more descriptive of modeling behaviors. See Reference: Pedretti and Early (eds). Foti, D: Activities of daily living.

78. (D) stenciling project on poster board. Stenciling on poster board is the safest craft choice, because it is free of sharp, toxic, and cordlike materials. A ceramic object (answer C) could be broken into sharp pieces that individuals could use to harm themselves. Craft projects that contain rope or cordlike materials that can be used for hanging (answers A and B) also should be avoided. See Reference: Early. Safety techniques.

79. (B) Instruct the client to take "one white and one blue pill" with the morning and even- ing meals. Cognitive disabilities' levels of function distinguish the types of assistance an individual needs to safely complete everyday tasks. An individual at cognitive level 4 can "...carry out familiar routines" (p. 247) and is able to attend to visible cues. Linking medications with meals helps the goal become routine and linking the visible cues of different colored pills to the routine also assists with training at this level of functioning. Answer A is consistent with cognitive level 5, answer C is consistent with level 3, and answer D is consistent with level 2. See Reference: Bruce and Borg. Cognitive disability frame of reference—acknowledging limitations.

80. (C) Introduce and discuss concepts of community living, and give clients an opportunity to voice their concerns. Clients who have not left the hospital in many years are likely to be anxious about moving into a new environment. Introducing and discussing concepts of community living (answer C), allows the staff to provide information and allows the client to voice concerns and ask questions. Visiting future community settings and developing goals (answers A and B) are important, but would follow later. Because the patients have been receiving OT in the hospital for many years, evaluation (answer D) should already have occurred. See Reference: Cottrell (ed). Baxley, S: Options for community practice: The Springfield Hospital model.

81. (A) short-term recall. This individual's inability to comb his hair without reminders suggests a deficit in short-term recall, which is the ability to recall all information that has just been received and to hold it in temporary use from 1 to 5 minutes or more. Judgment (answer B), the ability to make realistic and safe decisions based on available environmental information, would not be needed for this task. Since the person performed the first request, hearing (answer C) would seem to be intact. Abstraction (answer D) is the ability to extrapolate information from an idea to generalize to another situation and would not be needed to follow this direction. See Reference: Gillen and Burkardt (eds). Arnadottir, G: Impact of neurobehavioral deficits on activities of daily living.

82. (D) Attend an AA meeting. An individual who has recently been discharged from drug/alcohol rehabilitation is likely to need support (such as Alcoholics Anonymous) her first weekend at home. People in recovery should avoid situations, people, and places that lead to abuse of substances. Parties and clubs/concerts (answers A and B) are often closely associated with access to substances and should be avoided. A mini-vacation with the kids (answer C) would probably be too stressful for her first weekend at home. See Reference: Early. Understanding psychiatric diagnosis: The DSM-IV.

83. (C) Simple meal preparation group.
Obtaining food is a basic survival need and is often the focus of a homeless individual's day. Therefore, although all the above groups may meet a need, activities related to food are likely to be more highly valued by this individual. Craft groups (answer A) may be useful in developing healthy leisure interests. Volunteer activities (answer B) can help develop necessary work habits. Social skills groups (answer D) address interpersonal skills necessary for living in society. See Reference: Early. Who is the consumer?

84. (B) Confront the individual's behavior and ask, "Are you aware that your frequent interruptions prevent others from having a chance to contribute?"
In general, the group leader should try answers A, C, or D before confronting the individual who is monopolizing the conversation. However, considering that these more conservative attempts have failed the practitioner, answer B, confronting the behavior, would be the best approach for the OT to take to modify the behavior. See Reference: Posthuma. What to do if....

85. (B) Obtain as much information as possible from the chart.
By reviewing the individual's medical records before the interview (answer B) the OT practitioner can determine what information has already been obtained. This will enable the therapist to make the best use of the available time, and to avoid asking the individual to answer the same questions twice. With such a limited attention span, it would probably be more efficient to schedule two 15-minute sessions rather than one 30-minute session (answer A). Answers C and D are both essential to good interview technique, but would occur at the time of the actual interview after collecting data from the chart. See Reference: Early. Data collection and evaluation.

86. (B) the client will initiate one request to one other group member for sharing group materials within a 1-week period.
Reducing the number of requests and the variety or number of individuals the client is expected to interact with is the best way to simplify the initial goal. Extending the amount of time to accomplish the goal (answer A) does not make the goal easier to achieve. Increasing the number of individuals (answer C), and subsequently the number of requests, also makes the goal more difficult to achieve. Changing interactions to the group leader (answer D) moves the goal away from the original problem area of peer social conversation to authority conversations. See

Reference: Early. Analyzing, adapting, and grading activities.

87. (A) observe the individual's body language during group sessions.
By observing an individual's body language for behaviors such as fidgeting, nail biting, toe tapping, etc., the OT can determine whether an individual is experiencing anxiety during the group activity. Completion of a questionnaire (answer B) and feedback from group members (answer C) may not be practical or reliable alternatives for an individual with cognitive deficits. Answer D is an adaptive strategy, not a method for assessing anxiety. See Reference: Early. Responding to symptoms and behaviors.

88. (A) Give simple, step-by-step instructions, and physical guidance.
Answer A is correct because the severe memory impairment in individuals who have advanced Alzheimer's disease requires the use of "... simple one-step commands, step-by-step verbal cues, and physical guidance" (p. 711) during activities. Demonstration with multiple-step instructions (answer B) can be confusing because it provides too much stimulation. Multiple-step written instructions (answer C) are unlikely to be retained in the individual's short-term memory after reading or remembered in sequence. Also, written instructions could be lost if the individual puts them down. Verbally repeating directions over and over (answer D), or rehearsal, does not enable a person with Alzheimer's disease to retain information in the memory, and he or she may not repeat the instructions properly. See Reference: Pedretti and Early (eds). Glogoski, C: Degenerative diseases of the central nervous system: Section 2 Alzheimer's disease.

89. (B) The client will use facial expressions and gestures that are consistent with stated emotions during assertive, passive, and aggressive role-play situations.
Conversational skills (and effective communication) require the ability of an individual to express feelings and attitudes (p. 482) through appropriate and consistent verbal and nonverbal behaviors in a variety of social situations. Being able to vary one's expression during role playing (p. 484) of three different styles of expressing feelings is an example of this. Identifying pleasurable activities (answer A) will help to develop interests. Recognition of one's behaviors and consequences (answer C) relates to self-control. Identifying one's own assets and limitations (answer D) is related to self-concept. See Reference: Stein and Cutler. Leisure-time occupations, self-care, and social skills training.

90. (C) needs assessment. Needs assessment (answer C) is the necessary first step of gathering data about a population, treatment needs, and resources available. Program planning (answer A) involves establishing goals and objectives based on the results of the needs assessment. Program implementation (answer B) occurs following program planning and involves coordination, assessment, and intervention selection. Program evaluation (answer D) occurs after implementation, and involves systematic review and analysis of the program based on achievement of program goals. See Reference: Cottrell (ed). Grossman, J and Bortone, J: Program development.

91. (B) Discussing one's problems with an empathetic listener. One goal of stress management intervention is to identify "...behaviors that in the past have been effective in making us feel more relaxed, less anxious, and generally more secure about ourselves" (p. 437). Verbalization of stressful feelings and problems (answer B) is an effective stress coping strategy that also serves to reinforce connection with reality. Answers A and D, visual imagery and progressive relaxation of muscles, are effective relaxation techniques, but are typically performed with the eyes closed, which may increase psychosis and the effect of hallucinations. Engaging in a familiar activity may help relieve stressful feelings, but engaging in a new or too challenging activity (answer C) could add stress. See Reference: Stein and Cutler. Stress management, biofeedback, and relaxation techniques.

92. (B) Activities that encourage self-reflection and feedback. For a program designed to develop an individual's self-awareness, the most essential element, is the opportunity to verbalize one's ideas and feelings, and to receive feedback from others in a safe setting (answer B). Activities that emphasize the importance of self-awareness (answer A) are useful for motivation, but not as effective as self-reflection and feedback for gaining self-awareness. Problem-solving skills (answer C) and social interaction (answer D) are beneficial for developing other areas of psychosocial functioning, but these activities are not as critical to the process of gaining self-awareness as providing activities structured in a way to encourage increasing levels of self-reflection and feedback. See Reference: Early. Analyzing, adapting, and grading activities.

93. (B) remain matter of fact and consistent in approach. Individuals with borderline personality disorder demonstrate inconsistent behavior, have difficulty maintaining stable relationships, and have poor self-image. Practitioners usually need to work hard to remain consistent and trustworthy to those individuals. It is important in this case that the OT recognizes this behavior as part of the pathology and not take it personally. Because the accusation is a result of pathology, the OT has nothing to apologize for, and is unlikely to uncover any reasonable explanation for a misunderstanding (answer D). In addition, the practitioner should not complain of hurt feelings to a client (answer A). Delving into exploration of the individual's past (answer C) is not a recommended approach for occupational therapy. See Reference: Crepeau, Cohn, and Schell (eds). Ward, JD: Adults with mental illness.

94. (B) All group members construct one tower that incorporates all of the pieces provided in a set of constructional materials (e.g., Legos or Erector set). Activities used to evaluate performance in groups should require group collaboration and emphasize process rather than end product (answer B) The collage and crafts (answers A and D) are individual activities and do not demand group interaction. Making pizza for lunch (answer C) is an end product that serves the group as a whole. The pizza activity and format is typically not an evaluation group, but is better suited as a task-oriented group activity in which self-awareness and self-understanding are primary goals. See Reference: Bruce and Borg. Psychodynamic frame of reference-person perspective and meaning.

95. (D) in private, explain the nature of the client-therapist relationship. It is inappropriate for the OT practitioner to have more than a professional relationship with a client. While self-disclosing some information to clients can be a therapeutic tool, there is some information that would be misinterpreted or inappropriate (e.g., giving out personal information [Answer A]). Ignoring the client's request (answer B) constitutes avoidance on the therapist's part and is unprofessional. Though a difficult situation, the OT looses an opportunity to provide valuable feedback to her client. Whether the OT has a boyfriend or not (answer C), she should not use this as an excuse for not giving out her number. It would be an easy way out, but is unprofessional. See Reference: Early. Therapeutic use of self.

96. (C) topographical disorientation. Topographical disorientation is difficulty in finding one's way in familiar surroundings, or in learning new routes, and would be exhibited by the patient's inability to find the therapy clinic. Spatial relations disorders (answer A) would be exhibited as difficulties in relating objects to each other. Figure-ground discrimination deficits (answer B) would be exhibited as difficulty in differentiating objects in the foreground from the background. Form discrimination deficits (answer D) would be exhibited as the inability to distinguish between different types of forms. See Reference: Unsworth (ed). Arnadottir, G: Evaluation and intervention with complex perceptual impairment.

97. (D) respond to the emotional tone expressed by the words and provide extra attention and reassurance. Listening for the feelings behind the words will best help to identify and address the needs of the person who has lost the ability to use words effectively. The resident's searching for her mother may reflect a sense of loneliness. Explaining the factual truth (answer A) can have the effect of unnecessarily confronting the person with her deficits, and they may respond to the news as if hearing it for the first time. Telling the person to stop the behavior (answer B) will not address the need that is being expressed verbally. Answer C, telling a therapeutic fib, might work for a brief period of time, but may backfire if the person continues to question the story given, or if it causes sadness or anger. See Reference: Hellen. Communication: Understanding and being understood.

98. (A) Social relations skills. Appropriate social skills under the category of social relations requires individuals to conform to implicit and explicit social norms, assume a manner of acting that tries to establish a rapport with others, and to accommodate other people's reactions and requests, which means accommodating to other people's reactions and requests. (p. 622). While poor eye contact may indicate a difficulty with physical, nonverbal communication (answer B) and grabbing may indicate poor self-control (answer C), the combination of behaviors described is most indicative of poor social relations. By developing her interpersonal and coping skills (answer D), the individual may be able to demonstrate improved social conduct. See Reference: AOTA: Practice Framework. Table 2. Performance skills.

99. (A) Activities exploring one's perceptions of past, current, and future events and how they are connected. Answer A is correct because in the psychodynamic frame of reference, activities are used to provide "subjective experience and a catalyst for learning" (p. 41), and activities exploring one's perceptions of life events would provide this subjective element. Answer B, activities matched to the specific cognitive level of group members, reflects a cognitive disabilities approach. Answer C, activities that can serve as reinforcers for desired behaviors, would be used in a behavioral frame of reference.

Answer D, activities that can teach the use of problem-solving strategies, would be used within a cognitive behavioral context. See Reference: Bruce and Borg. Chapter 2. Person-activity/occupation-environment/context-occupational therapy practice variables.

100. (C) information on the definition and physiological signs of stress. It is important to have a basic understanding of stress to effectively develop stress-management skills. Answers A, B, and D are all effective stress-management techniques. Other techniques include healthy eating, assertiveness skills, changing attitudes, and balancing work, rest, and leisure. See Reference: Cottrell (ed). Mueller, S and Suto, M: Starting a stress management program.

101. (A) assist with skill development in the areas of life skills, leisure, and self-expression. In general, the areas of focus with OT intervention for individuals identified with substance abuse problems are the acquiring of social and occupational roles through skill development in life skills, alternative leisure time use, and improved expression of feelings. The approach described in answer B addresses the cognitive disability frame of reference approach, which is compensatory and does not provide any restoration of skills. Answers C and D may address specific needs of the individual with substance abuse problems, but not the overall needs of this population. See Reference: Early. Understanding psychiatric diagnosis: The DSM-IV.

102. (A) Perform a job analysis. A job analysis identifies essential functions of a particular job. Based on the results, the OT practitioner can then work with the individual to maximize performance or request reasonable accommodation (answer B). Activities that promote self-efficacy (answer C) are beneficial for individuals with depression, but should not be used at this stage of the individual's program. A weekly support group (answer D) may be an effective way for the individual to obtain support and can be recommended, but it is not the first action the OT practitioner would take. See Reference: Early. Work, homemaking, and childcare.

103. (B) Developing awareness about how thoughts and behaviors affect one's perceptions of and ability to cope with pain. All of the answers are aspects of the cognitive-behavioral process in addressing chronic pain. However, treatment begins with an educational approach that teaches clients, "...how their cognitions (thoughts) and behaviors impact pain perception and the ability to manage it" (p. 437) (answer B). Therapy should then move to learning alternative ways of responding to pain (answer A), followed by rehearsal of techniques (answer C), and finally implementation of techniques and coping strategies to decrease pain and stress during daily occupations (answer D). See Reference: Cara and MacRae (eds). Southam, M: Psychosocial aspects of chronic pain.

104. (C) ask the questions as they are stated on the interview sheet. A structured interview requires following the procedure, order, and wording of the questions to be asked. Answers A, B, and D are appropriate for semistructured interviews (e.g., in pursuit of more details and information). See Reference: Early. Data collection and evaluation.

105. (B) a cheese sandwich. The most basic level of meal preparation is accessing a prepared meal, which involves tasks such as opening a thermos and unwrapping a sandwich. When an individual becomes proficient at this level, he or she can, and should, progress to a higher level. More advanced meal preparation activities can be structured to increase in complexity in the following sequence: prepare a cold meal (answer B); prepare a hot one dish meal (answers A and C); and prepare a hot multi-dish meal (answer D). See Reference: Crepeau, Cohn, and Schell (eds). Rogers, JC and Holm, MB: Evaluation of areas of occupation; Section I: Activities of daily living and instrumental activities of daily living.

106. (C) Have the individual set down the utensil until the mouth is cleared. Having the individual learn to set down the utensil until the mouth is cleared is a method of imposing a restriction on the behavior which can then develop into an established routine to pace himself during feeding. Cutting the food into smaller pieces (answer A) and placing food in separate containers (answer D) are examples of environmental adaptations, not habit development. An impulsive person who eats too fast also will have difficulty counting slowly enough to have his mouth cleared by the time the count of 10 is reached (answer B). See Reference: Trombly and Radomski. Radomski, MV and Davis, ES: Optimizing cognitive abilities.

107. (C) applying grout to a tile trivet and waiting for it to dry. Activities provide a variety of opportunities for therapeutic gains depending upon the demands of the activity. Answer C is the best answer because the process of grouting a tile trivet involves covering the individual's tile design with a grout mixture (which tends to be very liquid in consistency) before setting up the material to dry. Waiting for the grout to dry requires an individual

to use self-control in delaying gratification of the finished product. Having a discussion on mosaic tile crafts (answer A) would present social demands. Selecting a tile design (answer B) would promote use of higher level cognitive functions such as decision making. Cleaning off the table (answer D) may promote self-esteem through the experience of success after a mess, but does not involve the concept of delaying gratification. See Reference: Crepeau, Cohn, and Schell (eds). Crepeau, EB: Analyzing occupation and activity: A way of thinking about occupational performance.

108. (A) Short-term memory. The onset of most dementias is slow and progressive. Cognitive abilities such as short-term memory are most often initially affected. Sensorimotor abilities used in functional activities, such as dressing, tend to follow. Superficial social abilities are often preserved until the last stages of dementia and may often hide the earlier cognitive and sensorimotor changes. See Reference: Crepeau, Cohn, and Schell (eds). Ward, JD: Psychiatric diagnoses and related intervention issues.

109. (B) Performing a clerical task such as sorting papers. The most appropriate type of activities to begin treatment for a person with severe depression are repetitive, structured, and simple enough to ensure success, such as "...housework, folding laundry, simple cooking, sanding, clerical tasks, and sewing" (p. 246). Engagement in leisure exploration (answer A), meditation (answer C), and stress management activities (answer D) would eventually be relevant intervention activities for a person with depression. However, in the early stages of depression, attention span, concentration, and energy level may to be too impaired to benefit from these types of activities. See Reference: Early. Responding to symptoms and behaviors.

110. (A) Use role plays that include practicing good table manners. A cognitive approach is best for individuals with memory and/or attention deficits, for those who must learn to do situational problem-solving, or when skills learned need to be generalized to other situations. Cognitive approaches include role playing, rehearsal, imagery, and memory enhancement techniques. Behavioral approaches include cause-effect associations, shaping, reinforcement, and behavior modification (answers B, C, and D). Behavioral approaches are recommended for individuals whose cognitive abilities are impaired by psychosis, who have normal attention span and memory abilities, or those living in a highly structured and consistent environment. See Reference:

Christiansen and Matuska (eds). Haertlein, CA and Stoffel, VC: Adaptive living strategies for people with psychiatric disabilities.

111. (B) Measuring ingredients for a recipe while there is music playing. The client demonstrated difficulty in attending to the activity because the presence of other environmental stimuli was distracting—this suggests a deficit in selective attention. Answer B, measuring ingredients for a recipe while there is music playing, is correct because it would provide the needed practice in concentrating on one set of stimuli while ignoring a competing stimuli to improve selective attention. Answer A, playing a repetitive card game, provides practice in maintaining sustained attention. Answer C, referring to a catalog while filling out a catalog form, would require the person to alternate attention from the catalog to the form. Answer D, playing a game where the person must walk and bounce a ball simultaneously, provides practice in dividing attention between to two activities at the same time. See Reference: Trombly and Radomski. Radomski, MV and Davis, ES: Optimizing cognitive abilities.

112. (B) interest checklist. An interest checklist is frequently used to initiate discussion of how a patient usually spends his leisure time and to identify areas of specific interest. Although the evaluations of living skills and self-care (answers A and D) address the use of leisure time, they are used primarily to assess skills in personal care, safety and health, money management, transportation, use of the telephone, and work. An activity configuration (answer C) is used to assess the patient's use of time and his feelings about all of the activities he performs in a typical day or week. See Reference: Early. Data gathering and evaluation.

113. (D) Family will demonstrate independence in current positioning and feeding techniques 50% of the time. Goals should be functional, measurable, and objective. In addition, short-term goals must relate to the long-term goal being addressed. Answer D meets those criteria. Answer A does not provide measurable criteria, nor does it directly relate to the long-term goal of family training. Answer B, while measurable, does not relate to the long-term goal. Answer C describes the long-term goal of family independence in the feeding program. See Reference: Borcherding. Writing functional and measurable goals and objectives.

114. (A) soft to hard to rough. The desensitization process involves applying a sequence of graded texture and force stimuli to the skin to reduce tactile hypersensitivity. Texture begins with soft, progresses

to hard, and moves to rough stimuli. Answer B is incorrect because the force of the stimuli begins at the level of touch, progresses to rub, and moves to tapping as tolerance for sensation increases. Light, medium, and heavy (answer C) do not specify what the texture and force of the stimuli would be during training. Answer D is incorrect because a person with hypersensitivity would be unable to tolerate stimuli beginning with a rough texture. See Reference: Crepeau, Cohn, and Schell (eds). Waylett-Rendall, J: Sensory reeducation.

115. (A) Velcro closures on front opening clothing. Parkinson's disease has five stages. In stage 1, a resting tremor appears and symptoms are mild and unilateral. In stage 2, problems develop with trunk mobility and postural reflexes, and symptoms are bilateral. Stage 3 results in mild-moderate functional disability with postural instability. Difficulty with manipulation and dexterity emerges in stage 4, as disability increases. Individuals in stage 5 are confined to a wheelchair or bed. Velcro closures on front-opening clothing (answer A) would require the least amount of dexterity, which becomes increasingly difficult for individuals in stage 4. Large buttons on front opening clothing (answer B) might be easier than smaller buttons, but would still require more manipulation than Velcro closures. Clothing slipped on over the head with no fasteners (answer C) would eliminate the need for dexterity, but having to raise the arms would be problematic because of the rigidity and stiffness of the limbs that typically accompanies Parkinson's disease. Though clothing which stretches freely is easier to put on than tightly constructed clothing, the need to tie the closures in the back of the garment (answer D) would be difficult for a person with upper extremity rigidity. See Reference: Trombly and Radomski. Copperman, LF, Forwell, SJ, and Hugos, L: Neurodegenerative diseases.

116. (B) Looped handle scissors. In order to open a plastic muffin mix bag, the OT would most likely recommend that the homemaker use looped handle scissors (answer B). This device would be much safer than the use of an electric knife, answer C, while compensating for the limited grip strength. Answer A, using a hand-powered mixer, does not address how the homemaker will open the muffin bag, while answer D does not coincide with the client's desire to make muffins rather than prepared slice cookies. See Reference: Trombly and Radomski. Fasoli, S: Restoring competence for homemaker and parent roles.

117. (C) Eat six small meals a day. An individual with ALS who becomes fatigued eating three full meals a day should attempt eating six smaller meals a day before resorting to tube feedings or pureed diets (answers A and D). Eating regular food is usually more enjoyable, and therefore is likely to enhance the quality of life. An upright position is optimal when feeding individuals with dysphagia. A semi-reclined position (answer B) can make swallowing more difficult or dangerous. See Reference: Pedretti and Early (eds). Schultz-Krohn, W, Foti, D, and Glogoski, C: Degenerative diseases of the central nervous system.

118. (A) Individual will purchase 10 items at the supermarket with supervision. Short-term goals must relate to the long-term goal being addressed. Because the long-term goal being addressed is independence in grocery shopping, the short-term goal must relate to grocery shopping. Answer D is an appropriate treatment intervention, but is written in a way that describes what the OT, not the individual, will do. Answers B and C describe activities related to the task of shopping, but not the shopping itself. See Reference: Borcherding. Writing functional and measurable goals and objectives.

119. (D) a weighted pen and weighted wrists. Weighting body parts and utensils (e.g., writing tools) is effective for individuals with ataxia to improve control during performance of a task. Hitting the keys on a keyboard (answer A) would be difficult for this individual, although weighting the wrists could make performance of the activity possible. A keyboard is a good alternative for individuals with difficulty writing due to weakness, limited range of motion, or incoordination. A universal cuff with a pencil holder attachment (answer B) would be appropriate for an individual with hand weakness who uses a universal cuff for other tasks. A balanced forearm orthosis (answer C) is appropriate for individuals with severe muscle weakness. In addition, individuals with muscle weakness find felt-tip pens easier to write with than ballpoint pens. See Reference: Pedretti and Early (eds). Gutman, SA: Traumatic brain injury.

120. (C) Data about overall occupational performance, activity needs, and health issues of clients. While day programs for adults offer a range of services, the primary focus is to provide, "...meaningful, structured activities designed to provide a safe environment so that people...can continue to live at home." (p. 935). The role of a consultant would be to recommend a program of, "general activities to meet the client's needs" (p. 935). To understand these needs, the consultant would need to learn about the kinds of activities provided by the setting and how the clients are engaged in activity to determine what kinds of additional activity programming would increase the general goals of increasing activity and social interaction level, enhancing health, and slowing decline. Answers A, B, and D would provide useful information when developing direct care programs for individuals or to determine goals for specific groups. See Reference: Crepeau, Cohn, and Schell (eds). Griswold, LA: Community-based practice arenas.

121. (A) make recommendations for ways of operating the technology. The OT practitioner on the assistive technology team typically determines which part of the body has sufficient motor control for operating the technology and then recommends the type of input access device (switch, keyword, software, etc.) that will best meet the client's needs. Answer B, assisting with vocational goals, is most often the job of the vocational rehabilitation counselor. A vocational rehabilitation agency typically assists in job placement (answer C). Answer D, solving mechanical and software problems, is usually the role of the rehabilitation engineer. See Reference: Cook and Hussey. Assistive technologies in the context of work.

122. (C) both sides of the individual's body. Answer C is correct because the individual must be able to transfer to both sides of the body. It is usually difficult, or impossible, to arrange the home and environment so that the all transfers can be done from one side only. For instance, if the toilet at home is close to the wall, getting on and off the toilet will require transfer first to one side of the body and then to the opposite side. The family also needs to know the different kinds, and amounts of support, they must use on each side of the individual's body. Thus, answers A, B, and D are incorrect because they all involve transfer to only one side. See Reference: Trombly and Radomski. Pierce, S: Restoring competence in mobility.

123. (C) Independent with use of a sliding board. Most individuals with paraplegia will be able to perform independent transfers, and will usually be able to perform car transfers with or without a sliding board to help bridge the distance between the car seat and wheelchair. Answer D, tenodesis, would not be implicated as a strategy to use with individuals with paraplegia. See Reference: Pedretti and Early (eds). Creel, TA, Adler, C, Tipton-Burton, M, and Lillie, SM: Mobility.

124. (D) The individual attempts to find coins in a pocket while occluding vision. According to Bentzel, "stereognosis—the ability to identify objects through proprioception, cognition and the sense of touch" such as identifying coins in a pocket (answer

D) would be the best choice. Answers A and B do not encourage the use of proprioception and touch while answer C, the use of theraputty, may be something used to increase strength; however, the goal of increasing strength was not identified in this question. See Reference: Trombly and Radomski. Bentzel, K: Assessing abilities and capacities: Sensation.

125. (A) coughing or choking. Coughing and choking are motor problems that are commonly noted in patients with dysphagia. Disorientation and confusion (answer B) are related to cognitive problems, and pain and decreased smell and taste (answer C and D, respectively), are related to sensory problems in patients with dysphagia. See Reference: Pedretti and Early (eds). Nelson, KL: Dysphagia: Evaluation and treatment.

126. (D) (1) gather shirt up at the back of the neck; (2) pull gathered back fabric off over head; (3) remove shirt from unaffected arm; and (4) remove shirt from affected arm. Answers A, B, and C are examples of incorrect sequences that would most likely result in failure to remove the shirt successfully. See Reference: Pedretti and Early (eds). Foti, D: Activities of daily living.

127. (A) A craft activity using increasingly heavy hand tools. Progressive resistive exercise is the most effective method for increasing strength in a muscle with fair plus strength. Mild resistance would be used initially, increasing resistance as appropriate. Mildly resistive activities that are stopped as soon as the individual begins to experience fatigue (answer B), are appropriate for maintaining or improving strength in individuals with conditions in which fatigue should be avoided (e.g., MS, ALS, and Guillain-Barré syndrome). Electric stimulation (answer C) is appropriate for increasing strength in very weak muscles. A craft activity that can be performed against increasing resistance for prolonged periods of time would be more effective than resisted active range of motion (answer D), which is usually only performed once or twice a day. See Reference: Dutton. Biomechanical postulates regarding intervention.

128. (B) Rubbing, tapping, or applying pressure. Desensitization techniques such as rubbing, tapping, and applying pressure are various ways to offer successful pain relief after wound closure of an amputation. Answer A, body mechanics, is a preventive technique that is not appropriate as an intervention for desensitization. Answers C and D, work simulation, PROM, and immobilization, are not activities typically related to pain management for chronic hypersensitivity conditions. See Refer-

ence: Pedretti and Early (eds). Keenan, DD and Morris, PA: Amputations and prosthetics.

129. (C) read the pulse oximeter. Oxygen saturation levels may drop during activity in individuals with compromised lung capacity. The use of oxygen may be required if oxygen saturation falls below 90% during activity. The instrument used to measure oxygen saturation is the pulse oximeter (answer C). Increased respirations and heart rate (answers A and B) may indicate the individual is not receiving enough oxygen, but they also occur normally with increased activity levels. It is important to note breathing patterns (answer D) when working with individuals with compromised lung capacity, such as fast and shallow breathing, holding breath, or shoulder elevation. While any of these behaviors may be indicative of decreased oxygen saturation, specific information about the saturation levels cannot be ascertained. See Reference: Trombly and Radomski. Huntley, N: Cardiac and pulmonary diseases.

130. (A) Remove all throw or scatter rugs. Regardless of whether an individual with instability walks with the help of a walker, cane, or no equipment, the floor should be cleared of any obstacles that could cause slipping or tripping. A person's foot or the tip of an assistive device may catch on scatter or throw rugs. Also, rugs may not be firmly taped down or secured with nonskid backing, causing a further safety hazard. Installing lever handles, a ramp, or a handheld shower (answers B, C, and D) would make certain tasks easier, but would not be necessary for safety. See Reference: Pedretti and Early (eds). Foti, D: Activities of daily living.

131. (C) impaired balance. "Effective balance requires adequate function in sensory and motor systems" (p. 509). Non-weight-bearing precautions must be observed in the days following a knee replacement, particularly while the individual remains in acute care. A loss of balance (answer C) was caused by the individual's inability to use the non-weight-bearing leg to adjust to the shift in the body's center of mass while showering. Unilateral neglect (answer A) might be observed in an individual following a CVA, and could result in impaired balance. Problems with gross motor coordination (answer D) or lower extremity weakness (answer B) are both factors that can contribute to balance impairment; however, the information provided does not lead us to conclude that these are the causes in this scenario. In addition, lower extremity weakness is best assessed by manual muscle test or a quick screen. See Reference: Trombly and Radomski. Sabari, JS: Optimizing motor control using the Carr and Shepherd approach.

132. (B) weight-bearing through the extremity in sitting or standing. Weight-bearing is the most effective way of normalizing tone, according to the NDT approach for adult hemiplegia. Placing a weighted cuff on the extremity (answer A) would have the effect of increasing muscle tone, making reaching more difficult. Answer C, using only the unaffected upper extremity, would accomplish the reaching task, but would not normalize muscle tone in the affected upper extremity. Answer D, "forced use," is a treatment concept used to encourage functional motor return in hemiplegic upper extremities, but is not a method designed to normalize muscle tone, nor is it a specific technique of the NDT approach. See Reference: Pedretti and Early (eds). Davis, JZ: Neurodevelopmental treatment of adult hemiplegia: The Bobath approach.

133. (B) Back up the body to the passenger seat, hold onto a stable section of the car, extend the involved leg, and slowly sit in the car. Answer B is the safest way to perform a car transfer after surgery for a total hip replacement. The posterolateral approach is the most frequently performed technique. The surgeon typically recommends that the individual avoid positions of hip adduction, internal rotation, and flexion. Answers A, C, and D are contraindicated due to their lack of adherence to total hip replacement precautions. See Reference: Pedretti and Early (eds). Coleman, S: Hip fractures and lower extremity joint replacement.

134. (D) observe for signs of visual deficits during daily living activities. Visual dysfunction in developmentally disabled adults can interfere with their ability to adapt to the environment. Observing for signs of visual deficits (answer D), such as poor acuity, difficulty with contrast sensitivity, and visual field deficits during functional activities, such as self-care and leisure activities would be the first step in identifying problems with vision. Answer A is incorrect because assessing and adapting lighting would be a method of environmental intervention, which would occur following the evaluation process. Administering formal assessments (answer B) would follow the screening procedure and would need to be performed by an OT practitioner or eye care professional skilled in giving these tests with specialized testing equipment. Answer C, referring the client to an eye care professional, such as an ophthalmologist, for further testing may or may not occur, but also would follow screening. See Reference: Ross and Bachner (eds). Williams, TA: Low-vision intervention for adults with developmental disabilities.

135. (C) take the bottom, supine position. Taking the bottom, supine position (answer C) requires the least amount of energy expenditure and should be the primary recommendation. In addition, the OT may encourage experimentation with a variety of positions (answer D). Having sex at times when there is most energy also would be beneficial, but the individual will most likely be more fatigued at the end of the day (answer A). See Reference: Pedretti and Early (eds). Burton, GU: Sexuality and physical dysfunction.

136. (C) place a foam wedge between the legs of the patient. A key aspect of the OT practitioner's plan when working with patients who have had hip replacement surgery is to provide positioning strategies to prevent postsurgical complications and maintain function. Patients who have had either posterolateral or anterolateral surgical approaches for hip replacement must avoid leg adduction past the midline (p. 919) as it is a position of instability for the healing joint. Placing a foam wedge between the legs of the patient (answer C) in sitting or supine is the correct answer because this positioning method helps to prevent leg adduction. Answer A, placing pillows on the lateral side of the hips, would not prevent hip adduction; elevating the foot on the side of the surgery, answer B, would increase hip flexion which is contraindicated, and placing a roll under the patient's knees, answer D, would also increase hip flexion. See Reference: Pedretti and Early (eds). Coleman, S: Hip Fractures and Lower Extremity Joint Replacement.

137. (D) present important principles in small units that are spaced at a slower than normal pace. According to learning principles for older adults, learning will be more effective if the information is presented in small units at a slower pace. Answer A is incorrect because learning will be impeded if information is presented too quickly and in large chunks. Answer B is incorrect because presentations that are highly organized will enhance retention of information more than loosely structured presentations. Attempts to persuade individuals on points that may not be in agreement with their preconceived ideas, values, or habits also may impede learning (answer C), whereas a more collaborative approach may result in better learning of concepts. See Reference: Bonder and Wagner (eds). Riley, KP: Cognitive development.

138. (D) swan neck deformity. A swan neck deformity (answer D) is typically characterized by PIP joint hyperextension and DIP joint flexion. Answer A, a boutonnière deformity, is characterized by PIP joint flexion and DIP joint hyperextension. Answer C is related to a deformity present at birth, and answer B, mallet deformity, is characterized by DIP joint flexion and loss of active extension. See Reference: Pedretti and Early (eds). Buckner, WS: Arthritis.

139. (A) Gentle, nonresistive activities. The initial phase of treatment for the individual with Guillain-Barré syndrome includes PROM and splinting, and positioning to protect weak muscles and prevent contractures. This should be followed by gentle, nonresistive activities and light ADL, as tolerated. Resistive exercises and activities (answers B and D) should be implemented after strength begins to improve. Activities within later treatment sessions should alternate between gross and fine motor (unlike answer C), and resistive and nonresistive types to avoid fatigue. See Reference: Pedretti and Early (eds). Lehman, RM and McCormack, GL: Neurogenic and myopathic dysfunction.

140. (D) Suggest furniture and accessories that promote better positioning at work. The best recommendation is for ergonomically correct furniture and accessories (answer D). Additional adaptations may include tool modification and the training of workers in appropriate positioning. Answers A and C, setting up stress management and work simulation activities, are not considered to be ergonomic interventions. Answer B is not an example of an ergonomic intervention, but is a treatment intervention. See Reference: Pedretti and Early (eds). Harlowe, D: Occupational therapy for prevention of injury and physical dysfunction.

141. (B) seating the individual upright on a firm surface with the chin slightly tucked. The best position for feeding an individual with a swallowing disorder is upright and symmetrical with the chin slightly tucked (answer B). Supine, semi-reclined, and side-lying positions (answers A, C, and D) all place the individual at greater risk for choking and aspiration. See Reference: Pedretti and Early (eds). Nelson-Jenks, K: Dysphagia.

142. (A) decrease joint stress and pain. It is very important to preserve joint integrity in individuals with arthritis by using adaptive equipment to avoid or reduce the wear and tear stresses on fragile joints. Adaptive equipment would not correct deformities (answer B) because deformities are only corrected by surgery or with orthotic devices that reposition the joints in correct alignment. Adaptive equipment allows activities to be completed but would not simplify work by eliminating steps to an activity (answer C). Another reason adaptive equipment is used is to increase (not decrease) independence (answer D). See Reference: Pedretti and Early (eds). Buckner, WS: Arthritis.

143. (C) repeated protecting of the joints while moving. An individual's protecting the joints while moving is an example of a motor response associated with chronic pain. Answer A, lack of concentration, is related to a cognitive function secondary to pain. Answer B, aching pain, can be associated with a sensory response to chronic pain, and answer D, the avoidance of certain ADL, is related to self-care responses to chronic pain. See Reference: Reed. Chronic pain.

144. (A) clearly direct a caregiver in preferred head position, food portion size, and choice of food to eat. An individual with C3 quadriplegia lacks the strength necessary to use an MAS or any cuff device (answers B, C, and D). It remains important for this individual to be able to instruct a caregiver how to assist with feeding in a manner that is pleasant and enjoyable. See Reference: Christiansen and Matuska (eds). Garber, SL, Gregorio-Torres, TL: Adaptive strategies following spinal cord injury.

145. (D) Suggest clothing modifications such as slip-on shoes, zipper pull, and pullover shirts. Instructing in the use of clothing modifications (answer D) would offer the best choice for dressing independently and efficiently. Answer A, showering in the morning to prevent joint stiffness, would be useful for individuals with arthritis. Training the spouse to assist with transfers (answer B) is not indicated at this point since trunk control and balance are not currently affected. Answer C, teaching range of motion exercises, is an important overall strategy to encourage general mobility and ease of movement, but does not directly address the goal of preparing for work. See Reference: Pedretti and Early (eds). Schultz-Krohn, Foti, D, Glogoski, C: Degenerative diseases of the central nervous system.

146. (B) flexed at all joints. When weight-bearing, the fingers should be flexed at all joints (the fisted position). This preserves the tenodesis function by protecting the finger flexors from overstretching. Another reason for this position is to prevent claw-hand deformity by protecting the intrinsic hand muscles from overstretching. See Reference: Trombly and Radomski. Atkins, MS: Spinal cord injury.

147. (D) provide a stockinette sleeve for the individual to wear inside the splint. A stockinette liner worn inside the splint will keep perspiration from irritating the skin by absorbing it through the liner. Stockinette also keeps the body part from direct contact with the plastic surface of the splint. Stockinette is inexpensive and can be washed easily with soap and water. Answer A, putting talcum powder in a splint, assists with odor control as a result of prolonged splint wear, but does not typically address the perspiration issue. In addition, it often requires frequent cleaning due to the accumulation of powder within the splint. While moleskin as a liner (answer B), may be comfortable, it does not clean well, hence it usually is removed because of the tendency to become soiled and odorous. Answer C, perforated material, will assist with ventilation, but the patient will typically continue to perspire, thus indicating the need to utilize alternative or additional methods to keep the splint from irritating the skin. See Reference: Trombly and Radomski. Callinan, N: Construction of hand splints.

148. (D) Loose-fitting clothing. Individuals with paraplegia can dress independently. The process is somewhat easier when loose-fitting clothing and dressing loops are used. Buttonhook zipper pull devices and clip-on ties (answers A and B) are useful for individuals without the hand function required to button, pull a zipper, or tie a tie. Individuals with C6 through C8 quadriplegia usually require assistance to put on shoes, but may be able to put on specially adapted shoes (answer C) independently. See Reference: Christiansen and Matuska (eds). Garber, SL, Gregorio-Torres, TL: Adaptive strategies following spinal cord injury.

149. (B) Playing Velcro checkers to tolerance. Gentle, repetitive, and resistive exercises such as playing Velcro checkers (answer B) help maintain strength and endurance in weakened muscles. A wrist support (answer A) compensates for loss of muscle strength, but does not help to maintain strength. Exercising without resistance once a day (answer C) also will not help maintain strength. Exercising against maximal resistance (answer D) is contraindicated for individuals with ALS. See Reference: Dutton. Biomechanical postulates regarding intervention.

150. (D) No equipment. An young adult with paraplegia at the T10 to L1 level or lower should not require any adaptive equipment for dressing. The client should demonstrate good trunk stability, fully intact intercostal, external oblique, and rectus abdominis function. Lower extremity paralysis will be present. See Reference: Trombly and Radomski. Section VI: Treatment to promote occupational function for selected diagnostic categories.

151. (B) boutonnière deformity. A boutonnière deformity is typically characterized by PIP joint flexion and DIP joint hyperextension. Answer A, a mallet deformity, is characterized by DIP joint flexion and a loss of active extension. Answer C is not a typical term used to describe a deformity. Answer D, swan neck deformity, is characterized by PIP joint hyperextension and DIP joint flexion. See Reference: Pedretti and Early (eds). Belkin, J and Yasuda, L: Orthotics.

152. (A) Complete independence with self-care and transfers. After rehabilitation, it is anticipated that an individual with T3 (or lower) paraplegia will most likely have the trunk balance and upper extremity strength and coordination to complete self-care and transfers independently. See Reference: Pedretti and Early (eds). Adler, C: Spinal cord injury.

153. (A) skin inspection. Visual inspection of an insensate area is essential for preventing pressure sores, which may develop when there are no sensory cues to alert a person to skin breakdown. Nail trimming (answer B) is an important issue to address with individuals with diabetes, but is secondary to skin inspection in importance. Many individuals with diabetes have abnormalities in nail growth, and instead of trimming their own nails, they have them trimmed by a podiatrist. Moreover, the nursing staff may address this issue with the patient. Retirement planning (answer C) and returning to work (answer D) are issues that may be addressed when discussing discharge plans. See Reference: Trombly and Radomski. Bentzel, K and Quintana, LA: Optimizing sensory abilities and capacities.

154. (C) flange the area around the ulnar styloid. Reddened areas indicate the splint is too tight in a particular spot. To reduce pressure, it is often helpful to flange splint edges to better contour the splint around the bony prominence. Lining the splint with any material, whether moleskin or foam (answers A and B), will only make a tight area tighter. Remaking the splint (answer D) is unnecessary and a waste of the OT practitioner's time. See Reference: Crepeau, Cohn, and Schell (eds). Emerson, S and Shafer, A: Splinting and orthotics.

155. (A) goniometer. A goniometer measures available joint movement. A pinch meter (answer C) is used to measure available thumb-to-finger pinch strength in all available positions. A dynamometer (answer B) measures grip strength in the hand. An aesthesiometer (answer D) measures two-point discrimination. See Reference: Trombly and Radomski. Trombly, CA and Podolski, CR: Assessing abilities and capacities: Range of motion, strength, and endurance.

156. (B) Functional-position resting splint. Bedridden individuals are often provided with splints to prevent the development of flexion contractures in the hand that can lead to problems with maintaining hygiene. A functional-position resting hand splint is most appropriate, because it will prevent flexion contractures from developing and allow the caregiver access to the hand for cleaning. Neither the dorsal nor volar wrist splints (answers A and C) would keep the fingers in extension, which is necessary to prevent development of finger contractures. Dynamic finger-extension splints (answer D) are appropriate for individuals who have active finger flexion, but limited active finger extension. See Reference: Pedretti and Early (eds). Belkin, J and Yasuda, L: Orthotics.

157. (B) Positioning, adaptive equipment, and patient education. Positioning and adaptive equipment are necessary to maintain the integrity of the musculoskeletal system and to prevent deformity. Patient education about the disease and ways of dealing with its effects also can be started at this stage. Resistive exercises (answer A) are not appropriate if there is joint swelling and inflammation, and are always used cautiously with individuals with RA because of the potential for tissue damage. Discharge planning would be more relevant at a later time (answer C). Surgical intervention (answer D) would not be needed in the early stages of rheumatoid arthritis. It may be offered later as a corrective measure for long-standing deformities. See Reference: Pedretti and Early (eds). Buckner, WS: Arthritis.

158. (B) Reposition the person in the wheelchair to allow optimal positioning. When a person in a wheelchair who uses an augmentative communication device suddenly begins making errors, it is necessary to first check the position of the individual. "The person and the control interface should both be positioned to maximize function...if inadequate positioning appears to be affecting the person's ability to control an interface, it should be addressed" (p. 221). Improper positioning could result in the wheelchair interfering with access or with range of motion needed to use the communication device. A person may eventually need to be referred to a physician for a physical examination (answer A). However, it is best for the therapist to first problem-solve and seek a solution if the person's medical status has not changed. The person's communication abilities would not be reassessed (answer C) until the person has been optimally positioned in the wheelchair. A communication device would only need to be replaced (answer D) if there were a mechanical problem within the system that could not be fixed. See Reference: Cook and Hussey. Control Interfaces for Assistive Technology.

159. (C) radial nerve. Injury to the radial nerve in the wrist area causes sensory damage only. This damage occurs to the radial two thirds of the dorsum of the hand. Damage to the median nerve at the wrist causes decreased thumb and prehensile strength and complete or partial loss of sensation in the distal portion of the second digit (index finger) and third digit (long finger) with some loss in the fourth digit (ring

finger). Damage to the ulnar nerve at the wrist causes decreased grip strength and complete or partial loss of sensation to half of the fourth digit (ring finger) and all of the fifth digit (little finger) as well as the proximal hypothenar region. The ulnar and median nerves are frequently entrapped together. A brachial plexus injury causes peripheral nerve damage to any or all of the fibers from C5 to T1. See Reference: Pedretti and Early (eds). Belkin, J and Yasuda, L: Orthotics.

160. (D) run a focus group comprising obese adults from the local community. For a program to be successful, it is important to determine what the targeted population perceive they need and want. Focus groups, interview, and surveys of members of the targeted population are all acceptable methods for obtaining this information. Collecting information concerning the incidence of obesity in the community and factors that contribute to the problem (answer A) is an important step toward developing the community profile. Information obtained from interviewing a hospital administrator or surveying doctors (answers B and C) may be helpful in identifying services that are already being provided, and may help to identify the needs as perceived by the administration and physicians, but not the population. See Reference: Fazio. Profiling the community, targeting the population, and assessing the need for services.

161. (B) Figure-ground discrimination. Figure-ground discrimination is the ability to visually separate an object from the surrounding background or from other objects. A problem with position in space (answer A) would be related to perception of relative orientation of clothing to the body and may be seen in dressing when a person overestimates or underestimates reach due to difficulty judging the relationship between the object and the body. Body image (answer C) is a mental picture of the person's body that includes how the person feels about their body. Visual closure (answer D) is the ability to recognize an object even though only part of it is seen, e.g., recognizing a partially covered button. See Reference: Pedretti and Early (eds). Wheatley, CJ: Evaluation and treatment of perceptual and perceptual motor deficits.

162. (D) compensation. When protective sensation is severely decreased or absent, the primary focus of intervention becomes protection of the insensate part through educational methods to increase awareness of potential dangers, teach safety procedures, and train in the use of vision to compensate for sensory loss. Sensory reeducation (answer A) is a remedial retraining technique that focuses on helping the patient correctly interpret sensory impulses through a program of graded sensory stimuli. Sensory desensitization (answer B) involves a program of graded sensory stimuli to gradually decrease hypersensitivity to sensory stimuli. Sensory bombardment (answer C) is a sensory retraining method of stimulating many senses. See Reference: Pedretti and Early (eds). Iyer, MB and Pedretti, LW: Evaluation of sensation and treatment of sensory dysfunction.

163. (B) use moderately heated water. Hot water may contribute to fatigue in individuals with MS, and therefore should be avoided. Moderate water temperature is recommended (answer B). Bathing in cool water (answer A) is unnecessary and may cause chilling and increase spasticity. Bathing rather than showering (answer C) is recommended for individuals with poor balance or standing tolerance, such as those with MS or COPD. Bathing at the sink (answer D) may be recommended for individuals who experience difficulty bending, such as those with hip or knee replacements or back pain. However, durable medical equipment is typically available for all of these diagnoses so bathing in the tub would be possible through the use of a tub bench and hand-held shower. See Reference: Trombly and Radomski. Copperman, LF, Forwell, SJ, and Hugos, L: Neuro-degenerative diseases.

164. (A) a cotton ball. When retesting, it is important to use the same method used initially in order to make an accurate comparison of status before and after treatment. In addition, evaluation results are more consistent when the individual who performed the initial evaluation performs subsequent reevaluations. An aesthesiometer (answer B) is used to measure two-point discrimination, not light touch. Semmes-Weinstein monofilaments (answer C) are a good tool for assessing light touch thresholds, but the results may not be as useful for comparison purposes. A pin or straightened paper clip (answer D) is used for testing superficial pain. See Reference: Pedretti and Early (eds). Pedretti, LW and Iyer, MB: Evaluation of sensation and treatment of sensory dysfunction.

165. (B) perform the evaluation over several sessions. Upper extremity evaluation is lengthy and can be fatiguing, and fatigue should be avoided with individuals with Guillain-Barré syndrome. In addition, results may be invalid if the individual is fatigued and not performing at the highest level possible. Strength, range of motion, and sensory testing (answers A, C, and D) are all important when evaluating an individual with Guillain-Barré syndrome, but must be administered using a method that will yield valid results. See Reference: Pedretti and Early (eds). Lehman, RM and McCormack, G: Neurogenic and myopathic dysfunction.

166. (C) Biomechanical. The biomechanical approach uses voluntary muscle control during performance of activities for individuals with deficits in strength, endurance, or range of motion. The biomechanical approach focuses on decreasing deficits in order to improve performance of daily activities. The neurophysiological approach (answer A) is applied to individuals with brain damage. Emphasis is on the nervous system and methods for eliciting desired responses. The neurodevelopmental approach (answer B) also focuses on the nervous system, but emphasizes eliciting responses in a developmental sequence. The rehabilitative approach (answer D) teaches an individual how to compensate for a deficit on either a temporary or permanent basis. See Reference: Pedretti and Early (eds). Breines, EB: Therapeutic occupations and modalities.

167. (B) flaccidity. Flaccidity or hypotonicity (answer B) is often present immediately after a stroke and may later change to spasticity (answer D) or increased muscle tone. The flaccid extremity feels heavy and hangs limply at the individual's side. The weight of the arm may eventually pull the humerus out of the glenohumeral joint, resulting in subluxation (answer C). Neither flaccidity, spasticity, nor subluxation are normal (answer A). See Reference: Pedretti and Early (eds). Preston, LA: Motor control.

168. (C) fair plus (3+). An individual with strength of fair or fair minus would be unable to tolerate resistance. An individual with strength of fair plus can tolerate minimal resistance, such as a lightweight can of deodorant. An individual whose strength is good minus can tolerate less than moderate resistance, but more than minimal resistance. See Reference: Pedretti and Early (eds). Pedretti, LW: Muscle strength.

169. (B) Increase the number of towels from 10 to 20. Endurance is improved by increasing the number of repetitions so the muscle has to work over a longer period of time. Placing towels on a higher shelf (answer A) would help to increase range of motion. Placing towels on a lower shelf (answer C) decreases the difficulty of the activity, and does not lengthen the period of time needed to improve endurance by providing more repetitions. The arm could be strengthened by adding a 1 pound weight (answer D), but that would not increase the repetitions needed to improve endurance. See Reference: Pedretti and Early (eds). Breines, EB: Therapeutic occupations and modalities.

170. (D) incoordination. A person who has tremors or poor coordination could eliminate much instability by stabilizing the limb proximally before working distally. Stabilization adds a secure base of support from which to work. Reduced vision, poor endurance, and impaired fine motor performance would not require stabilization when writing, but they would require stronger contrast of guiding lines or ink on paper, more frequent rests, or built-up writing tools. See Reference: Trombly and Radomski. Trombly, CA: Restoring the role of independent person.

171. (A) Plaster cylindrical splint. A plaster cylindrical splint would encourage a static stretch of the PIP joint contracture. Answer B is a form of PIP extension and is considered to be a dynamic splint. Answer C is used to isolate tendon and joint range of motion. Answer D also is a form of dynamic splinting. See Reference: Pedretti and Early (eds). Belkin, J and Yasuda, L: Orthotics.

172. (D) Maintain a neutral spine, slowly shifting feet as the turn is completed. A correct transfer is performed slowly with the knees bent and the feet a shoulder width apart, while the normal curve of the back is maintained, and the lifting is performed with the legs. The body should not be twisted at the trunk (answer A), as this could cause back injury. Lifting with the arms (answer B), instead of the legs, also could injure the therapist's back. Another cause of back injury during a transfer is to keep the feet planted when moving (answer C), because this causes twisting of the back and may damage the knees. See Reference: Pedretti and Early (eds). Creel, TA, Adler, C, Tipton-Burton, M, and Lillie, SM: Mobility.

173. (D) "Pt. has improved significantly in his ability to work at the computer by using periodic stretch breaks." The assessment section of a discharge summary identifies the functional performance deficits and indicates whether they have been resolved or, if they still exist, to what degree. Answer C is a subjective report. Answer A is an example of a statement that belongs in the objective section of a discharge summary. Answer B belongs in the plan section. See Reference: Borcherding. Appendix.

174. (A) Loosening nuts and bolts by hand. Loosening nuts and bolts by hand is the activity that most closely resembles a tip or lateral prehension activity. Prehension is a hand position that permits finger and thumb contact, while facilitating the manipulation of objects. Answers B, C, and D are more closely related to grasping activities, which encourage contact of an object against the palm and the flexed digits. See Reference: Pedretti and Early (eds). Breines, EB: Therapeutic occupations and modalities.

175. (B) bend both knees, keep the back straight, and bring the object close to the body. Bending with both knees while keeping the back straight and the object close to the body (answer B) will prevent low back bending and strain. Answers A, C, and D are all incorrect methods for lifting and carrying objects. Answers A and C will actually increase an individual's chance of increasing low back strain. See Reference: Pedretti and Early (eds). Smithline, J and Dunlop, LE: Low back pain.

176. (A) strength in the deltoid, brachialis, biceps, and brachioradialis muscles. Erb's Palsy, a type of brachial plexus injury, "is indicative of lesions to the fifth and sixth brachial plexus roots" (p. 798), which innervate the deltoid, brachialis, biceps, and brachioradialis muscles. Injury to the eighth cervical and first thoracic brachial plexus roots would affect the hand, and evaluation of sensation and fine motor coordination (answers B and D) would be indicated. Sitting balance (answer C) would not be affected by a brachial plexus injury. See Reference: Pedretti and Early (eds). Lehman RM and McCormack, GL: Neurogenic and myopathic dysfunction.

177. (C) a subacute facility. The most appropriate recommendation for this person is to receive rehabilitation in a subacute facility because the patient requires rehabilitation services provided at a lower level of intensity, but has the goal of returning home. An acute rehabilitation program (answer A) requires a person to tolerate 3 hours minimum per day, which would be unlikely for this patient. Answer B, extending the patient's stay in the acute care hospital, is not possible because the length of stay is usually determined by third-party payers, and patients are discharged once medically stable. This individual requires assistance with ADLs and is not ready to return home alone, even with home health-care services (answer D). See Reference: Pedretti and Early (eds). Matthews, MM and Tipton-Burton, M: Treatment contexts.

178. (A) Biofeedback, distraction, and relaxation techniques Biofeedback, distraction, and relaxation techniques are all examples of psychosocial measures that can be introduced to manage pain. Answers B and C, specific skill training and endurance building, are not directly related to pain management techniques and are often associated with cognitive or motor limitations. Answer D, cognitive retraining techniques, also are not directly related to pain management techniques. See Reference: Crepeau, Cohn, and Schell (eds). Engel, JM: Pain management.

179. (D) Lock the brakes. Brakes should be locked first to stabilize the wheelchair. Answers A, B, and C involve movements that could cause loss of balance or wheelchair movement unless the brakes are locked. See Reference: Pedretti and Early (eds). Adler, C and Tipton-Burton, M: Wheelchair assessment and transfers.

180. (C) an aquatic therapy class. Many community centers offer aquatic therapy programs for individuals with physical disabilities. In a warm water environment, people with arthritis can perform AROM further, and with less pain, than on land. The group format also provides excellent opportunities for socialization and information sharing. A weightlifting program (answer A) would be contraindicated for individuals with RA. Providing and instructing in the use of adaptive equipment (answer B) is very important for this population, as is education in energy conservation and joint protection (answer D). However, these options do not address the physical fitness and socialization components required. See Reference: Pedretti and Early (eds). Buckner, WS: Arthritis.

181. (B) pain, edema, skin temperature and skin color. Answer B is correct because this diagnosis describes a group of disorders marked by severe pain that seems out of proportion to the initiating injury, along with edema, coolness of the hand, and blotchy, shiny skin. Answer A describes the symptoms of carpal tunnel syndrome, a nerve compression disorder. Answer C describes a quick motor function test for ulnar nerve paralysis. Answer D, decreased range of motion and strength, are common features of many hand conditions and are not specific symptom indicators of complex regional pain syndrome. See Reference: Pedretti and Early (eds). Kasch, MC and Nickerson, E: Hand and upper extremity injuries.

182. (D) 5 feet by 5 feet. An outward opening door needs a space of 5 feet by 5 feet to allow for a wheelchair to be maneuvered around the door. A standard wheelchair requires 5 feet of turning space for a 180 or 360 degree turn. An area that is 3 feet by 5 feet (answer A), 4 feet by 4 feet (answer B), or 4.5 feet by 3 feet (answer C), would not provide enough space to allow the wheelchair to be turned. See Reference: Pedretti and Early (eds). Smith, P: Americans with disabilities act: Accommodating persons with disabilities.

183. (D) resume the homemaker role. The Commission on Accreditation of Rehabilitation Facilities defines work hardening as "a highly structured, goal oriented, individualized treatment program designed to maximize a person's ability to return to work" (p. 553). A homemaker's job is working in the home. A work-hardening program would not focus on obtaining employment outside the home (answer A), nor resuming leisure activities (answer B) for this individual. Although a work-hardening program may help to reduce pain levels (answer C), the emphasis is on a return to work in this case, resuming the homemaker role (answer D). See Reference: Pedretti and Early (eds). Burt, CM: Work evaluation and work hardening.

184. (A) A frame with crossbar folding construction. A folding or crossbar folding construction chair is needed when a wheelchair will be frequently lifted in and out of a car trunk or back seat, and folded to fit into the space. This is much easier on the individual or family member who will be lifting the wheelchair. Answers B, C, and D will add a great deal of weight and bulk, which makes the wheelchair much more difficult to lift. This in turn may cause an individual or family member to be more reluctant to go on a community outing. See Reference: Cook and Hussey. Technologies that enable mobility.

185. (D) Carpal tunnel and chronic cervical tension. Carpal tunnel syndrome and chronic cervical tension are just some of the work-related occurrences secondary to the arrival of visual display terminals and specialized technology that require repetition and unusual body positioning. Answers A and C are injuries typically not associated with repetitive motion or cumulative trauma disorders. Answer B, edema and paresthesias, are typical symptoms (not injuries) of repetitive motion and cumulative trauma disorders. See Reference: Crepeau, Cohn, and Schell (eds). Kasch, MC and Nickerson, E: Hand and upper extremity injuries.

186. (A) tip of the index finger. The correct position for tip pinch is the thumb against the tip of the index finger. The thumb against the side of the index finger (answer B) describes the position for lateral pinch. The thumb against the tips of the index and middle fingers (answer C) describes the test position for three-jaw chuck, or palmar pinch. The thumb against the tips of all the fingers (answer D) is not a standard test position. See Reference: Trombly and Radomski. Trombly, CA and Podolski, CR: Assessing abilities and capacities: Range of motion, strength, and endurance.

187. (D) use brochures, posters, videotapes, and films available from the AOTA to enhance the presentation. The emphasis of this question is that it is every OT practitioner's responsibility to promote the profession. Simple, daily public relations activities occur each time an OT practitioner describes the services to be provided to patients and families. More complex public relations may include developing a plan to promote community awareness regarding the profession. A public relations program is designed to increase public awareness about the role and importance of OT services. See Reference: Sladyk, K (ed). Bowler, DF: OT and political action.

188. (C) instrument reliability. According to Polgar, "an instrument is considered to be reliable when a similar score is achieved on repeated administration...when an instrument is reliable, it is expected that on subsequent testing an individual will achieve scores that are consistent with, but not necessarily identical to, previously achieved scores" (p. 303). Supervisory feedback (answer A) and evidence of competence in the ability to competently administer the evaluation (answer B) also may be reasons for a student or new practitioner to ask the supervisor to check her results, but not for an experienced therapist. Answer D, evidence of incompetence in performing this skill, would be unlikely. See Reference: Crepeau, Cohn, and Schell (eds). Polgar, JM: Critiquing assessments.

189. (C) interpreting results of assessments for the purposes of treatment planning. Interpretation of assessment results for purposes of treatment planning must be performed by the OTR. The functions noted in answers A, B, and D may all be performed by the COTA in a long-term care facility. See Reference: AOTA: Guidelines for Supervision, roles, and responsibilities during the delivery of occupational therapy services.

190. (A) obtain services from a home health OT. Home health-care services, which may include nursing, OT, PT, and speech therapy are provided in the patient's home. Individuals who require continued care following discharge from the hospital may be appropriate for home health-care services if they are unable to travel to the hospital for outpatient services. If the decision to discharge the person has already been made, recommendations for a continued stay in the acute care hospital or transfer to a rehabilitation center (answer B and C) are not appropriate. The person's weakness and continuing requirement for intravenous drug therapy would make it extremely difficult for the patient to return to the hospital for outpatient therapy (answer D). See Reference: Piersol and Ehrlich (eds). Zahoransky, M: The system and its players.

191. (C) Decline the current offer, ask if company can wait to hire, and apply for a tempo- **rary license.** All OT practitioners must hold a current, updated state license if residing in a licensed state. According to AOTA's Standards of practice (1998), "an occupational therapy practitioner maintains current licensure, registration, or certification as required by laws or regulations" (p. 3). Students completing fieldwork II placements should apply for a temporary license prior to beginning their job search. It is essential that all practitioners maintain a high level of professional standards. See Reference: AOTA: Standards of practice for occupational therapy.

192. (D) Treat the client with the student observing the session. Occupational therapy practitioners should always respect the recipients of their services. According to the Occupational Therapy Code of Ethics (2000), under Principle 3d, "occupational therapy personnel shall respect the individual's right to refuse professional services or involvement in research or educational activities." Attempts to persuade the client (answer A) would conflict with this principle. Canceling the session (answer B) would be punitive. Consulting with other fieldwork educators (answer C) may help the OT develop strategies for facilitating student involvement. See Reference: AOTA: Occupational Therapy Code of Ethics.

193. (D) Interdisciplinary care improvement teams. Health-care professionals who are part of an interdisciplinary care improvement team work together to "address such issues as patient flow, the discharge process, patient outreach, and promotion and cost-efficiencies" (p. 47). Quality improvement (answer A) is a systematic approach to monitoring patient care. Peer review (answer B) is a component of quality improvement. Cost accounting (answer C) is a method of tracking the costs of specific services or costs incurred by diagnosis-specific groups. See Reference: Jacobs and Logigian (eds). Logigian, MK: Cost management.

194. (A) total quality management. Total quality management (answer A) "encourages health care institutions to move away from a focus on compliance to standards and refocus on improvement goals in an effort to deliver high quality care" (p. 121). Answers B, C, and D, are all concepts that contribute to the model of total quality management and include finance, marketing, and operations. See Reference: Jacobs and Logigian (eds). Logigian, MK: Quality management.

195.: (B) No, it violates the AOTA's Position Paper on modalities. Despite the level of training she has achieved, according to the position paper it is still necessary for the COTA to demonstrate service competency in order to administer PAMs. Service competency in this area includes the theoretical background and technical skills for the safe and effective use of the modality. Although study and practice are necessary to establish service competency, they are not by themselves sufficient; an OTR must determine that the COTA is competent before she can administer PAMs (answers A and C). Having an OTR on duty in the facility (answer D) does not make it acceptable for a COTA to administer a modality if the COTA has not demonstrated service competency. See Reference: AOTA: Physical Agent Modalities: A Position Paper.

196. (D) Transdisciplinary. In the transdisciplinary method of teamwork, one member provides the direct intervention and other team members function in collaborative consultant roles. This allows the family to interact with one service provider rather than several. Answer A is incorrect because a unidisciplinary team is not really a team; as the term implies, there is only one member. Answer B is not correct because the multidisciplinary team uses several disciplines, but they may not work in a collaborative manner. Answer C also is incorrect because in the interdisciplinary team, although it has group consensus regarding program planning, the members carry out their programs in their own environments. See Reference: Case-Smith (ed). Stephens, LC, and Tauber, SK: Early intervention.

197. (A) Contact administration to let them know of the unforeseen change in service delivery and make appropriate adjustments to billing. Occupational therapy practitioners are ethically bound to charge fairly and accurately for services. Billing is a form of documentation and should reflect skilled services that are actually provided. While patient education can and should be considered an appropriate skilled intervention under the right circumstances, time spent coaxing a client to participate (answer C) does not fall under this activity. Answers B and D both involve fraud and are unethical. See Reference: Crepeau, Cohn, and Schell (eds). Perinchief, JM: Documentation and management of occupational therapy services.

198. (B) have at least 1 year of experience as a certified OT practitioner. An individual who passes the NBCOT examination becomes a certified OT practitioner. In order to be a primary supervisor for a level-II OT student, the individual must be a registered OT with at least 1 year of experience. To supervisor level-II OTA students, the individual must be a certified OT practitioner with at least 1 year of experience. There is no minimum experience requirement for supervising level-I students. Although it may help to develop supervisory skills to work with a level-I student before taking a level-II student (answer D), there is no such requirement. See Reference: AOTA: Standards for an accredited educational program for the occupational therapist.

199. (B) Medicaid. Medicaid is a joint federal and state program. Because it is a joint program, benefits vary widely from state to state. In each state, the Medicaid program must include Aid to Families with Dependent Children (AFDC) and Supplementary Security Income (SSI). Coverage for occupational therapy varies from setting to setting. Medicare (answer A) is a federal program that funds health coverage for individuals 65 years of age or older, disabled individuals, and people in the end stages of renal disease. Workers' compensation (answer C) is a state-supported program funded by employer contributions. Beneficiaries receive coverage for services identified as covered within their respective states. The Education for All Handicapped Children Act (answer D) mandates programs funded in part through state and federal grants. It does not fund health care, but requires any school receiving federal assistance to provide handicapped children with a free, appropriate education in the least restrictive environment. See Reference: McCormack, Jaffe, and Goodman-Lavey (Eds). Thomas, VJ: Reimbursement.

200. (A) collecting chart review information. After a certified OT has demonstrated service competency, it is appropriate for him or her to complete data collection through record reviews, interviews, general observations, and behavior checklists. Answers B, C, and D require interpretive and analytical skills in which OTs have received additional training. A certified OT assistant can collaborate with an occupational therapist, but it is inappropriate to have a COTA complete these portions independently. See Reference: AOTA: Guidelines for Supervision, roles, and responsibilities during the delivery of occupational therapy services.

Bibliography

American Occupational Therapy Association Inc.: Enforcement procedures for occupational therapy code of ethics. Am J Occup Ther 58:655–662, 2004.

American Occupational Therapy Association Inc.: Guidelines for supervision, roles, and responsibilities during the delivery of occupational therapy services. Am J Occup Ther 58:663–667, 2004.

American Occupational Therapy Association, Inc. Occupational Therapy Code of Ethics. Am J Occup Ther 54:614–616, 2000b.

American Occupational Therapy Association, Inc.: Occupational therapy practice framework: Domain and process. Am J Occup Ther 56:609–639, 2002.

American Occupational Therapy Association Inc.: Physical agent modalities: A position paper. Am J Occup Ther 57:650–651, 2003.

American Occupational Therapy Association Inc.: Standards for an accredited educational program for the occupational therapist. Am J Occup Ther 53:575–582, 1999.

American Occupational Therapy Association Inc.: Standards of practice for occupational therapy. Am J Occup Ther 52:866–869, 1998.

Bonder, BR and Wagner, MB (eds): Functional Performance in Older Adults, ed. 2. FA Davis, Philadelphia, 2001.

Borcherding, S: Documentation Manual for Writing SOAP Notes in Occupational Therapy. Slack, Thorofare, NJ, 2000.

Breines, EB: Occupational Therapy Activities from Clay to Computers: Theory and Practice. FA Davis, Philadelphia, 1995.

Bruce, MAG and Borg, BA: Psychosocial frames of reference: Core for occupation-based practice, ed. 3. Slack, Thorofare, NJ, 2002.

Bundy, AC, Lane, SJ, and Murray, EA (eds): Sensory Integration: Theory and Practice, ed. 2. FA Davis, Philadelphia, 2002.

Cara, E and MacRae, A (eds): Psychosocial Occupational Therapy: A Clinical Practice, ed. 2. Thompson Delmar Learning, Clifton Park, NY, 2005.

Case-Smith, J (ed): Occupational Therapy for Children, ed. 4. CV Mosby, St. Louis, 2001.

Christiansen, C and Baum, C (eds): Occupational Therapy: Enabling Function and Well-Being, ed. 2. Slack, Thorofare, NJ, 1997.

Christiansen, C and Matuska, KM (eds): Ways of Living: Adaptive Strategies for Special Needs, ed. 3. American Occupational Therapy Association, Bethesda, MD, 2004.

Cook, AM and Hussey, SM: Assistive Technologies: Principles and Practice, ed. 2. CV Mosby, St. Louis, 2002.

Cottrell, RP (ed): Proactive Approaches in Psychosocial Occupational Therapy. Slack, Thorofare, NJ, 2000.

Creek, J (ed): Occupational Therapy and Mental Health, ed. 3. Churchill Livingstone, New York, 2002.

Crepeau, EB, Cohn, ES, and Schell, BA (eds): Williard and Spackman's Occupational Therapy, ed. 10. Lippincott Williams & Wilkins, Philadelphia, 2003.

Dutton, R: Clinical Reasoning in Physical Disabilities. Williams & Wilkins, Baltimore, 1995.

Early, MB: Mental Health Concepts and Techniques for the Occupational Therapy Assistant, ed. 3. Lippincott Williams & Wilkins, Philadelphia, 2000.

Fazio, L: Developing Occupation-Centered Programs for the Community: A Workbook for Students and Professionals. Prentice Hall, Upper Saddle River, NJ, 2001.

Gillen, G and Burkardt, A (eds): Stroke Rehabilitation: A Function-Based Approach. CV Mosby, St. Louis, 2004.

Hellen, CR: Alzheimer's Disease: Activity-Focused Care, ed. 2. Butterworth-Heinemann, Boston, 1998.

Jacobs, K and Logigian, M (eds): Functions of a Manager in Occupational Therapy, ed. 3. Slack, Thorofare, NJ, 1999.

Kornblau, BL and Starling, SP: Ethics in Rehabilitation: A Clinical Perspective. Slack, Thorofare, NJ, 2000.

Kramer, P and Hinojosa, J (eds): Frames of Reference for Pediatric Occupational Therapy, ed. 2. Lippincott Williams & Wilkins, Philadelphia, 1999.

Mackin, EJ, Callahan, AD, Skirven, TM, Schneider, LH, and Osterman, AL (eds): Hunter, Mackin and Callahan's Rehabilitation of the Hand and Upper Extremity, ed. 5. CV Mosby, Philadelphia, 2002.

McCormack, GL, Jaffe, EG, and Goodman-Lavey, M (eds): The Occupational Therapy Manager, ed. 4. AOTA Press, Bethesda, MD, 2003.

Miller-Kuhaneck, H: Autism: A Comprehensive Occupational Therapy Approach, ed. 2, AOTA Press, Bethesda, MD. 2004.

Mulligan, S: Occupational Therapy Evaluation for Children: A Pocket Guide. Lippincott Williams & Wilkins, Philadelphia, 2003.

Pape, L and Ryba, K: Practical Considerations for

School-Based Occupational Therapists. American Occupational Therapy Association, Bethesda, MD, 2004.

Pedretti, LW and Early, ME (eds): Occupational Therapy: Practice Skills for Physical Dysfunction, ed 5. CV Mosby, St. Louis, 2001.

Piersol, CV and Ehrlich, PL (eds): Home Health Practice: A Guide for the Occupational Therapist. Imaginart, Bisbee, AZ, 2000.

Posthuma, BW: Small Groups in Counseling and Therapy: Process and Leadership, ed. 4. Allyn & Bacon, Boston, 2002

Reed, KL: Quick Reference to Occupational Therapy, ed. 2. Aspen, Gaithersburg, MD, 2001.

Ross, M and Bachner, S (eds): Adults with Developmental Disabilities: Current Approaches in Occupational Therapy (revised edition). American Occupational Therapy Association, Bethesda, MD, 2004.

Scaffa, ME (ed): Occupational Therapy in Community-Based Practice Settings. FA Davis, Philadelphia, 2001.

Sladyk, K (ed): OT Student Primer: A Guide to College Success. Slack, Thorofare, NJ, 1997.

Sladyk, K and Ryan, SE (eds): Ryan's Occupational Therapy Assistant: Principles, Practice Issues, and Techniques, ed. 3. Slack, Thorofare, NJ, 2001.

Solomon, JW (ed): Pediatric Skills for Occupational Therapy Assistants. CV Mosby, St. Louis, 2000.

Stein, F and Cutler, SK: Psychosocial Occupational Therapy: A Holistic Approach, ed. 2. Singular Publishing Group, Inc., Delmar, NY, 2002.

Trombly, CA and Radomski, MV: Occupational Therapy for Physical Dysfunction, ed. 5. Lippincott Williams & Wilkins, Philadelphia, 2002.

Unsworth, C (ed): Cognitive and Perceptual Dysfunction: A Clinical Reasoning Approach to Evaluation and Intervention. FA Davis, Philadelphia, 1999.